Advanced Praise for *There's a Mushroom for That!*

Finally, a comprehensive resource for two of the most important topics for forward-thinking, wellness-oriented pet parents: using cannabis (CBD) and mushrooms for medicinal purposes. These plants and fungi have incredible health benefits and a long track record of use in the animal kingdom, but they come with so much confusion and fear. The protocols in this all-in-one resource were assembled by Dr. Silver, one of the leading veterinary experts on both subjects. His 40+ years of career experience and advocacy for plant medicine and natural therapies make him exceptionally well-qualified to relay the exciting science he's included in this book.

Dr. Karen Becker, co-author of
The Forever Dog and *The Forever Dog Life*

There's a Mushroom for That! is a must-read for any pet parent wanting to improve their pets' healthspan and lifespan. Dr. Robert Silver provides in-depth descriptions, including scientific background, on the use of mushrooms, herbs, and healthy diets for both dogs and cats. Dr. Rob is a brilliant healer but provides explanations that any pet parent can understand and use immediately. Highly recommended!

Judy Morgan, DVM, CVA, CVCP, CVFT

A groundbreaking journey into the future of veterinary care! Dr. Silver seamlessly blends passion and expertise in *There's a Mushroom for That!*, revealing the untapped potential of mushrooms and cannabis compounds for our beloved pets. A must-have for every pet parent and animal lover.

Lee Carroll, BSc, BHSc (whm), MNHAA
Chief Medical Herbalist Real Mushrooms

Doc Rob Silver is a nationally recognized holistic veterinarian and educator. His great depth of knowledge regarding the holistic use of cannabis and medicinal mushrooms in pets is now available in his latest book, *There's a Mushroom for That!* This easy to read and scientifically comprehensive book presents both the real life evidence and the information that supports the effective use of medicinal mushrooms and cannabis to provide new ways of preventing and treating a number of medical problems. I believe this book will help open doors of perception around these emerging therapies, and I heartily recommend it for pet parents and veterinarians alike.

Ihor Basko, DVM, CVA
All Creatures Great and Small Veterinary Services

In my 50 years of experience as a holistic vet, it is such a pleasure to find a book such as *There's a Mushroom for That!*, which provides detailed treatment plans for the use of cannabis, mushrooms, and health supplements for dogs and cats. This is one of the very few books available that provide these details specifically to address a number of difficult-to-treat medical conditions of our dogs and cats. Dr. Silver understands very well how vitally important cannabis, medicinal mushrooms, and other supplements are in providing optimal health and quality of life for our four-legged family members. Dr. Silver has nailed it with the proper understanding, science and practical know-how in this true masterpiece of a book, *There's a Mushroom for That!* Thank you Doc Rob!

Marty Goldstein, DVM

THERE'S A
MUSHROOM
FOR THAT!

YOUR HEALTHY PET GUIDE

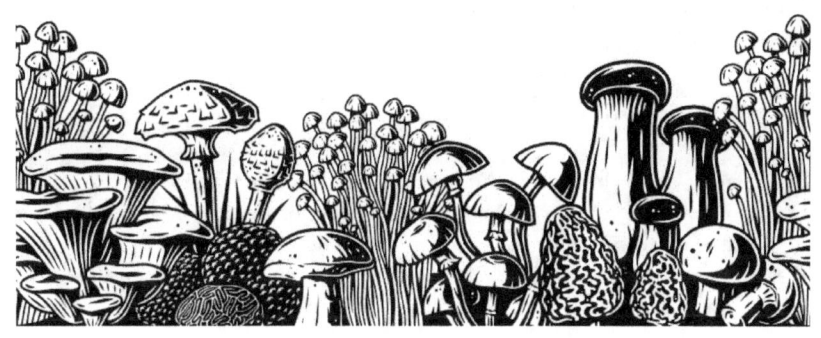

Learn How Mushrooms, Cannabis, and Integrative Medicine Help Your Pets Live Long and Healthy Lives

Dr. Robert Silver, DVM, MS, FACVBM

ISBN: 979-8-9910951-0-5

Cover Design by Hailey Schulz
hailey.wellpet@gmail.com

Cover Illustrations by Megan Nolte
www.instagram.com/megannolteart

Author Photography by Lucy Tuck
www.lucytuckphotography.com

Published by Holistic Wellness Publishing

The content of this book is for informational purposes only and is not intended to diagnose, treat, cure, or prevent any condition or disease. This book is not intended as a substitute for consultation with a licensed veterinary practitioner. Please consult with your own veterinarian regarding the suggestions and recommendations made in this book. The use of this book implies your acceptance of this disclaimer.

Nothing herein contained shall be construed as creating a veterinarian-patient relationship nor a personal diagnostic consultation between the author and any individual, regarding his or her animal, nor shall any information presented herein be deemed to be providing professional veterinary medical advice or treatment recommendations for any specific animal.

The publisher and the author are providing this book and its contents on an "as is" basis and make no representations or warranties of any kind with respect to this book or its contents.

The publisher and the author disclaim all such representations and warranties, including but not limited to warranties of veterinary healthcare for a particular purpose. In addition, the publisher and the author assume no responsibility for errors, inaccuracies, omissions, or any other inconsistencies herein.

Doc Rob's
Favorite Quotes About Dogs

"Sharing your life with a dog is to know the meaning of LOVE without words."

Anonymous

"*Everything I know I learned from dogs.*"
Nora Roberts, author of *The Search*

"It's not the size of the dog in the fight, it's the size of the fight in the dog."

Mark Twain, author of
The Adventures of Huckleberry Finn

"Dogs do speak, but only to those who know how to listen."

Orhan Pamuk, author of *My Name is Red*

"Everyone thinks they have the best dog. And none of them are wrong."

W.R. Purche

"The poor dog, in life the firmest friend. The first to welcome, foremost to defend."

Lord Byron,
poet of "Epitaph to a Dog"

"Petting, scratching, and cuddling a dog could be as soothing to the mind and heart as deep meditation and almost as good for the soul as prayer."

Dean Koontz, author of *False Memory*

"Dogs are better than human beings because they know but do not tell."

Emily Dickinson, poet of
"Hope is the Thing with Feathers"

"Dogs love their friends and bite their enemies, quite unlike people, who are incapable of pure love and always have to mix love and hate."

Sigmund Freud, psychoanalyst

"A bone to the dog is not charity. Charity is the bone shared with the dog when you are just as hungry as the dog."

Jack London, author of *The Call of the Wild*

Doc Rob's
Favorite Quotes About Cats

"Dogs come when called. Cats take a message
and get back to you."

Anonymous

"Time spent with cats is never wasted."

Sigmund Freud, psychoanalyst

"I have felt cats rubbing their faces against mine and
touching my cheek with claws carefully sheathed.
These things, to me, are expressions of love."

James Herriot, UK Veterinarian,
author of *All Creatures Great and Small*

"Like all pure creatures, cats are practical."

William S. Burroughs, author of *Naked Lunch*

"The smallest feline is a masterpiece."

Leonardo da Vinci, artist, scientist,
engineer, sculptor, and architect

"Cats choose us, we do not own them."

Kristin Cast, author of
the *House of Night* series

"In ancient times cats were worshipped as gods;
they have not forgotten this."

Terry Pratchett, author of *Good Omens*

"One cat just leads to another."

Ernest Hemingway, author,
received the Nobel Prize for Literature in 1954

"There are two means of refuge from the miseries of life: music and cats."

Albert Schweitzer,
received Nobel Peace Prize in 1952

"How we behave towards cats here below determines our status in heaven."

Robert Heinlein, author of
Stranger in a Strange Land

"The phrase 'domestic cat' is an oxymoron."

George Will,
received Pulitzer Prize for Commentary in 1977

"I had been told that the training procedure with cats was difficult. It's not. Mine had me trained in two days."

Bill Dana, comedian

"As anyone who has ever been around a cat for any length of time well knows, cats have enormous patience with the limitations of humankind."

Cleveland Amory, author of
The Cat Who Came for Christmas

DEDICATION

To the four-legged teachers in my life who have shaped and inspired my journey as a veterinarian.

To the herbalists and mycologists I have met on my path who have embedded in me both the love and the knowledge to use these gentle earth remedies for the good of our four-legged companions.

And to Hannah, my wife and my rock; and to Callejune, my daughter: The flame that ignites my inspiration.

Without their loving support, this book could not exist.

Rob Silver,
August 2024

CONTENTS

PREFACE 1

AUTHOR'S FOREWORD:
WHY YOU SHOULD READ THIS BOOK 5

Section One: A Journey Into the World of
Medicinal Fungi, Our Marvelous Mushroom Friends........... 6

Section Two: Your Healthy Pet Guide –
Real-Life Stories of Healing 6

Learn Important Integrative Medicine Tools...................... 10

How to Use This Book to Help Your Pet............................ 11

SECTION ONE:
OUR MARVELOUS MUSHROOMS 15

Chapter One: Introduction to the Fungal Kingdom 17

The History of Mushroom Use 20

The Nutritional Value of Mushrooms 22

Chapter Two: What Is a Mushroom? 26

The Fungal Life Cycle 27

How Mushrooms Are Grown... 29

Mushroom Quality Product Analysis Study......................... 30

Chapter Three: Active Mushroom Compounds 35

    Beta-glucans 35

    Terpenes 36

    Ergothioneine 38

    Ergosterol 39

    Cholesterol Statins 40

    Nucleosides 41

    Psilocin (Psilocybin) 42

Chapter Four: Important Mushrooms for a Healthy Pet, What They *Are* and What They Are *For* 44

    Quick Reference Guide to Uses of Mushrooms for Pets 45

    Agaricus 46

    Chaga 51

    Cordyceps 56

    Lion's Mane 62

    Maitake Mushroom 67

    Oyster Mushroom 72

    Psilocybin 75

    Reishi 78

    Shiitake Mushroom 85

    Snow Mushroom 90

    Turkey Tail 94

Chapter Five: How to Give Mushrooms to Your Pet 101

    Establishing an Effective Amount to Give Your Pet 102

    How to Select an Effective Mushroom 105

**SECTION TWO: YOUR HEALTHY PET GUIDE—
THERE'S A MUSHROOM FOR THAT!**..........................**111**

Chapter Six: Allergies and Inflammatory Dermatitis 113

Allergies in a Dog: "Poochie" Smith's Allergic Dermatitis...113

Poochie's Allergy Supplements 116

About Skin Allergies in Pets 122

Conventional Approaches to Allergies in Pets....................124

Integrative/Holistic Treatments...131

**Chapter Seven: Anxiety and Behavioral Problems
in Dogs and Cats...139**

Cat Anxiety 139

Example of Dog Anxiety: Ollie's PTSD
and Anxiety as a Rescue Dog..141

Anxiety and Behavioral Problems Explained 148

Conventional Approaches to Anxiety 149

Dog Issues 150

Cat Issues..151

Integrative/Holistic Approaches to
Anxiety and Behavioral Problems in Pets............................153

CBD 153

CBG 155

Lion's Mane Mushroom Extracts.....................................155

Example of a Proprietary Product Formulation for
Behavioral Issues...156

Alternative Therapy Calming Devices.............................157

Calming Supplements...158

Diet: "You Are What You Eat"...160

Lifestyle Modifications 161

Chapter Eight: Arthritis (and Other Painful Conditions) ... 162

Arthritis in a Dog: Chester 162

Chester's Arthritis Plan... 164

Understanding and Detecting Arthritis in Your Pet 165

Conventional Approaches to Treat Arthritis.................... 169

Integrative/Holistic Approaches 172

Cannabinoid Therapies:
Cannabis, CBD, and Other Cannabinoids..................... 172

Medicinal Mushrooms and Arthritis:
Anti-inflammatory and Immune Support..................... 175

Joint Supplements 176

Diet – Feeding the Arthritic Dog............................ 179

High Carbohydrate Diets Are Pro-inflammatory
and Add "Empty" Calories. 180

Exercise and Activity Considerations 181

Manual Therapies and Physical Rehabilitation............. 182

Chapter Nine: Cancer and Cancer Therapy Side Effects 187

Cancer in a Dog: The Sudden Collapse of Grover............... 187

Grover's Plan for His Hemangiosarcoma............................ 195

How Did Grover Do On This Program? 198

Why Did Grover Do So Well Surviving with
This Aggressively Terminal Cancer Diagnosis?................... 202

Supplements That Made a Difference with Grover 203

How Do You Know When It's Time?................................ 206

What Is Cancer? What Causes It? How Is It Treated?..... 209

Conventional Approaches.. 211

Diagnostics for Cancer.. 211

Is Chemotherapy Right for Your Pet's Cancer? 214

Turkey Tail Study of Hemangiosarcoma in Dogs.........216

Integrative/Holistic Approaches for Cancer 220

    Using Cannabis to Treat Cancer 220

    CBD 221

    Ratio Products with CBD:THC....................................224

    DIY Ratio Products – When Ratio Products
    Are Not Available Locally 225

    How to Create the Ratio Product Your Pet Needs.......228

    Medicinal Mushrooms for Cancer 229

    Other Supplements for Cancer Patients 231

    Antioxidants..232

    Immune System Modifiers..235

    Beta-glucans 237

    Vitamin D 237

    Curcuminoids (*Curcuma longa*) 238

    Polysaccharides 239

    Adaptogens..240

    Chinese Herbal Formulations for Cancer 241

    Alternative Cancer Therapies 245

    Diets for Cancer Patients 247

Chapter Ten: Digestive Disorders 252

    Digestive Problems in a Dog 252

    Tawny's Unrelenting Diarrhea....................................252

    Understanding the Digestive System 257

    Causes of Bowel Problems 258

    Integrative/Holistic Approaches to Digestive Disorders ..260

    Cannabis and the Digestive System 261

    Medicinal Mushrooms and Healthy Bowel Function ...266

    Dietary Supplements = Digestion "Boosters"................267

    Digestive Herbs and Nutraceuticals 271

Conventional Pharmaceutical Approaches...........................278

Diet – The Most Important Thing to
Change with Digestive Problems 281

Food Sensitivity and Allergy Testing................................283

Home Prepared Meals (and Raw Versus Cooked)........286

Doc Silver's Home-Prepared Meal Guidelines 288

Canine Nutrient Profiles 290

Feline Nutrient Profiles.......................................295

Sources of Healthy Fatty Acids 296

How Much to Feed?..299

Determining the Body Condition Score (BCS) 300

Introducing the New Diet....................................303

Making the Diet as "Complete"
and Balanced as Possible....................................304

Is Raw Food Safe to Feed? 306

Meal-Balancing Supplements 308

Limited Antigen Diets 310

**Chapter Eleven: Epilepsy
and Other Neurologic Disorders** 312

Treatment-Resistant Canine Idiopathic Epilepsy: Crystal... 312

About Treating Neurologic Conditions 320

Understanding Canine Idiopathic *and/or*
Treatment-Resistant Epilepsy.................................322

Conventional Approaches.....................................327

Integrative/Holistic Approaches 329

Supplements for Epilepsy and
Other Neurodegenerative Conditions 332

Traditional Chinese Veterinary Medicine for Epilepsy ..333

Vitamin D and Vitamin E.....................................334

Medicinal Mushrooms...335

Acupuncture for Epilepsy...336

Ketogenic Diet..337

Chapter Twelve: Ollie's Healthy Pet Wellness Program 340

12-Point Wellness Program for Your Dog or Cat 342

How to Achieve Wellness for Your Pet:
A Simple Summary...343

Ollie's Wellness Program...345

Wellness Program Additions Specifically for Cats............ 349

**SUMMARY: DOC ROB'S WELLNESS PROGRAM
FOR YOUR FOUR-LEGGED FAMILY MEMBER.............. 353**

Note to the Reader 355

RESOURCE GUIDE.. 356

Find a Holistic Vet 356

List of Pet Nutrition Consultants....................................357

Books 358

INDEX.. 362

REFERENCES 392

PREFACE

Mark J. Plotkin, PhD
Ethnobotanist
Amazon Conservation Team

W e live in an age that has been deemed "The Psychedelic Renaissance." One of the most significant recent developments in the field of human medicine is the integration of mind-altering plants and fungi into mainstream Western medical practices. From time immemorial, these substances have served as the tools of healers who have skillfully utilized plants and fungi as intricate instruments for exploring, diagnosing, treating, and curing a myriad of ailments. It was only with the advent of modern chemistry and technology, over the course of the past century, that we have reduced or sometimes eliminated Mother Nature as our primary source of therapeutic compounds.

The utilization of these psychoactive compounds is rapidly gaining recognition within conventional clinical settings. Yet, it would be a mistake to believe that these psychoactive compounds are valuable solely for their mind-altering capabilities. These chemicals cause a variety of changes in the body, not just the inducement of hallucinations. One concrete manifestation of that is the burgeoning field of microdosing, which entails ingesting miniscule amounts of these molecules in the belief that they can enhance creativity, slow the aging process, and improve hand-eye coordination.

Meanwhile, medicinal fungi are repeatedly being prized and

utilized for treating and sometimes curing a variety of challenging afflictions. Mycologist and herbal clinician, Dr. Christopher Hobbs, author of the classic, *Medicinal Mushrooms: An Exploration of Tradition, Healing, & Culture*, and his recently published, *Medicinal Mushrooms: The Essential Guide*, recently told me that fungi can be effective for the prevention and treatment of cardiovascular issues, respiratory problems, and immune support.

So, if these compounds can be used to treat human ailments and infirmities, why would they not work on our beloved pets as well?

A fast-developing field in the biology world is the science of "zoopharmacognosy," the study of how animals use plants and other substances to self-medicate. Initially launched by the great Jane Goodall, we now know that creatures from fruit flies to chimps to elephants ingest botanical materials to treat everything from skin infections to intestinal parasites. Further field study will undoubtedly reveal more plants and fungi used by animals for therapeutic purposes!

It should therefore come as no surprise that plants and fungi can heal our own furry friends as well as they can heal us.

The challenge this book addresses is how best to employ fungi and cannabis products for this purpose. It is indeed ironic that these "new" medicines are in fact two of the oldest remedies employed by the human (and, possibly, pre-human) species. There are 7,000-year-old carvings of medicinal mushrooms at the Tassilli site in southeastern Algeria. And mycologist Paul Stamets has recently identified magic mushroom wall carvings in Pharaonic tombs in ancient Egypt.

Similarly, cannabis is demonstrably one of our most ancient plant companions. The earliest written records are from China, where the plant was originally employed as a fiber. Shortly thereafter, however, it was widely used in both China and India for a variety of therapeutic purposes.

Meanwhile, as the Western world increasingly appreciates both the utility and versatility of these once "banished" organisms, new discoveries and uses are happening all the time. Fungal mycelia are being used to manufacture everything from acoustic panels to yoga mats. Cannabis fiber is being turned into auto parts, leather, and high-end fashion.

So can all of us animal lovers know how (and how much) mushrooms and cannabis can best be used to tone and heal our four-legged friends?

The good news is that both the general public and the veterinary and human medical establishments are more interested in incorporating these compounds into the lives of their pets (and sometimes their own lives) as never before. Where there is money to be made—lots of money as the veterinary medical field may be worth in excess of 10 billion dollars on an annual basis—all sorts of people will have an interest. Given how recent is the interest on the part of pet doctors, very little formal instruction and reliable references are available, while well-meaning amateurs are now cranking out articles, books, and websites addressing the issue based on little reliable research and studies.

Into this niche steps Dr. Rob Silver, a veterinarian of deep learning and experience and even deeper compassion. Rob has been working on these issues and with these substances for decades, giving him an almost unique perspective that he shares with us in this book. I observed Rob's wisdom and empathy first-hand when he treated a beloved pet and family member, a case history he shares in this book.

If you have ever wanted to learn more about employing plants or fungi for pet care—whether you are a 10-year-old with your first puppy or a vet of long experience confronting a difficult case—then this book is for you. In clear and compelling language, and with ample examples of case histories, Rob draws on his decades of work as a clinician and researcher to make suggestions and point the way, always based on what he knows, what he has seen, and what he has done for and with his patients and their human companions.

As such, this book is destined to be a landmark in the field, the equivalent of the famous *Physician's Desk Reference*—except unlike the *PDR*, it will be on the desk of every veterinarian and the bookshelf of many if not most pet owners.

I give it my highest recommendation!

Mark J. Plotkin, PhD.
Ethnobotanist
Amazon Conservation Team

WHY YOU SHOULD READ THIS BOOK

As a veterinarian, I have dedicated my life to the care and well-being of animals. Throughout my career, I have witnessed the remarkable bond that exists between pets and their human companions, and I have strived to provide the best possible care for our beloved animal friends. In my journey, I have seen the landscape of veterinary medicine evolve, incorporating innovative approaches and treatments to improve the lives of pets.

The book you are about to delve into is a testament to the ever-evolving field of veterinary medicine. *There's a Mushroom for That!* explores the potential of mushrooms and cannabis compounds for pet health. It is a pioneering work that sheds light on a fascinating and relatively uncharted territory within the veterinary profession, and it addresses a subject that has garnered increased attention in recent years: the use of mushrooms and cannabis compounds to get pets healthy and keep them that way.

This exploration of these emerging pet treatments is driven by a fundamental truth: our pets, like us, can suffer from a myriad of health issues, some very serious and life-threatening. From chronic pain and anxiety to debilitating diseases, the spectrum of conditions that affect our furry companions can be vast and complex. As a veterinarian, it is my duty to seek out new and effective ways to alleviate animal suffering to enhance their quality of life.

SECTION ONE: OUR MARVELOUS MUSHROOMS

In Section One, you will embark upon a journey into the amazing world of our marvelous mushrooms and fantastic fungi. Here you will learn how mushrooms grow, and find out how the way they are grown can affect their potency, and more importantly, their ability to help your pet. Mushrooms have a rich history of use in human health care, dating back millennia, but are only recently being used for animal health care.

Here, I describe in great depth and detail 11 of the most important medicinal mushrooms that can help your four-legged companion. It's likely that as you read these mushroom profiles, you will find some that you should consider giving your pet for a longer and happier life with you.

Cannabis, and CBD, like mushrooms, are equally exciting and important emerging natural therapies for pets. The therapeutic benefits of these unique compounds found in cannabis for pets, including CBD and THC, are explained in simple to understand terms. You will find a better understanding of the science behind these substances is crucial to appreciating their potential for your pet's health.

SECTION TWO: YOUR HEALTHY PET GUIDE—
THERE'S A MUSHROOM FOR THAT!

Mushrooms have long been revered for their healing properties. In the second section of this book, you will discover how mushroom species can boost the immune system, reduce inflammation, and even slow the progression of cancer in pets. We explore the beneficial relationship between mushrooms and animals in nature, shedding light on the innate connection between these organisms and the potential they hold for veterinary medicine.

I have provided eight stories from patients I have seen in my 40-plus-year career in veterinary practice that will guide you to use medicinal mushrooms, cannabis, and integrative medicine to support and help your four-legged friend with one of these conditions:

- **Allergies**
- **Anxiety**
- **Arthritis**
- **Cancer**
- **Digestive Disorders**
- **Epilepsy**
- **Wellness**

Throughout Section Two, each chapter tells the story of some of my most interesting patients, and I then describe my understanding of their medical concerns. I define and describe that medical condition and the conventional approach to that condition. Finally, I explain, in simple terminology, the best integrative approach to that condition, and specifically, how much of which mushrooms and cannabis I used to help that patient's concerns.

It is important here to emphasize the necessity of responsible and informed use when considering these treatments for your pets. Although my advice in this book is solid, it is important that you partner with a veterinarian you trust who you can work with. Collaboration with a knowledgeable veterinarian is essential to ensure the health and safety of your furry friends. In the Resource section at the end of this book, I've provided links to several holistic veterinary organizations that offer directories of their members, which can help you find a holistic partner for this healing journey with your pet.

Your Healthy Pet Guide is based on years of research into the scientific literature and my own hands-on 40+ years of experience in practice as a veterinarian to provide a comprehensive health reference and guide for the dedicated and compassionate pet parent. In this book, I have presented how and when these novel and powerful natural products can and should be used.

The anticipated reader for this book is the dedicated and concerned pet parent looking to discover every possible health-enhancing tool that could benefit the health of their pets and contribute to their longevity and quality of life.

Your Healthy Pet Guide can also serve as a good entry-level source text for veterinarians looking to understand more of the practical aspects, and the foundations of the science, for the veterinary use of medicinal mushrooms and cannabis.

This book provides **guidance and inspiration to those veterinarians** aspiring to practice integrative medicine who are looking for practical instructions from one who has been *down that road* many times.

Although they are quite potent therapeutics, cannabis and mushrooms are not panaceas, curing anything and everything in their path. Often, they are most effective as part of a comprehensive program blended with conventional therapeutics using an integrative medicine approach.

Your Healthy Pet Guide gives the loving pet parent tools they can use to help their pets suffering from serious chronic disease problems, such as allergies, arthritis, cancer, digestive disorders, epilepsy, and dermatologic issues. This easy-to-read book also contains a section that discusses several strategies for creating and maintaining health and wellness in your pet.

Each of these six common, yet difficult-to-treat problems, is explained in easy-to-understand language that expertly guides you in the effective use of medicinal mushrooms, cannabis, home-prepared diets, and dietary supplements. This book also contains information about the conventional diagnostics, pharmaceuticals, and procedures that your vet may suggest for your pet for one of the six conditions discussed.

This information will better help you understand what the vet was saying to you in the exam room so you can make an intelligent and informed decision when choosing veterinary care for your beloved four-legged furry family member.

Your Healthy Pet Guide gives you detailed information to help you make the right decisions about your pet's care. For instance, you may have just returned from seeing your vet, where you got a frightening diagnosis for your pet, like cancer or epilepsy. **Not to worry**, you can reach for this book and read through it to better understand your pet's problem.

You will learn which alternative therapies to use in an effective healthcare program—one that you can get started right away. It will also guide you in understanding what drugs or surgical therapies your conventionally-minded veterinarian has recommended for your pet so you can approve of their use or discuss further options with your vet.

The sooner you start **Your Healthy Pet's Wellness Program,** *as described in this book, the sooner your pet will experience improved health.*

If you are a citizen-scientist pet parent, then you will enjoy the sections of the book explaining how mushrooms and cannabis work to create good health and wellness. Each medical condition is explained in depth so you can better understand the problems and the DIY solutions this book offers you and your "fur baby."

LEARN IMPORTANT INTEGRATIVE MEDICINE TOOLS

- How to prepare **home-made diets**, including the **ketogenic** diet

- How to provide **healthy mushrooms** as part of your pet's diet and daily supplement program for better immune and nervous system health

- How to select the best **cannabis** product for your **pet**

- How to navigate the many products found in dispensaries to the **few products that are safe for your pet**

- How to **introduce dispensary products** to your pet, as recommended in this book, to avoid potential problems

- How to **help your pet** with cannabis, mushrooms, and integrative medicine for the seven conditions covered by this book

- How to find **resources for more information**, and how to find a skilled integrative veterinarian to help you with your pet's problems.

- Learn what to do when **cancer** strikes your pet

- Learn to better manage your pet's **anxiety**

- Help your pained pet have better **mobility** and **quality of life**

- Use supplements for **healthy skin and haircoat** and to help reduce **allergic** symptoms

- Consider trying CBD for idiopathic **epilepsy** and see if it can be a true game-changer in helping your pet's misery

This book is an invaluable tool for you to use over your pet's lifetime to help guide you in effective ways to keep your pet happy and healthy.

HOW TO USE THIS BOOK TO HELP YOUR PET

If you are reading this book, you are one of many pet parents who are wondering if medicinal mushrooms, CBD, and cannabis can help their pets in a natural way without the often-nasty side effects that we see with many drug therapies.

I'm a vet, so I know how expenses can escalate even with simple medical problems. If mushrooms, CBD, or cannabis can help keep an animal healthy, I'm all for that. Vets have plenty of animals to care for, so if one stays healthy by taking a safe and simple plant or mushroom extract, then so much the better.

These are some of the questions I get asked all the time about using CBD, cannabis, and mushrooms in pets:

- **What's it for?**

- Is it **safe?**

- Will it **work** for my pet's unique problem?

- How do I **find** a product that is effective but not contaminated with something toxic to my pet?

- **How much** should I give to my pet for its size or problem?

- What about the **drugs and other supplements** my dog may be on—will it be a problem if I use them at the same time?

These questions and more will be answered in this book so you can learn how to best help your pet safely and effectively with mushrooms and cannabis. Each chapter will build a foundation for the next chapter but can also be used as a stand-alone chapter providing information on a topic. You can read this book from cover to cover or use the table of contents or index to find the exact topic you need.

Your Healthy Pet Guide will provide you with all you need to know about using mushrooms, CBD, and cannabis for your pet. This information comes from an expert in medicinal mushrooms and cannabis for pets, who has years of experience understanding the clinical applications of mushrooms, cannabis, and CBD in animals.

Holistic treatments, such as supplements, dietary changes, Chinese herbal therapies, cannabis, and medicinal mushrooms, are commonly used to improve the quality of life and longevity of many pets diagnosed with difficult-to-treat diseases like cancer, epilepsy, or allergies. Or even anxiety and IBD.

In my long career, my most successful cases are those that come to me early enough that there is still some "life" left. When I see a patient who is in the end stages of their cancer or some other problem, it's much more difficult to try and muster up reserve-healing capacity in that pet whose life force is totally depleted. So don't delay addressing your pets' problems, and find a good holistic vet to be your partner on the journey to health with your pet.

I've also found that even with what seemed to be impossible cases, success is possible when the pet's parents fought tooth and nail to manage that disease. They would fix home-prepared meals, administer supplements several times daily, provide physical therapy and rehab treatments, or acupuncture and/or chiropractic treatments for their ailing pet, as well as other tasks and treatments. I found that it's the dedicated pet parent who always seemed to have the best results for their pets.

I remember one case where a cat named "Cow" had a fungal infection of his nose that was extremely severe. The vets before me had tried to treat Cow with antifungal medications. But they did not help. In fact, these strong medications caused his liver to react with elevated enzyme levels.

I thought about fighting a fungal infection with a fungus, fighting fire with fire, so to speak. In homeopathy, we say that **"Like Cures Like."** With this strategy in mind, I tried using medicinal mushrooms to improve his immune system response to the infection. I also used ozone therapy in an attempt to stop the growth of this fungus that had nearly eaten away all of his nasal tissue. Ozone is "super-oxygen, and can kill many types of disease-causing microbes, like fungi, bacteria, and yeast, and can be used to treat cancer as well."

Unfortunately, it was too late to help this cat. I was really sad about this. In my short time treating Cow, I had bonded with her; she was so sweet and loving. It seems like the nicest animals get the worst conditions. It's just not fair!

Throughout my career as a veterinarian, I have concentrated on using these alternative cancer therapies in combination with conventional cancer therapies to bring quality of life and extended life spans to my patients. Many of my own patients have far exceeded the survival statistics for cancer and other terminal diseases with the use of integrative medicine.

In this book, you will find eight stories about pets I have treated for the seven conditions that are most commonly treated with cannabis and mushrooms. I chose these stories because they are good examples of how to treat each of these conditions. If your pet has one of these conditions, you will learn from the stories about how to get started with your pet's problem(s).

SECTION ONE

OUR MARVELOUS MUSHROOMS

Since pet CBD became a big thing, mushrooms have now become the next big focus of interest for pet parents and veterinarians. This is why I want to provide plenty of information to help you understand what mushrooms are and how to best use them for your pets.

Mushrooms have health benefits for our dogs, cats, and horses to maintain health and wellness and to address difficult-to-manage problems, such as cancer; dementia; stress; anxiety; seasonal allergies; viral, bacterial, fungal, and yeast infections; and kidney, liver, and lung support. Mushrooms also help with providing more energy and improving stamina and performance. That's just to name just a few of the many potential applications for mushrooms!

The huge popularity of the Netflix documentary *Fantastic Fungi*™ is just one example of this current "mushroom madness." This interest in mushrooms began with people finding great benefits with their own use of mushrooms. The search for products that protect against viral diseases during the pandemic led to the increased use of medicinal mushrooms. It is, therefore, a natural progression that folks would want to give their beloved pet family members the same benefits they were experiencing.

The first event that boosted popular interest in giving mushrooms to one's pet occurred in 2012 when the University of Pennsylvania published a pilot study in dogs with hemangiosarcoma, a very aggressive malignancy of the spleen and heart. They were using an extract from turkey tail (*Trametes versicolor*), and the results were astounding![1]

All of the dogs in this small study had already had their spleens removed, which is done to prevent the splenic cancer from spreading further. But these dogs' parents had also refused chemotherapy and instead had opted to try this mushroom extract. This study tested different doses of the turkey tail extract to see which had the best benefits. There were five dogs in each of the three dosage tiers.

This study found that the dogs who received the highest dose of the mushroom extract lived far longer than dogs who were splenectomized and receiving chemotherapy. The study shocked the world of oncology, as it showed that a natural product could succeed where conventional pharmaceuticals failed. As a result of this study, sales of turkey tail increased astronomically as pet parents sourced this mushroom for their own pets' cancer.

Pet parents and veterinarians are interested in offering their pets and patients the health benefits that mushrooms provide, but first, four questions will be answered in the pages that follow, so you can know how to best use them:

First, what is it in mushrooms that has these benefits? Is it one compound or multiple compounds like we find with cannabis?

Second, are mushrooms safe for pets, and can they be used with other supplements and pharmaceuticals a pet may be on?

Third, how much do you give your pet?

And finally, are there differences in the effects of the different mushrooms? There are many mushrooms that have health significance. How do I choose the right mushroom for my pet?

INTRODUCTION TO THE FUNGAL KINGDOM

Fungi are a separate kingdom, different and apart from the kingdom of plants and the kingdom of animals. Fungi are ubiquitous on our planet; they are everywhere! It has been estimated that there are approximately 1.5 to 3.8 million species of fungi globally.[2] Fungi can be found in our stratosphere, on the bottom of the Dead Sea, in Antarctic glaciers, and in arid deserts. They have been identified in the digestive system of insects and in deep oceanic sediments. Evidence shows that some mushrooms growing 320 million years ago are very similar to the mushrooms we see today.

Studies in evolutionary biology support the idea that fungal organisms share a common ancestor with animals, a single-celled organism with a whip-like "flagella." This means the DNA of fungi is more alike with our own animal DNA than with plant DNA.[3] This may explain why fungal infections can be so pathogenic and difficult to treat. It may also explain why the active molecules found in fungi are so effective in supporting the health of humans and animals.

Fungi are significantly involved in our global "geochemistry" by recycling carbon and releasing nitrogen, phosphorus, and other bio-elements. They provide intrinsic support to the plant kingdom in the form of *endophytes* and *mycorrhizae*.

"*Endophytes*" are bacteria or fungi that live within a plant for at least part of its life cycle without causing disease. Endophytes are widespread and have been found in all species of plants. Some endophytes may enhance host growth and nutrient acquisition and improve the plant's ability to tolerate environmental stresses, such as drought. They can decrease stresses caused by insects, pathogens, and plant-eating animals.

Endophytes may produce biologically active constituents that are attributed to the plant when, in fact, these molecules are derived from the fungal endophyte. One example is the chemotherapy agent Taxol, which is produced by the fungal endophyte that lives on the bark of the Pacific yew tree (*Taxus brevifolia*) that has been considered the source of the useful therapeutic agent.

"*Mycorrhizae*," like endophytes, are another symbiotic association between a plant and a fungus. Mycorrhizae are fungal mycelium that grow around the roots of plants and improve their ability to absorb nutrients for growth and contribute to soil biology and soil chemistry.

The plant provides organic molecules like sugars from photosynthesis to the fungus, and the fungus supplies water and mineral nutrients, such as phosphorus from the soil. A few mycorrhizae have a parasitic relationship with the plant. Evolutionarily, before plants developed root systems, fungal mycorrhizae were needed to provide the plant with nutrients.

Fungi play many important roles in keeping our planet healthy:

1. Fungi have provided humans and the animals they steward with fermented foods and beverages, as well as medicines and compounds that have important industrial applications.

2. Fungi are an essential source of food, either from the mushroom itself or from the fermentation of mycelium digesting soybeans, for instance, in the case of Tempeh, or tea in the

case of the kombucha fungus, or vegetables, in the case of kimchee and sauerkraut.

3. Fungal materials are being used in the production of clothing and building materials.

Fungi aren't always beneficial. For instance, fungal pathogens are some of the most toxic on the planet and can destroy food supplies and entire species of plants and animals.

Lately, quite a bit of ecological interest has been focused on the impact that mushrooms, particularly their mycelium, have on the health of our planet. As recyclers, the fungal mycelium consumes dead and dying plant and animal materials and elaborates strong enzymes that digest these biological materials that they break down into basic nutrients. They provide nourishment for themselves, as well as support the growth of plants and animals, which, when they die, are then digested and recycled by the fungal mycelium.

Fungi and mushrooms, in particular, are key players in the micro-ecology and macro-ecology of the earth. Interest in this mycelial network is high. Mycelial networks can spread through very large areas. One fungal mycelial network in Oregon has been measured to be 2,385 acres in size! This mycelial network is likened to the circulatory and nervous system of an animal, providing a path for the movement and distribution of the digested nutrients and of "information" communicated throughout the network.

This extensive system is thought to have an "intelligence" in how it transfers information and nutrients throughout it. The mycelial network intertwines with the root systems in forests and interfaces with the forest this way. Mycelia, as the vegetative stage of the fungal lifecycle, have very powerful ecological properties, which are similar, yet different, to the powerful properties of the fruiting stage of the life cycle: the mushroom.[4]

THE HISTORY OF MUSHROOM USE

Mushrooms have played an important role in the development of human civilization. They have been of interest to people for millennia. In addition to their nutritional value as a food, many edible mushrooms have also been valued for their medicinal properties. Some mushrooms, too woody to be edible, can also have potent medicinal properties.

Anthropological data supporting the use of mushrooms for medicinal purposes goes back to about 10,000 years ago (8000 B.C.E.)! Prehistoric humans used mushrooms collected in the wild as food and medicines. "Ötzi," an early human from circa 5000 B.C.E, was found frozen in a melting glacier in the Italian Alps in the 1990s. He had two species of medicinal mushrooms found on him. Pieces of the birch polypore (*Piptoporus betulinus*) were strung on a leather thong. This mushroom was also found in his digestive system, so we know he was taking this medicinal mushroom. This mushroom is known as an anti-parasite, anti-infection medicine with anti-inflammatory and fever-reducing properties. Ötzi's digestive system was found to be riddled with parasites.

The other mushroom found on Ötzi was the tinder polypore (*Fomes fomentarius*), also known as "tinder conk." Like the birch polypore, it is also commonly found on birch trees. These bracket-like fungi are used with flint and steel as a fire starter. They can be pounded into a felt-like material that keeps embers smoldering and thus was used to carry fire safely. It also can be used as a kind of mushroom "leather" for hats, belts, and packs. This mushroom, like the birch polypore, also has traditional uses as a medicine for its anti-inflammatory and antibacterial properties used in the cauterization of wounds and for treating cancer.[5]

Early civilizations of Greeks, Egyptians, Romans, Chinese, Mexicans, Central Americans, and South Americans thought of mushrooms as a delicacy, understood their therapeutic value, and used them in religious ceremonies. In these cultures, mushrooms were considered "flesh of the gods." This was especially true with the mushrooms that provide a psychotropic or spiritual experience, such as the mushroom species that produce psilocybin.

Mushroom cultivation began in 600 A.D. with the cultivation of the popular wood ear mushroom (*Auricularia auricula*) in China. Shiitake was first cultivated in 1000 A.D., and the button mushroom (*Agaricus bisporus*) was first cultivated in France around 1600 A.D.[6]

Over the millennia, mushrooms have provided an easily harvested forest edible that has been cultivated and commercialized into the multi-billion-dollar global industry it is today. Mushrooms have been used for food and health as long as they have been collected. They have served as medicines prior to the age of pharmaceuticals. Mushrooms still play an important role in many indigenous people's way of life.

Mushrooms today are having a resurgence in public interest as food and medicine. Social media groups and mushroom foraging clubs are forming around the country where people get together to walk in areas where mushrooms grow, such as forests and urban parks. These gatherings allow people to learn how to identify mushrooms. Some mushrooms are quite poisonous and look similar to edible mushrooms. It's vital to be able to identify a mushroom correctly to avoid toxicity. These "mushrooming" groups serve both an educational and social purpose in bringing people together to share their knowledge and experience.

THE NUTRITIONAL VALUE OF MUSHROOMS

Mushrooms provide a ready-to-eat source of nutrition. It is estimated that globally there are around 140,000 mushrooms out of
1-2 million fungal species. Of these 140,000 mushrooms, only
about 10% (14,000) have been identified. Of this 10%, 50% are
considered "edible," 21% are considered to be "prime" edible, 15%
are medicinal, and it's estimated that 1-10% are toxic.[7]

NUMBERS & TYPES OF MUSHROOMS

Total Number Fungal Species Globally	1-2 Million
Total Number of Mushrooms Estimated Globally	140,000
Number of Mushrooms Currently Known	14,000
Number of Edible Mushroom Species	7,000 total edibles 3,000 prime edible
Number of Medicinal Species, Estimated	2,000
Number of Toxic Species	~1% of all mushrooms

Mushrooms have a very high moisture content when fresh, containing anywhere from 70-95% water. They are low in calories,
sugars, and fats (2-8%) and high in fiber and polysaccharides (50-
65%). Mushrooms are rich sources of protein (35%), vitamins,
and minerals. They have a naturally low content of starch, which
is the digestible carbohydrate (<10%), and a high non-digestible

carbohydrate content (50-65%) that is made up primarily of poly-saccharides and fiber—the beta-glucans and chitin from their sturdy cell walls.[8]

Due to their low starch content, mushrooms have a very low glycemic index and, as such, have little to no negative nutritional influence on blood glucose and insulin regulation. Medicinally, though, mushrooms are known to help regulate blood sugar through their active constituents. They are considered to be true *functional foods* with excellent nutritional and medicinal proper-ties.

The mushroom cell wall contains mostly non-digestible fiber and polysaccharides. For this reason, all mushrooms need to be cooked before eating. Some mushrooms may also contain slightly toxic compounds that are destroyed by heating. To completely break down the fiber in mushrooms, which releases their bioactive components, mushrooms benefit from being cooked for several hours. Longer cook times are preferable, but at minimum, mush-rooms must be cooked for at least 15-30 minutes before consuming.

White button mushrooms (*Agaricus bisporus*), that are so commonly found at the grocery store, contain hydrazine com-pounds, such as agaritine. These are relatively low-toxicity com-pounds. One can still eat a small amount of button mushrooms raw, if that is to your taste, and not worry about toxicity. You would have to eat a lot of raw button mushrooms for an extended period of time for there to be any actual toxicity. Cooking the mushrooms will further reduce the amount of agaritine in the raw mushroom. When white button mushrooms are kept refrigerated for 7 days or more, the agaritine content reduces naturally over this time period. Toxicity studies have not been able to definitively define this compound's risk to humans. Mycelium also contains agaritine.

NUTRITIONAL VALUE OF MUSHROOMS[9]

Mushroom Species	Oyster	Shiitake	Maitake	Agaricus	Lion's Mane	Average
kcal	41 kcal	44 kcal	38 kcal	31 kcal	43 kcal	39.4 kcal
Protein	2.9 g	2.4 g	2.2 g	2.9 g	2.5 g	2.6 g
Starch	6.94 g	8.17 g	6.6 g	6.94 g	7.59 g	7.25 g
Fat	0.20 g	0.20 g	0.30 g	0.20 g	0.30 g	0.32 g
H_2O	89.2 g	88.6 g	90.4 g	91.8 g	88.6 g	89.7 g
Dietary Fiber	2.9 g	4.2 g	3.1 g	1.7 g	4.4 g	3.26 g
Ash	0.73 g	0.62 g	0.56 g	0.83 g	1.08 g	0.76 g
Beta-glucans	3.0 g	2.8 g	2.5 g	0.75 g	2.4 g	2.3 g
Ergothioneine	14 mg	11 mg	2 mg	4 mg	17 mg	9.6 mg

CHAPTER ONE SUMMARY

In Chapter One, we learned that the fungal kingdom and its mushrooms range from easily harvested forest edibles to medicinal, psychotropic, or even toxic in nature. Mushrooms have played an important role throughout human history dated back before recorded time. This is due, in part, to their rich nutritional value; mushrooms contain substantial high-quality protein and healthy fiber. This is also due to the critical role mushrooms have in maintaining both the health of our planet and the people and animals that live on Earth.

In Chapter Two, we will "dig down" further and learn much more about the biological aspects of mushrooms. We will discover why the mushroom, as the birthplace of the spores, is such an important part of the three-part fungal life cycle, as well as cover the growing procedures, and the importance of quality analysis in modern-day mushroom products.

WHAT IS A MUSHROOM?

Mushrooms are called the "fruiting body" because, in an analogy with plants, the mushroom is like the fruit, and the spores are like the seeds inside the fruit. The definition of mushroom includes those fungal structures that can be either above ground or below ground and are large enough to be seen with the naked eye and to be picked by hand.[10] Mushrooms can be edible, inedible, medicinal, toxic, or "spiritual" in terms of their activity.

Mushrooms take on a variety of different shapes, but the most common shape is an umbrella-like cap (pileus) and a stem (stipe). Some have a ring around the stipe, and some have a cup (volva) around the base.

MUSHROOM ANATOMY

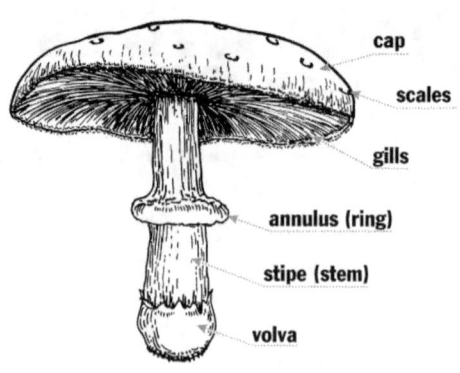

cap

scales

gills

annulus (ring)

stipe (stem)

volva

Other shapes that mushroom fruiting bodies can assume include:

- Pliable cups
- Round like golf balls
- Small clubs
- Coral
- Jelly-like globs
- Human ear resemblance
- Bracket or shelf

THE FUNGAL LIFE CYCLE

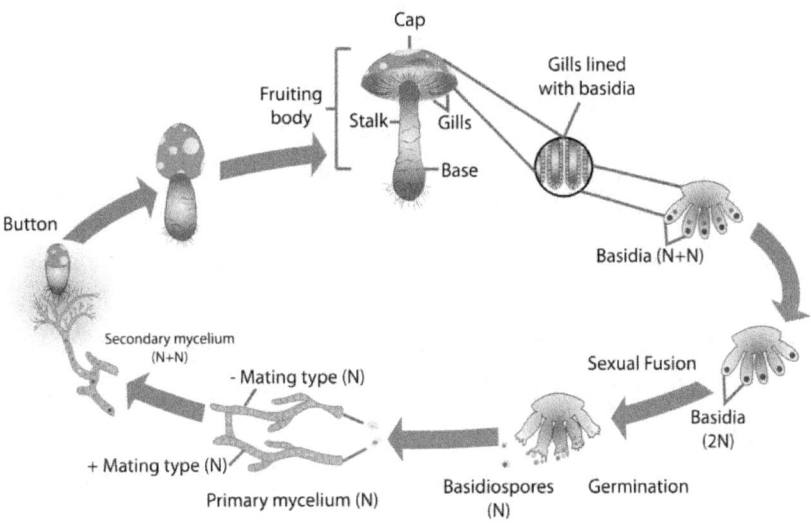

Mushrooms have a life cycle, and the mushroom, also known as the "fruiting body" or "sporocarp," is produced when the fungus needs to reproduce. This occurs when environmental conditions are appropriate in terms of temperature, moisture, and the waning presence of nutrients in the substrate material from which they are feeding.

The mushroom produces the spores, which, as mentioned, are like the seeds of a plant. Technically, they are more like sperm or ova because they only have half the total chromosomes, which is why once they germinate into their hyphal tube (see below), they need to find a "compatible" hyphal tube that is made up of the other set of chromosomes.

When the mushroom releases the spores, they are disseminated by the wind, or if an animal eats the mushroom, the spores may pass undigested through the stool and then be able to grow in a location away from where the animal ate the mushroom.

When spores germinate, they produce a "hyphal tube," a thin-walled tubular structure that grows and feeds off of the material on which it is growing. The hyphal tubes join with other compatible hyphal tubes to form the "mycelium."

The mycelium is a mass of joined hyphal tubes that is the "vegetative" part of the fungal life cycle. During the vegetative part of the fungal life cycle, the mycelium is nourished by the digested material it is growing on. The mycelium produces powerful digestive enzymes that can digest almost anything.

Common materials from which mushrooms derive nourishment (known as "substrates") are dead and decaying wood, leaf litter, compost, manure, or an insect (more on insect substrates later when I discuss the *Cordyceps sinensis* mushroom).

Mycelium grows until environmental conditions change sufficiently for the vegetative stage, which is the mycelium, to transform itself into the mushroom stage. The mushroom then produces spores (reproductive phase) and releases them when conditions are favorable. As mentioned, another name for the mushroom is the fruiting body, because it produces the spores. Yet another name is "sporocarp" because it contains the spores. The use of the word "mushroom" refers to this stage of the fungal life cycle. Some people, in error, say mushroom mycelium and mushroom spores, when in fact, the mushroom is just one of three fungal forms of this life cycle. This cycle repeats itself over and over again, as the spores germinate into hyphal tubes, mycelium, and then the mushroom.

HOW MUSHROOMS ARE GROWN

In the commercial cultivation of mushrooms, spores are germinated on agar in petri dishes. The resultant pure growth of mycelium on the agar is then transferred to sterile grain. Rye is commonly used, but other grains, such as milo, oats, millet, and rice may also be used. The mycelium grows throughout the grain, digesting it for nourishment. When completely myceliated, 30% of the grain still remains.

This "myceliated grain" is known in the commercial mushroom industry as "grain spawn." It is used to "seed" the mushroom growth on its natural substrate. For most mushrooms, the substrate is dead and decaying wood. Some species, like the button mushroom, *Agaricus bisporus*, and many of the *psilocybin* species, grow best on compost.

A newer technique for the cultivation of mushrooms doesn't actually grow mushrooms. It grows the mycelium on grain, as with the grain spawn. However, instead of seeding the substrate with the myceliated grain so mushrooms will form, they just dry the grain and mycelium, powder it, and sell that as medicinal mushrooms.

There are few, if any, mushrooms in this powder. It is more than 50% carbohydrates from grain and less than 25% mycelium. When the beta-glucan content of this grain spawn is measured, it typically is less than 10%, and when digestible starch is measured in this grain spawn, it can be as high as 66%. Beta-glucans in mushrooms are measured to be around 25-50%. The digestible starch content (sugars and glycogen) in mushrooms is usually less than 10%.

MUSHROOM QUALITY PRODUCT ANALYSIS STUDY
(which products are grain-free?)

I conducted a study in 2022 in which I purchased 10 pet products from the internet that all stated on their labels that they contained turkey tail mushrooms. I analyzed these products for both beta-glucan content and starch content. When I reviewed this data, presented in the table below, out of 10 products tested, only four were actually from mushrooms. The rest were all myceliated grain products!

If you are using mushrooms to treat your pet's cancer, you will want to give your pet as much potency as possible in order to have a better chance of a successful outcome for your pet. By giving the myceliated grain, you will not be giving your pet the best that mushrooms have to offer. Instead, you will be giving them a lot of grain carbohydrates and very few immune-potent beta-glucans. You may even be feeding your dog a grain-free diet. These grain spawn products contain a lot of grain, which defeats your purpose in avoiding grain for your pet.

It is essential for you to read the label of your mushroom product. Not all mushroom products are labeled with transparency or honesty, but some are. If it has myceliated grain in it, some companies are disclosing that and using this phrase to describe their grain spawn: "mycelial biomass." They may also tell you what the grain substrate was, whether it was rice flour, oats, millet, or milo.

If it says the product has "primordia" or "fruiting bodies" in it, be aware that the amount of these fungal life stages in these products is quite low, less than 5% of the total amount. Primordia are the early stages of mushroom formation and contain very little beta-glucans. The beta-glucan content of the product in which you are interested is directly related to the amount of mushroom they contain, not primordia and not mycelium grown on grain (MOG).

I am the Chief Veterinary Officer for Real Mushrooms (www.realmushooms.com). This Canadian company uses no grain fillers. They contain absolutely no myceliated grain in their products. They manufacture a 100% whole mushroom product, and they are organically grown. This is why I joined them: their integrity and transparency speak for themselves. They are the leading mushroom grower and retailer in the world!

ANALYSIS OF 10 COMMERCIAL MUSHROOM PRODUCTS FOR BETA-GLUCAN AND STARCH

BRAND	Label Claim of Type of Fungal Extract: Mushroom/ Mycelium	Product Label Potency Claim	Measured Beta-glucan% *(Immune-active)*	Measured Alpha-glucan % *(Starch)*	Is This a Mushroom Product or Mycelium on Grain?
PET-001	Turkey Tail, Reishi, Maitake, Shiitake Mushrooms	150 mg Turkey Tail/4 grams	1.8%	19.5%	Mycelium on grain
PET-002	Turkey Tail mycelium biomass cultivated on organic oats/1,000 mg of "mycelium and fruit body"	100 mg Turkey Tail/1,000 mg	3.1%	39.2%	Mycelium on grain
PET-003	Organic Mushroom Blend, containing 10 mushroom extracts including Turkey Tail	500 mg/serving size of 10 mushrooms	40.4%	2.3%	Mushroom

BRAND	Label Claim of Type of Fungal Extract: Mushroom/ Mycelium	Product Label Potency Claim	Measured Beta-glucan% (Immune-active)	Measured Alpha-glucan % (Starch)	Is This a Mushroom Product or Mycelium on Grain?
PET-004	Mushroom Complex containing Turkey Tail (500 mg); Maitake (100 mg); Reishi (100 mg); Shiitake (100 mg); no attribution to mushroom or mycelium other than the name of the product	500 mg Turkey Tail/1,000 mg scoop	8.1%	21.8%	Mushroom
PET-005	Turkey Tail mushroom (243 mg) with Chaga mushroom extract (243 mg); Cordyceps mushroom extract (243 mg); Phellinus mushroom extract (243 mg); Maitake mushroom extract (243 mg); Reishi mushroom extract (243 mg); Shiitake mushroom extract (243 mg)	243 mg Turkey Tail/1,700 mg/serving size	35.7%	2%	Mycelium on grain
PET-006	Turkey Tail Organic Turkey Tail Mushrooms; Back panel reads: Active: Organic Turkey Tail/Inactive: Myceliated Brown Rice	1,000 mg/1,000 mg scoop	10.3%	15.7%	Mycelium on grain

BRAND	Label Claim of Type of Fungal Extract: Mushroom/ Mycelium	Product Label Potency Claim	Measured Beta-glucan% (Immune-active)	Measured Alpha-glucan % (Starch)	Is This a Mushroom Product or Mycelium on Grain?
PET-007	Turkey Tail Certified Organic Mushroom Powder Blend: Active: Organic Turkey Tail mycelial biomass and primordia; Organic myceliated Oats; Inactive: NONE	1,000 mg/1,000 mg scoop	7%	24.7%	Mycelium on grain
PET-008	No front panel claim for Turkey Tail; Back panel reads: Proprietary Blend: Organic Turkey Tail plus 6 other species (all consist of mycelium, primordia, fruit bodies and extracellular compounds; Other ingredients: vegetarian capsule; organic white milo growing substrate.	500 mg/capsule	1.1%	66.6%	Mycelium on grain
PET-009	Turkey Tail Mushroom claim on front panel of label	½ teaspoon contains 1,000 mg Turkey Tail	38.2%	6.2%	Mushroom
PET-010	Turkey Tail plus 4 other species identified as mushroom on the front panel	½ teaspoon contains Turkey Tail plus 4 other species	25%	5.5%	Mushroom

CHAPTER TWO SUMMARY

The definition of a mushroom is very specific, referring to the part of the fungal life cycle that creates and releases the spores so future generations of the fungus can survive. It plays an important role in the reproduction and preservation of the fungal species, but no less important than the role played by both the mycelium and spores.

In todays' mushroom marketplace, many companies are growing a different part of the fungal life cycle than has been cultivated for hundreds of years, mycelium grown on grain. Unfortunately for the consumer, these companies are identifying these products as mushrooms, when in fact, they contain very little mushroom mass, if any.

In Chapter Three, we will learn about the many active compounds found in mushrooms, which are not always found in mycelium or spores. Mycelium, however, can be a very valuable source of some powerful immune-modulating ingredients, which we will discuss further in the next chapter.

CHAPTER THREE

ACTIVE MUSHROOM COMPOUNDS

Mushrooms contain many different potent compounds that have substantial health benefits. Any single compound would be powerful enough to be a healthy influence, but each mushroom contains multiple active compounds. It is the synergy among these multiple compounds in the mushroom that creates its strong activity to support health and address disease.

This chapter will detail for you these active compounds, starting with the best known compound and the one that is most commonly associated with mushroom medicinal activity, the beta-glucans.

BETA-GLUCANS[11]

Beta-glucans are structural components of the cell walls of fungi and yeast and are also found in the cell walls of seaweed, algae, and grains. Beta-glucans are chains (polymers) of the glucose molecule, and the "classic" beta-glucan contains just glucose molecules.

The potency of beta-glucans is enhanced by the number and type of side chains to the main chain of sugar molecules. Many mushrooms produce beta-glucans that aren't the classic format with just glucose molecules. Variations in these sugar molecules that make up the beta-glucan also contribute to increased potency.

Beta-glucans signal our white blood cells, especially the dendritic cells, monocytes, and mast cells, to become more immunologically active. Dendritic cells travel around the body, collecting information about pathogens and allergens, for instance.

It is thought that one reason mushrooms are so good for cancer is, in part, because of the ability of their beta-glucans to stimulate the immune system to kill off the cancer cells.

Some mushrooms produce beta-glucans that also have an amino acid group or a peptide or protein molecule attached to the glucan chain. The presence of these peptides increases the immune-enhancing effect of the beta-glucan molecule. These are the types of beta-glucans found in I'mYunity™ and Krestin™. Both of these are single molecular isolates of this peptide-enhanced beta-glucan that is manufactured from the turkey tail mycelium grown in a liquid culture medium. Note that when mycelium is grown in a liquid culture, it can be separated from the liquid culture, unlike when mycelium is grown on grain, which cannot be separated. Mycelium grown in a liquid culture is a pharmaceutical method to derive new drugs from the mycelial culture.

Other compounds in the mushroom may also have anti-cancer effects, such as the terpenes found in turkey tail, shiitake, reishi, chaga, and other mushrooms. *(See next section below.)*

TERPENES
(Triterpenes, Diterpenes, Sesquiterpenes, and Sesterpenes)[12]

Terpenes are chains (polymers) of a hydrocarbon molecule called an isoprene group. They are very bioactive and provide food and herbs with their taste and aroma. They are fat soluble, so they cross the blood-brain barrier and can have a strong effect on the brain in terms of calming or reducing inflammation, or even with seizures and epilepsy. In cannabis, terpenes interact with the cannabinoids and membrane receptors to increase the effectiveness of the cannabis extract. They provide a similar synergism to enhance the medicinal benefit of mushrooms.

Most mushrooms contain terpenes, although each mushroom has its own unique terpenes that give the mushroom its specific medicinal activity. Certain terpenes in reishi and chaga are known to have an antihistamine-like effect, whereas other terpenes in lion's mane are known to benefit cognition and reduction of stress. Turkey tail mushrooms have the highest concentration of terpenes and the highest number of variations in beta-glucan structures, which may be one reason for their potent anti-cancer reputation.

Terpenes can have quite a bitter taste, especially the larger terpenes, such as the triterpenes found in the reishi mushroom. Reishi triterpenes have the following medicinal properties, though:

- Calming

- Anti-inflammatory

- Antioxidant

- Hepatoprotective

- Inhibition of histamine release by mast cells

- Lipid-lowering, cholesterol-lowering

- Synergistic effect on immune activation in combination with beta-glucans

One of the important terpenes found in chaga is a lanostanic triterpene called "*inotodiol.*" It has an anti-allergy effect by its inhibition of the release of histamine from mast cells following allergic stimulation. It has strong anti-inflammatory properties. Inotodiol's potent anti-cancer properties inhibit cell migration and invasion and induce apoptosis, thus killing cancer cells.

Apoptosis is defined as "programmed cell death." All cells live out their life span and then die to give room to new cells being formed. With cancer, these cells are immortal, they never die, they just keep dividing and destroying the tissue they arise from. Cancer cells need to die, and apoptosis is the process whereby they perish.

Another important terpene found in chaga is betulinic acid. Chaga is a fungal mycelium that grows into the bark of the birch tree. The betulinic acid is derived from the birch tree and other trees as well. This pentacyclic triterpenoid has a wide range of pharmacological activities, including anti-viral, anti-tumor, anti-diabetic, anti-hyperlipidemic, and anti-inflammatory. The turkey tail mushroom contains this same triterpenoid.[13]

ERGOTHIONEINE

Ergothioneine ("ERGO") is a sulfur-containing amino acid antioxidant, very similar in structure to glutathione, the major antioxidant that all mammals produce. Glutathione is also naturally occurring in mushrooms. Sources of ERGO are fungi and soil bacteria, like the cyanobacteria and mycobacteria. It cannot be manufactured by the mammalian body. ERGO is strictly derived from nutritional sources. Plants and the animals that eat them, contain ERGO derived from the soil bacteria where they grow.

A lower intake of dietary ERGO has been associated with a greater prevalence of chronic neurological diseases of aging and lower life expectancies.[14] In a study using data from the WHO, the consumption of ERGO is negatively associated with total mortality and mortality from neurological disorders and positively associated with greater longevity.[15]

Preclinical studies of "ERGO" have determined a role in reducing oxidative stress, cardiovascular disease, neurodegenerative disease, sickle cell anemia, and improving the health of the skin.[16] In a study of Parkinson's disease (PD) patients, ERGO levels were found to be lower than in age-matched individuals without PD.[17] ERGO has been found to cross the blood-brain barrier, which helps to explain its potency for neurodegenerative conditions.[18]

A study found that blood levels of ERGO decline with age and that it declined faster in individuals who show cognitive impairment as compared to those humans who did not have signs of cognitive impairment.[19]

ERGOSTEROL

One sterol found in mushrooms is ergosterol, a compound found in all fungi, not just mushrooms. Testing for ergosterol is one way to document that there may be fungal contamination of grain. Ergosterol is a precursor in the formation of vitamin D_2. It is transformed into ergocalciferol when exposed to UVB light. Ergocalciferol is the dietary source of vitamin D_2. The liver then further transforms the ergocalciferol into the circulating form of vitamin D_2, 25(OH) vitamin D_2.

Dogs and cats are unable to convert cholesterol in their skin with UVB from sunlight into sufficient circulating vitamin D_3 to maintain healthy vitamin D levels.[20] For this reason, dogs and cats are dependent upon dietary sources of vitamin D to maintain healthy vitamin D levels.[21] Shiitake (*Lentinus edodes*), maitake (*Grifola frondosa*), and button (*Agaricus bisporus*) mushroom powder that has been exposed to UVB will contain substantial amounts of ergocalciferol.

This mushroom source of Vitamin D_2 is gaining a lot of traction in the natural health industry as a healthier source of vitamin D for people and pets. As a non-animal source of vitamin D, it may provide a more hypoallergenic, organic, and vegan alternative to animal-sourced vitamin D_3. Mushroom vitamin D powder is an organically grown source of D_2 that also contains beta-glucans and other bioactive molecules naturally occurring in the mushroom.

Early studies found that both vitamin D_2 and D_3 can reverse rickets, the vitamin D deficiency disease that affects bone formation and growth. Studies comparing the relative efficacy and potency in dogs and cats of Vitamin D_2, as compared to Vitamin D_3, found that, for a given dosage, Vitamin D_2 had less potency than vitamin D_3. It is recommended when supplementing with mushroom vitamin D_2 to analyze for levels of vitamin D_2 in order to determine the most effective amount to give of Vitamin D_2.[22]

In most other species (pigs, chickens, horses, fish, and primates) vitamin D_3 is more potent in comparison to vitamin D_2 as with dogs and cats. The one exception is the rat, for whom vitamin D_2 is more potent than Vitamin D_3.

By increasing the dose of vitamin D_2 by about 30% in these species you can improve the efficacy of the D_2 to be comparable to vitamin D_3.[23]

CHOLESTEROL STATINS

Mushrooms, such as the oyster mushroom (*Pleurotus spp.*), as well as other mushroom species, have been found to contain cholesterol-lowering enzymes that are naturally-occurring in the mushroom. This cholesterol-lowering effect is caused by *mevinolin*, which is a secondary metabolite found in many fungi and all medicinal basidiomycetes.

Ergosterol, which is found in all mushrooms and is essential for their survival, is nearly identical to the cholesterol molecule. Simply put, the enzymes that mushrooms create to metabolize their ergosterol will also work on cholesterol.

Mevinolin is now patented under the trade name Lovastatin™ as a cholesterol-lowering drug.[24] The cholesterol-lowering effect of mevinolin is in addition to the effect of beta-glucan compounds as found in oats, barley, and fungi to lower cholesterol by a mechanism of action that involves the effect of these compounds on bile acid and cholesterol metabolism.

The shiitake mushroom has a compound found exclusively in it called *"eritadenine,"* which has a cholesterol-lowering effect through a different mechanism of action than mevinolin and beta-glucans.

NUCLEOSIDES

Nucleosides are molecules that make up the base pairs of DNA. Individually, they can also activate their specific membrane receptors to have a biological effect. Nucleosides such as adenosine, guanosine, uridine, and cytidine are found in varying amounts in most mushrooms.

One of the active molecules in the medicinal mushroom *Cordyceps spp.* is a nucleoside-like compound called cordycepin. Cordycepin is what is called a nucleoside "analog," which means that it is very similar in chemical structure to the nucleoside, adenosine, differing in structure only by a single side chain.

The nucleoside adenosine is found in both *Cordyceps militaris* and *Ophiocordyceps sinensis*. It plays a key role in managing cellular energy production. This contributes to cordyceps' benefit to athletic performance and its ability to maintain tissue oxygenation in diseased organs. Due to the one side chain that is different for cordycepin versus adenosine, cordycepin can also block DNA synthesis in rapidly dividing cells like cancer cells, which can have a toxic effect on the cancer. Cordycepin binding to the adenosine receptor also has a beneficial effect on lung function, and is one mechanism of action whereby cordyceps benefits patients with asthma.[25]

PSILOCIN (PSILOCYBIN)

Psilocin is the main active hallucinogenic component in the *Psilocybe* mushroom, also known as the "magic mushroom." It is converted from psilocybin in the liver rapidly once the mushroom is ingested. This molecule is an indole alkaloid. Psilocin is fat-soluble as compared to psilocybin, so it will cross the blood-brain barrier easily in order for it to affect the brain, its target organ.

Psilocin is very similar to the 5-HT (the active form of tryptophan) molecule that is known popularly as serotonin. The technical, chemical name for these compounds is dialkyl tryptamines. All of these psychoactive compounds will activate the serotonin receptors.[26]

The amount of these hallucinogenic compounds will vary depending on the mushroom species and the growing conditions. Reported ranges for psilocin are from about 0.5% to 0.7%. Some species are naturally higher in psilocybin than others.[27]

Safety studies have found that of all the hallucinogenic substances, psilocybin/psilocin have the most favorable safety profile. The psilocybin mushroom has been used for thousands of years by indigenous peoples in spiritual and religious ceremonies.[28]

Recently, scientists have found that the hallucinogenic molecules of psilocybin can effectively treat mood and anxiety disorders more effectively than existing pharmaceutical interventions. Applications in mental health and substance abuse disorders, such as depression, anxiety-related disorders, bipolar disorder, autism, psychoses like schizophrenia, and substance-dependence disorders are being explored clinically with very encouraging results.[29,30]

CHAPTER THREE SUMMARY

Mushrooms are powerhouses of potent molecules. When these active compounds are combined together in a full-spectrum extract of a mushroom, the end result is increased potency due to their synergy.

In fact, when multiple mushrooms are combined in one formula, there is increased synergy, not just among the individual compounds found in each mushroom, but also between the many individual compounds in each of the mushrooms in the formula.

In Chapter Four, which is one of the longer chapters in this book, we will go into great depth and detail to help you understand the individual characteristics and applications for 11 of the most important functional mushrooms that have been in use historically for medicinal purposes.

IMPORTANT MUSHROOMS FOR A HEALTHY PET, WHAT THEY *ARE* AND WHAT THEY ARE *FOR*

This chapter covers 11 of the most popular and powerful mushrooms in the world in depth. Much of this information is quite technical. I've included many details about each mushroom in this section to provide you with a ready reference, should you ever need it.

You will find information about how the mushroom is named; where it is commonly found; the classification of the mushroom biologically and functionally; what it was used for historically in traditional indigenous systems of healing; a listing of its active ingredients categorized by type of molecule (i.e., beta-glucan, triterpene, nucleoside); how it is described in Traditional Chinese Veterinary Medicine; potential applications in veterinary species; and a summary of published studies of that mushroom, if available, in veterinary species.

Many modern mushroom products contain more than a single mushroom species. Some have as many as 10-15 different mushrooms in the blend. This is an attempt to create a "shotgun" approach to the use of mushrooms. This is potentially a good way to get a little bit of each mushroom's "goodness" to create a comprehensive product.

The problem with using a multiple mushroom blend containing as many as 10-15 mushrooms per blend is that the individual amount of each mushroom in the blend may not be enough to have any value unless you substantially increase the amount of that blend given to increase the amount given of each individual mushroom in that formula.

Generally, with mushroom blends, look for products containing 3-7 individual mushrooms so that each mushroom will be present in sufficient amounts to make a real difference for your pet.

A QUICK REFERENCE GUIDE TO USES OF MUSHROOMS FOR PETS

Cancer Support
- Turkey Tail
- Reishi
- Shiitake
- Chaga
- Maitake
- Cordyceps
- Lion's Mane
- White Button mushrooms

Cardiac Issues
- Reishi
- Shiitake
- Cordyceps
- Oyster
- Maitake

Cognition-Mentation-Memory Support
- Lion's Mane
- Reishi
- Tremella

Immune Support
- Turkey Tail
- Reishi
- Shiitake

Infectious Diseases
- Shiitake
- Chaga
- Reishi
- Agaricus

Kidney Support
- Cordyceps
- Reishi

Liver Support
- Reishi
- Shiitake

Energy/Mood/Stress
- Cordyceps
- Lion's Mane
- Reishi

Neurological Support (e.g., epilepsy)
- Reishi
- Lion's Mane
- Tremella

AGARICUS (A COMMON COMMERCIALLY AVAILABLE MUSHROOM)

If you've ever had mushrooms in a meal, they probably were the common white button mushroom. Or perhaps you've had a portobello mushroom prepared like a hamburger. This common mushroom species comes in a variety of shapes and sizes, but they all have in common their edible tastiness and their many beneficial medical properties.

Mushroom Scientific Name: *Agaricus spp.*

Mushroom Common Names
- Crimini (*Agaricus bisporus*)
- Field mushroom (*Agaricus campestris*)
- Horse mushroom (*Agaricus arvensis*)
- Portobello (*Agaricus bisporus*)

- Royal Sun Agaricus (*Agaricus blazeii*; also known as *A. subrufescens*)
- White button mushroom (*Agaricus bisporus*)

Where This Mushroom Grows
- Widespread globally for the genus Agaricus, geographically local for specific species like *A. blazeii* found in the south-eastern U.S., Brazil, and Japan.

Type of Mushroom: Agaric (gilled) Basidiomycete

Traditional & Historical Uses[31]
Medical use first described in 4th century A.D.
Used in the Unani, Chinese, and Eclectic ethnobotanical systems
- Anti-viral
- Antimicrobial
- Sinusitis
- Colds
- Cough
- Weakness
- Debility
- Treats several types of cancer (especially breast cancer)
- Infections (especially abscesses)
- Increases milk production in nursing mothers
- Indigestion
- Benefits microbiome
- Supports healthy metabolism
  o Lowers cholesterol
  o Helps regulate blood sugar for diabetics and metabolic syndrome

- o Hyperlipidemia is reduced
  (high triglycerides in the blood)
- Improves appetite

Active Ingredients

- Beta-glucans
- Proteoglycans (beta-glucans with amino acids attached)
- Novel anti-neoplastic fractions:
  - o LM
  - o ISY-15
  - o AB-P
  - o ATOM
  - o AB-FP
- Ergosterol
- Ergothioneine
- Lectins
- Vitamins
- Healthy fats, like conjugated linolenic acid (CLA)
- Agaratines (1%)
  - o Hydrazine compounds that are converted to car-cinogens but are destroyed (25%) by cooking—another reason to cook your mushrooms.
  - o Recently it has been found that storage under re-frigeration for 7 days or more will also reduce sub-stantially the agaritine content.
  - o At this low level in cooked Agaricus (white button mushrooms), it does not pose a risk, especially with the many anti-cancer compounds also in this mushroom.

Key Power: Tasty mushroom medicine
- Immune
    - Anti-cancer
    - Anti-viral
    - Anti-microbial
- GI & metabolism
    - Lowers cholesterol
    - Supports healthy blood sugar levels for diabetes
    - Supports healthy pancreatic functions
    - Lowers triglycerides in *Hyperlipidemia*

Traditional Chinese Veterinary Medicine Characteristics
- Organ Affinity
    - Spleen
    - Stomach
    - Liver
- Taste
    - Sweet
    - Bland
- Actions
    - Regulates Qi
    - Removes Phlegm
    - Supports the Stomach and Spleen

Potential Applications for Veterinary Species
- Anti-cancer
    - Throat cancer
    - Lung
    - Breast
    - Utero-cervical
    - Colon
    - Liver

- Hepatoprotective
- Supports healthy digestion
- Cancer therapy side effects improved
    - Less hair loss with chemotherapy
    - Less weak, better emotional stability
    - Appetite improvement
- Support a healthy microbiome
- Supportive of pancreas
- Immune enhancement
- Sinusitis
- Colds
- Cough
- Anti-viral
- Anti-bacterial
- Good for abscesses
- Anti-hypertensive
- Anti-cholesterol
- Reduces excess fats in blood (hyperlipidemia)
- Blood sugar regulating (help manage diabetes)
- Antioxidant

Results of Studies in Veterinary Species for this Mushroom
- No studies in species other than chickens and bees
- Mushrooms fed to broiler chickens improved their intestinal health[32]
- Bees fed an Agaricus syrup had fewer Nosema fungal infections[33]

- Three studies found that human breast cancer incidence reduction (50%-65%) associated with the consumption of 10 grams of mushrooms about ½ a button) daily along with green tea.[34]

Synergistic Pairings with Other Mushrooms
- w/shiitake, chaga, and/or lion's mane for digestive support
- w/turkey tail, chaga, or maitake for cancer support

CHAGA (THE BIRCH TREE FUNGUS)

This mushroom is not really a mushroom. It is a fungus, for sure, but the mycelium never develops into the fruiting body that is what we call a "mushroom." Chaga is actually a parasitic fungal mycelium that infects a tree's bark. Birch trees are most commonly affected. The tree reacts to the mycelium growing into its outer bark by growing its bark out and around it into what looks like a tumorous cancer growing on the tree. It forms what is called a "canker" (tree cancer).

Early humans believed that the appearance of a plant, or mushroom, told you something about what it was for. Chaga, because it is associated with that tree cancer/canker, traditionally has been used to treat cancer in humans. It can also be used for your pet with cancer. Another example is lion's mane, which looks like a brain, and that's what it's for, although it has other uses as well—for instance, with gastritis.

What is really interesting about chaga is that when it grows into the birch tree, it absorbs some of the biologically active molecules that the birch tree manufactures for its own health. These triterpenes, including betulinic acid, betulin, lanosterols, and inotodiol, give chaga its incredible potency.

Because the mycelium is growing into the bark, the levels of beta-glucans in chaga are lower than as found in true mushrooms, but these other chaga active molecules are so potent that chaga works great even with a lower beta-glucan content. The beta-glucan content of chaga is still greater than the beta-glucan we measure in mycelium grown on grain.

The famous Nobel Prize-winning author Alexander Solzhenitsyn wrote about his successful use of chaga to treat the cancer he developed while incarcerated in the Russian Gulag prison.

Mushroom Scientific Name: *Inonotus obliquus*

Mushroom Common Names
- Chaga
- *Polyporus obliquus*
- *Poria obliqua*
- Clinker polypore

Where This Mushroom Grows
- Northern latitudes
   o Siberia
   o Russia
   o Canada
   o Scandinavia

Type of Mushroom
- Not a "mushroom" but actually a fungal mycelium causing exuberant growth reaction from the birch tree it's growing on. (It is a "canker")

Traditional & Historical Uses

- Anti-tumor
  - Breast
  - Lung
  - Cervical
  - Stomach
  - Liver
- Anti-viral
- Anti-tuberculosis
- GI support
- Gastritis
- Inflammatory bowel disease
- Diabetes
- Ulcers
- Cardiovascular support
  - Reduces cholesterol levels
- Anti-hyperlipidemic
- Liver support
- Psoriasis

Active Ingredients

- Beta-glucans
- Protein-bound polysaccharides
- Ergosterol
- Lanosteroid triterpenoids
- Trametenolic acid
- Sterols
- Betulin
- Betulinic acid
- Lanosterols

- Lactones
- Inotodiol
- Inositol
- Melanin

Key Power: Birch tree molecules
- Swiss army knife "shroom" with many applications
  o Cancer
  o Allergies
  o GI issues
  o Fatigue

Traditional Chinese Veterinary Medicine Characteristics
- Organ Affinity
  o Liver
  o Stomach
  o Spleen
  o Kidney
- Taste
  o Sweet
  o Bitter
- Actions
  o Supports Zheng Qi
  o Tonifies deficiency
  o Tonifies Kidney/adrenals
  o Strengthens Spleen
  o Dispels toxins

Potential Applications for Veterinary Species

- Gastrointestinal support
- Gastritis
- Pancreatitis
- Inflammatory Bowel Disease
- Diabetes support
- Anti-fatigue
- Antioxidant
- Anti-inflammatory
- Analgesic
- Anti-cancer
- Immune support
- Anti-viral
- Anti-parasitic
- Anti-aging
- Anti-cholesterol
- Antihistamine effect from its triterpenoids (similar to reishi's anti-histaminic effect)
  - Mast cell tumors
  - Atopic dermatitis
  - Food sensitivities and intolerances

Results of Studies in Veterinary Species for this Mushroom

- **None** in veterinary species
- Multiple studies support:
  - Mast cell degranulation properties
  - Anti-neoplastic properties
  - Activation of NKT cells
  - Benefits lower urinary tract disease (LUTD)
  - Bronchial asthma

  o Fibromyalgia
  o Hypertension
  o Allergic rhinitis

Synergistic Pairings with Other Mushrooms
- w/lion's mane for gastritis and inflammatory bowel disease
- w/turkey tail for cancer
- w/reishi for allergies

CORDYCEPS (THE CATERPILLAR MUSHROOM)

Cordyceps are in the same class of mushrooms as the very tasty truffles and morels. They taste a bit like toast to my palate. Cordyceps have an unusual life cycle. Most mushroom mycelium will grow through natural substrate that is usually dead or decaying wood, compost, leaf litter, or manure. Cordyceps are in the family of fungi that infect insects.

One member of this family of fungi infects an ant, and it takes over the ant's nervous system to cause it to climb to the top leaf of a bush and bite into the leaf at the top just before it dies from the parasitic fungus. That way, they release their spores into the wind as high as possible for the best dissemination and distribution to spread their growth as widely as possible.

Cordyceps infect the caterpillar stage of a moth's life cycle while the caterpillar is in its pupa stage, and it buries itself in the soil. The fungal mycelium grows throughout the caterpillar body, killing it. When conditions are right, the mycelium sends up a fruiting body above the soil to release its spores to infect the next generation of caterpillars. Thus, the life cycle continues on and on. The cordyceps mushroom that grows wild is found only in the highlands of Nepal, Tibet, and Bhutan. It is reputed to have aphrodisiac properties, so the mushrooms collected in the wild fetch a high price of over $15,000 per kilogram!

Fortunately, we can now cultivate the cordyceps mushroom on a rice substrate. Since the mushroom grows on the top of the rice growth medium, it can be separated from the grain so that the extract can be a grain-free fruiting body with optimal potency.

Cordyceps is known to support the kidneys and lungs, according to Chinese medicine. Studies have proven that cordyceps can help improve kidney function and can help with the chronic cough associated with asthma or chronic bronchitis. The beta-glucans in cordyceps are high and can help regulate the immune system inflammation associated with asthma and chronic bronchitis.

Cats have a strong tendency to develop chronic kidney disease. The use of cordyceps prophylactically in cats can support their kidney function and help improve their longevity through the prevention and modulation of chronic kidney disease (CKD). Because they are so bland yet tasty, cordyceps make an even better fit for your feline friend.

It's said that horses are all legs and lungs. The support that cordyceps give to the lungs and the healthy generation of energy in the body can provide the equine athlete an edge in competition. At this point in time, cordyceps is not tested in competitive riding.

Mushroom Scientific Names
- Cultivated = *Cordyceps militaris*
- Wild = *Ophiocordyceps sinensis*

Mushroom Common Names
- Caterpillar fungus
- Dong Chong Xia Cao
  - "Summer grass, Winter worm"
- Yartsa Gunbu

Where This Mushroom Grows
- Tibet
- Nepal
- Bhutan

Type of Mushroom: Ascomycete (spores in sacs)

Traditional & Historical Uses
- Provides energy, vitality, and endurance
- Restores immune function
- Aphrodisiac
  - Influences testosterone levels
- Fertility
- Diabetes
- Hepatoprotective
- Renoprotective (kidney support)
- Cardiotonic
- Anti-fatigue
- Anti-fibrotic
- Adaptogen
- Cancer
  - Gastric
  - Cervical
  - Oral
  - Reduces metastasis
  - Radiation protective
- Anti-viral
  - Hepatitis B or C
- Asthma/bronchial/lung inflammation
- Protects the kidneys

- Lung tonic for weak lung function
- Stops coughing and wheezing
- Good for recovery from anesthesia
- Elderly tonic

Active Ingredients
- Polysaccharides
- Beta-glucans
- Cordycepin
- Nucleosides
- Ergosterol
- Ergothioneine

Key Power: Energy support for increased stamina and athletic performance
- Enhances metabolic energy production by increasing cellular ATP stores
- Supports
  - Kidney
  - Lungs
  - Liver
- FELINE FRIENDLY
  - Kidney support and bland, toasty taste that is ideal for our feline friends
- EQUINE FRIENDLY
  - Lung support, energy support, and stress support through the pituitary and adrenal glands is ideal for our equine friends
- Anti-aging
- Longevity
- Adrenal support for stress

- Immune modulating
- Cardiovascular support

Traditional Chinese Veterinary Medicine Characteristics
- Organ Affinity
  - Kidney
  - Lung
  - Liver
- Taste
  - Sweet
  - Bland
- Temperature
  - Slightly warming
- Actions
  - Stops chronic cough
  - Stops hemorrhage
  - Strengthens Kidney Qi, yang, and *jing*
  - Builds marrow and benefits the brain
  - Nourishes blood
  - Promotes circulation
  - Transforms phlegm
  - Supports *Wei Qi*
  - Nourishes Lung yin

Potential Applications for Veterinary Species
- Geriatric support
- Immune support
- Cancer
  - Lung
  - Liver
  - Kidney

- Asthma
- Protective for radiation and chemotherapy
    - Supports stem cell regeneration in bone marrow
- Anti-leukemia
- Anti-viral
- Anti-bacterial
- Anti-fungal
- Anti-Lyme's disease
- Cardiovascular support
- Cardiotonic
- Supports liver detoxification
- Hepatoprotective
- Renoprotective
- Chronic kidney disease
- Lung disorders
    - Asthma
    - Chronic cough,
    - COPD
    - Pulmonary inflammation
    - Mucolytic
    - Relaxes bronchiolar constriction
- Bronchitis
- Supports athletic activity
    - Performance competition
    - Agility
    - Search and rescue
    - Hiking
    - Dock jumping
- Reproductive support

Results of Studies in Veterinary Species for this Mushroom

- **None** in veterinary species
- Multiple studies in humans and laboratory animals support:
    - Chronic kidney disease support
    - Cancer patient benefits
    - Asthma and respiratory support
    - Anti-inflammatory activity
    - Analgesic properties
    - Activity enhancement

Synergistic Pairings with Other Mushrooms

- w/chaga, shiitake, and/or lion's mane for fatigue support
- w/turkey tail, reishi, chaga, or maitake for cancer support
- w/reishi for liver protection and support, bronchial asthma, and allergic bronchitis support

LION'S MANE
(IT'S GOOD FOR THE BRAIN AND THE BOWEL)

This prized edible mushroom has an appearance like a hedgehog, brain, or coral. It is the only medicinal mushroom with teeth-like spore-bearing structures, which creates its very unusual appearance. The doctrine of signatures describes the health association of the appearance of something like a mushroom or a plant with the organ or body part it most looks like. For instance, kidney beans would be good for the kidneys, and for lion's mane, the brain or bowel. The spines also look like the lining of the gut—the microvilli.

Currently, lion's mane is the most popular mushroom in the U.S. due to its ability to reduce stress, improve memory, and help with cognition. There are reports of its benefit to human patients with Alzheimer's disease and Parkinson's disease. Our pets need help with their stresses just as we do. Life in the 21st Century is hectic, confusing, stressful, and sometimes dangerous. Lion's mane, although not a panacea, can help reduce these stressors.

When combined with cannabinoids like CBD, CBG, or CBN, lion's mane's calming effects are synergistically enhanced without causing profound sedation. Like cordyceps, lion's mane is a very bland but tasty mushroom extract. Some say it has a slightly fishy taste. I think that is more of its umami flavor coming through.

Older pets suffer from their own geriatric cognitive failures. This condition is much like dementia in humans. Reports from pet owners and vets support the use of lion's mane for this senior dementia in dogs. Veterinary behaviorists have given a name to this problem in older dogs. They call it "canine cognitive disorder," or abbreviated, CCD.

Traditionally, lion's mane had been used for its ability to address gastritis and esophageal and gastric cancers. It can also help with inflammatory bowel disease. It is only recently that researchers have discovered unique triterpenes and diterpenes in the lion's mane mushroom and the mycelia grown in a liquid culture. These molecules can stimulate brain-derived nerve growth factor (bNGF) production in the central nervous system, which helps to regenerate damaged neurons and support the growth of new nerve cells.

Mushroom Scientific Name: *Hericium erinaceus*

Mushroom Common Names
- Lion's mane
- Monkey's head
- Yamabushitake
- Houtou

Where This Mushroom Grows
- Widespread global distribution
  - North America
  - Europe
  - China
  - Japan

Type of Mushroom: Teethed Basidiomycete

Traditional & Historical Uses
- Tonic effect on nerves and neurasthenia
  - Neuro-protective
  - Neuro-regenerative
  - Improves cognition and mobility
  - Improves memory and learning
  - Delays degenerative aging in the brain
- Helps with general debility
- Stomach ailments
  - Gastritis
  - Ulcers
- Prevention of cancer in the GI tract
- Anti-cancer
  - Leukemia
  - Esophageal
  - Gastric
- Renoprotective (kidney support)
- Hepatoprotective
- Cardioprotective
- Metabolic support for blood sugar and blood fats
- Microbiome support
- Anti-microbial

Active Ingredients

- Cyanthane derivatives
- Ergostane derivatives
- Erinacines
- Hericenones
- GABA
- Beta-glucans
- Polysaccharides
- Ergosterol

Key Power: Neurologic and cognitive support

- Senior senility/dementia
  - Canine cognitive disorder (CCD)
- Stress management
- Nerve growth factor support
- Immune support
- Neuroprotection
  - Alzheimer's disease
  - Parkinson's disease
  - MS
- Nerve tonic
- Microbiome support
- GI support
  - Gastritis
  - Esophagitis
  - IBS/IBD
- Anti-cancer

Traditional Chinese Veterinary Medicine Characteristics

- Organ Affinity
    - Spleen
    - Stomach
    - Heart
- Taste
    - Sweet
    - Bland taste
- Actions
    - Strengthens the Stomach/Spleen
    - Benefits digestion and metabolism
    - Nourishes the Lung
    - Regulates Qi
    - Nourishes the Kidneys
    - Calms the Shen
    - Strengthens the Marrow (brain)

Potential Applications Veterinary Species

- Geriatric support
- Cognitive dysfunction
    - Canine cognitive disorder (CCD)
- Calming and adaptogenic support
- Neurological disease/injury
- Anxiety/depression
- Gastritis
- Cancer support
    - GI
    - Brain

Results of Studies in Veterinary Species for this Mushroom

- **None** in veterinary species
- Multiple studies support
  - Cognition
  - Dementia
  - Anxiety
  - Depression
  - Cancer prevention and intervention

Synergistic Pairings with Other Mushrooms

- w/reishi for enhanced calming and neurological support
- w/turkey tail, chaga, or maitake for cancer support, especially of the GI tract or nervous system (brain)
- w/chaga for digestive support

MAITAKE MUSHROOM (A TASTY AND POTENT MUSHROOM)

The maitake mushroom (*Grifola frondosa*), also known popularly as "hen of the woods" or "sheep's head," is a polypore that is highly regarded for its flavor as an edible mushroom. It can be found growing in many locations around our planet, but modern cultivation technology has allowed it to be widely cultivated and commercialized as a food. Its popularity is so great that for cultures where it is harvested from its natural habitat (wild-crafting), families would pass down, as their legacy to their family, from one generation to the next, the well-guarded and top-secret locations where this mushroom could be wild-crafted, year after year.

Wild-growing maitake mushrooms can be quite large, often weighing as much as 50 pounds! Ethical wildcrafters understand the need to conserve their harvest sufficiently so as to not adversely affect mushrooms growing from a given area and to be able to maintain and not deplete the wild supply. With modern cultivation techniques, wildcrafting has become a less important source of this prized edible mushroom. Cultivation of this mushroom has also allowed for a more standardized supply of the mushroom for its medicinal applications.

The maitake mushroom fruiting body, the source of its popular edible and functional food properties, contains the precursor to Vitamin D_2, ergosterol, which, when exposed to ultraviolet light, converts to ergocalciferol, the dietary form of this essential vitamin. Analysis of the maitake fruiting body has consistently found about 40% protein content, 15% fiber, 8% fats, and 9% minerals.[35]

Maitake is rich in its unique beta-glucans (26%), which are highly branched, thus contributing to its powerful immune-modulating properties. Each mushroom species has a unique pattern of branching and cross-branching that contributes, along with its other bioactive molecules (triterpenes and flavonoids), to its unique potency and range of applications.

Mushroom Scientific Name: *Grifola frondosa*

Mushroom Common Names

- Maitake ("maitake" means "dancing mushroom" from its appearance or by the dance someone does when they find this prized edible mushroom)
- Kumotake ("cloud mushroom")
- Mushikusa
- Hui Shu Hua
- Hen-of-the-Woods
- Grifola means "braided fungus"

Where This Mushroom Grows

- Northern, northeastern, mid-Atlantic states and Canada, temperate deciduous forests
- Northeastern Japan
- Temperate hardwood regions of China and Europe
- Grows on stumps or at the base of dead or dying deciduous hardwoods (oak, elm, maple, black gum, beech, larch)

Type of Mushroom: Polypore; Basidiomycete

Traditional & Historical Uses

- Immune modulating
- Inhibits tumor growth
- Diuretic
- Fever
- Anti-microbial
  - Gonorrhea
  - Anti-viral
- Stomach/spleen conditions
  - Hemorrhoids
- Neuroprotective
  - Neuralgia
  - Palsy
- Hepatoprotective
- Stress support
- Microbiome support
- Helps regulate healthy blood sugar levels for diabetics
- Enhances memory
- Anti-depressant
- Anti-cancer

- Anti-inflammatory
- Antioxidant
- Supports healthy immune response to skin inflammation
- Cholesterol-regulating
- Arthritis

Active Ingredients
- Beta-glucans
  - Grifolan
  - Grifolan-LE
  - D-fraction™ (beta-glucan with 30% protein)
- Polysaccharides
- Triterpenes
- Ergosterol
  - after exposure to UVB for >3 hours vitamin D_2 increases from 460 IU to 32,000 IU

Key Power: Tasty, anti-cancer edible

Traditional Chinese Veterinary Medicine Characteristics
- Organ Affinity
  - Lungs
  - Spleen
  - Liver
  - Heart
- Taste
  - Sweet
  - Bland
- Actions
  - Strengthens digestion
  - Moistens the Lungs
  - Protects the Liver
  - Supports the Stomach/Heart

Potential Applications for Veterinary Species

- Cancer
- Diabetes
- Fevers
- Anti-hypertensive
- Anti-obesity
- Anti-viral
- Anti-arthritic/analgetic = COX1 and COX2 inhibition
- Hepatoprotective

Results of Studies in Veterinary Species for this Mushroom

- Two studies have been published using maitake mushroom extracts (D-fraction) for canine cancer cell lines or as a clinical trial of dogs with malignant lymphoma.

    o The canine cancer cell line study found cytotoxicity of maitake extracts in all five lines (lymphoma, breast cancer, connective tissue cancer). Lymphoma cells were killed better by the D-fraction than the other two cell lines.[36]

    o The clinical trial in dogs with lymphoma was not successful. The dosage was too low, and they chose dogs that were close to death from the lymphoma.[37]

- Multiple other studies of maitake mushroom and cancer have been performed in laboratory animals with experimentally-induced tumors.[38]

Pairings with other Mushrooms

- w/turkey tail for cancer support
- w/cordyceps for mobility support
- w/lion's Mane for calming

OYSTER MUSHROOM
(SOURCE OF STATINS AND GOOD EATING)

The oyster mushroom is an edible mushroom with a very pleasant taste that grows widely around our planet. With a distinctive trumpet-like shape, oyster mushrooms are easy to cultivate and easy to eat, and at the same time, they provide many valuable health benefits for ourselves and our four-legged friends. Oyster mushrooms provided the first anti-cholesterol medication, mevinolin, which has since been patented as Lovistatin™. Oyster mushrooms, like maitake and shiitake, when exposed to sunlight's UVB for several hours, will transform their ergosterol into the active precursor to vitamin D_2, ergocalciferol.

Oyster mushroom's beta-glucan extracts were used in two Eastern European studies of immunocompromised puppies that were in humane shelters. When puppies are immunocompromised from the stresses of being strays or abandoned, their vaccinations may not be effective. The vaccine doesn't create a protective antibody titer in the puppy against important and potentially life-threatening diseases, such as canine distemper, parvovirus, and especially rabies.

Oyster mushroom's beta-glucans improved these puppies' response to the vaccine such that they were able to, after preconditioning with the beta-glucans, achieve protective titers for rabies, distemper, and parvovirus. Any beta-glucan from any mushroom can improve immune response as well as oyster beta-glucans.

Mushroom Scientific Names
- *Pleurotus ostreatus*
- *P. citrinopileatus* (golden oyster)
- *P. salmoneostramineus* (pink oyster)
- *P. eryngii* (king oyster)
- and more…

Mushroom Common Names

- Oyster mushroom
- King trumpet
- King oyster
- Pink oyster
- Golden oyster
- Hiratake
- Ping Gu

Where This Mushroom Grows

- Common throughout the northern hemisphere and temperate and tropical forests of the world

Type of Mushroom: Agaric (gilled) Basidiomycota

Traditional & Historical Uses

- Edible
- Metabolism and cholesterol
- Immune benefits

Active Ingredients

- Ergosterol
- Beta-glucans
- Mevinolin
- Ergothioneine
- Glutathione
- Carotenoids
- SOD
- Catalase
- Copper and zinc levels are higher than other mushrooms (caution required in copper liver storage disease patients)

Key Power: Tasty, metabolic mushroom medicine

Traditional Chinese Veterinary Medicine Characteristics
- Organ Affinity
    - Spleen
    - Stomach
    - Liver
- Taste
    - Sweet
    - Bland
- Energy
    - Slightly warming
- Actions
    - Strengthens Spleen
    - Boosts metabolism and
    - Immune function
    - Regulates fluids
        - Mild diuretic (safe)
    - Supports the Liver
        - Soothes sinews, ligaments, and tendons
    - Invigorates Blood
        - Promotes circulation
    - Regulates intestines
        - Moistening, helps prevent constipation

Potential Applications for Veterinary Species
- Hyperlipidemia (high levels of fat in the blood)
- Immune modulation
    - Protective vaccine titers
- Anti-infective benefits

- Disease prevention
  - Beta-glucans protect against upper respiratory illnesses
- Longevity
- Anti-aging
- Whole body support

Results of Studies in Veterinary Species for this Mushroom

- Immune-enhanced rescue puppies who were immuno-compromised from being abandoned and strays to be able to achieve protective vaccine antibody titers.[39]
- In a study in dogs, 8 mg/kg/day of mevinolin for three weeks resulted in a 30% reduction in serum cholesterol.[40]

Synergistic Pairings with Other Mushrooms

- w/shiitake for digestive and metabolic support
- w/turkey tail for cancer
- w/maitake for immune support

PSILOCYBIN
(AN EMERGING THERAPY FOR MENTAL HEALTH)

When the word "cannabis" is mentioned, the first thing that comes to most people's minds is THC or "marijuana." So, too, for mushrooms, the first thing that most people think of are the "magic mushrooms" or psilocybin species. The animated version of *Alice in Wonderland* with a hookah-smoking caterpillar sitting on top of a huge mushroom (*Amanita muscaria* with its red cap spotted with white dots) did a lot to promote the world of magic mushrooms to our modern generations.

Psilocybin mushrooms have been in use by most cultures around the world since the days of pre-history, and they are still being used by a number of indigenous people in their shamanic ceremonies, especially in Mexico, Central America, and South America.

Recently, magic mushrooms have gained a very positive reputation for their ability to help humans with generalized anxiety disorders, post-traumatic stress disorder (PTSD), severe depression, OCD, and other mental health problems.

The two Netflix documentaries, *The Fantastic Fungi*, which popularized the use of mushrooms, including magic mushrooms, and Michael Pollens' *How to Change Your Mind*, which featured the use of psilocybin mushrooms in therapy sessions for people with serious mental health issues, have helped immensely in promoting the use of these mushrooms for mental health.

Many people are now taking the psilocybin mushroom in very small "microdoses" that they claim improve their creativity, cognition, and mental stability, and help them with day-to-day challenges to their anxiety and mental calm.

It sounds like psilocybin mushrooms could also be good for those dogs with PTSD, generalized anxiety disorders, and other difficult-to-address mental health conditions that we see in our domestic dog population. Unfortunately, there is very little experience with the use of psilocybin in dogs as of this writing.

Once we gain more experience and learn how to better provide doses of the psilocybin that are therapeutic and do not pose a problem, we may start to see psilocybin used more commonly and effectively for these difficult-to-treat mental health conditions in our dogs.

Mushroom Scientific Names

- *Psilocybe cubensis*
- *P. cyanescens*
- *P. semilanceata*
- *P. azurescens*
- *P. caerulescens*
- *Paneolus cyanescens*
- *Gymnopilus junonius*

Mushroom Common Names

- Magic mushroom
- Liberty cap
- Laughing mushroom
- Psilocybin

Where This Mushroom Grows

- Worldwide distribution

Type of Mushroom: Agaric (gilled) Basidiomycota

Traditional & Modern Uses[41]

- Shamanic medicine
- Behavioral disorders (OCD)
- Cancer-related anxiety and depression
- Major depressive disorder
- Addiction treatment and recovery
- Spiritual journeys
- Cluster headaches
- Neurogenesis (stimulates nerve growth)
- Reduced fear response

Active Ingredients
- Beta-glucans
- Ergosterol
- Psilocybin
- Psilocin

Key Power: Visionary/emotional support

Potential Applications for Veterinary Species
- Anxiety disorders
- PTSD

Results of Studies in Veterinary Species for this Mushroom
- **None** in veterinary species as of this writing
- Multiple studies in humans
- See "Modern Uses" above

Synergistic Pairings with Other Mushrooms
- w/reishi for "grounding"
- w/lion's mane for grounding and digestive support
- w/chaga for digestive support

REISHI (THE MUSHROOM OF IMMORTALITY)

This mushroom is one of the most well-known mushrooms, with one of the oldest history of use by humans, dating back thousands of years. In China, people who would find large and beautiful specimens of this mushroom growing in the wild would harvest them and present them to the emperor, which was thought to convey longevity and good health for the emperor. It was an honor for the person who found it and gifted it. This mushroom is still very popular today, and that popularity is reflected in annual U.S. sales of well over two billion dollars.

This specific species, called red reishi, or *Ganoderma lucidum*, is also known as *Ganoderma lingzhi*. There are many other species of Ganoderma found growing naturally around the world with similar but different actions than reishi.

Reishi contains over 130 active ingredients, with its beta-glucan and triterpenoid content providing most of its medicinal activity. The beta-glucans are water soluble and need to be extracted with hot water at 90° C (194° F) for several hours to release the chitin and beta-glucan content in its fibrous cell wall. The triterpenoids are responsible for the very bitter taste of reishi but also account for many of its medicinal properties, such as its antihistamine and calming effects.

These large terpenes are fat-soluble molecules and do not extract very well in hot water extractions used for the beta-glucans. Terpenes need to be extracted in alcohol to provide the highest concentration of them. This is why you may find reishi extract described as "dual extraction." Both hot water and alcohol are used to remove most of the beta-glucans and triterpenoids in a dual extraction.

Mushroom Scientific Name(s)
- *Ganoderma lingzhi* (reishi)
- *Ganoderma lucidum* (reishi)

Other species of Ganoderma that are not reishi include:
- G. *applanatum* (artist's conk)
- G. *tsugae* (varnished conk)
- G. *oregonese* (western varnished conk)
- G. *resinaceum* (varnish shelf)

Mushroom Common Names

- Ganoderma is from the Latin meaning "shiny skin."
- *Ling zhi* is the Chinese name for this mushroom and means "spirit plant" or "tree of life mushroom."
- "Reishi" is from the Japanese tradition and means "divine" or "spiritual mushroom."
- *Mannetake, also* from the Japanese tradition, means "10,000-year mushroom" or the "mushroom of immortality."
- "Red reishi" is the common name for G. *lingzhi.*
  - o Interchangeable with G. *lucidum*
- Each species of Ganoderma, as listed above, also has a common name associated with it, which is in parentheses.

Where This Mushroom Grows

- Ganoderma species are found worldwide; some species have specific geographical distributions, such as G. *oregonensis,* which is found in Oregon.
- Commercially available Ganoderma is cultivated worldwide.

Type of Mushroom: Polypore; Basidiomycete

Traditional & Historical Uses (used in Asia for over 4,000 years)

- Hepatitis
- Nephritis
- Hypertension
- Arthritis
- Asthma
- Gastric ulcers
- Neurasthenia (weakness and fatigue)
- Longevity
- Cancer

Active Compounds and What They Do

(over 130 active constituents identified)

- Beta-glucans
    - Immuno-Modulating
    - Anti-tumor
- Ergosterol
    - Vitamin D_2 precursor
- Beta-sitosterol
    - Immune-modulating
    - Anti-inflammatory
- Ganoderic acids A, B, C, D, R, S, F, H, K, S, Y, Mf (triterpenoids)
    - Inhibit histamine release
    - Anti-hepatotoxic
    - Anti-hypertensive
    - Inhibit cholesterol synthesis
- Ganoderans A, B, C (triterpenoids)
    - Hypoglycemic
- Ganodosterone
    - Anti-hepatotoxic
- Ganodermadiol
    - Anti-hypertensive
- Ganodermic acid
    - Inhibits cholesterol synthesis
- Cyclooctasulphur
    - Inhibits histamine release
- LZ-8
    - Broad spectrum anti-allergic, immune-modulator, anti-neoplastic
    - Similar to PSP Coriolus
- Oleic acid
    - Inhibits histamine release

Key Power

Reishi is truly the most studied and most used mushroom over the years due to the many real as well as potential clinical uses it possesses.

- Longevity/anti-aging
  - The mushroom of immortality and longevity
- Supports
  - Liver
  - Lungs
- Immune support
- Inflammation
- Cancer
- Vaccine titers
- Allergy support
  - Immune modulation reducing allergy (beta-glucans)
  - Antihistamine-like action (triterpenes)
- Benefits the cardiovascular system with its influence in reducing cholesterol levels and hypertension
- Microbiome support
- Supports neurological function
  - Neuroprotective
  - Stroke
  - Traumatic injury to the brain or spinal cord
  - Neurodegenerative conditions
  - Parkinson's disease
  - Alzheimer's disease
  - Epilepsy
  - Depression
  - Calming influence (used by Zen Masters as a meditation aid)

Traditional Chinese Veterinary Medicine Characteristics

- Organ Affinity
  - Heart
  - Liver
  - Lung
- Taste
  - Sweet
  - Slightly bitter
- Energy
  - Neutral
  - Slightly warm
- Actions
  - Tonifies Qi
  - Nourishes blood
  - Calms the Shen
  - Transforms phlegm
  - Stops cough

Potential Applications for Veterinary Species

- Anti-cancer
- Reduces side effects from radiation and chemotherapy
- Allergies
- Rhinitis
- Upper respiratory infections
- Chronic infections like FIV/FIP/FELV
- Conjunctivitis
- Autoimmune disease
- Hypertension
- Antioxidant
- Anti-viral

- Anti-anxiety
- Sleep aid
- Hepatoprotection: protects and supports healthy liver function
- Renoprotective: protects and supports healthy kidney function
- Neuroprotective
  - Epilepsy
  - Stroke injury
  - Neurodegenerative conditions
- Supports healthy wound healing
- Anti-inflammatory
- Mildly analgesic to reduce pain and discomfort
- Anti-depressant
- Anti-aging
- Helps to control blood sugar for diabetes
- Microbiome support
- Anti-aging
- Longevity

Results of Studies in Veterinary Species for this Mushroom

- No published studies in veterinary species but many studies in humans and laboratory animals.

Pairings with other Mushrooms

- w/lion's mane for calming and neurological conditions
- w/turkey tail for cancer
- w/chaga for allergies

SHIITAKE MUSHROOM (MEDICINALLY-POWERFUL PREMIER EDIBLE MUSHROOM)

The shiitake mushroom is second only to the white button mushroom (*Agaricus bisporus*) in global sales. It is a very tasty, very popular, edible mushroom that also possesses substantial medicinal benefits, from managing cholesterol levels to supporting a weak immune system while also providing substantial benefits for patients with certain types of cancer or difficult-to-treat viral diseases. It is also one of the best-studied mushrooms in terms of its medicinal applications.

Millennia ago, this mushroom was discovered growing on the Japanese evergreen oak tree, the "Shiia tree." So, in English, it is the "oak mushroom." Currently, shiitake mushrooms are cultivated commercially on logs throughout the world. Like all mushrooms, shiitake needs to be cooked in order to release its nutritional and medicinal benefits.

Shiitake are extremely safe since they have been ingested for centuries by humans with minimal side effects. A few individuals have been found to have an allergic reaction to shiitake, although it may take repeated ingestion for a week or two for the reaction to occur based on published reports.[42]

Mushroom Scientific Name: *Lentinula edodes*

Mushroom Common Names
- Shiitake
- *Xiang gu*
- Black Forest mushroom

Where This Mushroom Grows

- Native to Japan, China, and other temperate Asian countries
- Grows on the native evergreen oak in Japan called the Shiia tree, as well as other fallen broadleaf trees, such as: chestnut, beech, oak, Japanese alder, sweet gum, maple, walnut, and mulberry.
- Cultivated worldwide on logs

Type of Mushroom: Agaric (gilled) Basidiomycete

Traditional & Historical Uses

- Increase stamina and circulation
- Arthritis/anti-inflammation
- Reduces cholesterol
- Diabetes
- Cancer
- Anti-aging
- Hepatoprotective
- Renoprotective
- Immune deficiency

Active Compounds and What They Do

- Beta-glucans
  - Lentinan is a commercial product in Japan used to treat cancers
  - Used as an injectable and orally
  - Lowers cholesterol
  - Anti-microbial

- Eritadenine
    - A polysaccharide that reduces cholesterol, triglycerides, and phospholipids
    - Anti-viral properties
    - Anti-hypertensive
- LEM: Lentinula edodes mycelium is a protein-bound polysaccharide
    - Anti-viral
        - HIV
        - Herpes simplex
        - Western equine encephalitis
- AHCC
    - Active Hexose Correlated Compound
        - Derived from the liquid culture of mycelium
        - Acetylated beta-glucan increases potency
        - Stimulates immune cell activation
        - Increases production of cytokines
            - Interferon
            - IL-12
            - Tumor necrosis factor (TNF)
        - Anti-viral
        - Anti-cancer

Key Power: Tasty, anti-cancer, immune-modulating, and metabolism balancing

Traditional Chinese Veterinary Medicine Characteristics

- Organ Affinity
  - o Stomach
  - o Spleen
  - o Lung
- Taste
  - o Sweet
- Energetics
  - o Neutral
- Actions
  - o Tonifies Qi and Blood

Potential Applications for Veterinary Species

- Metabolic disorders
  - o Hyperlipidemia (high fat in the blood)
- Chronic infections
  - o Upper respiratory
  - o Urinary infections
  - o Viral infections like Feline Immunodeficiency Virus (FIV)
- Hepatoprotective
- Renoprotective
- Anti-aging tonic
- Anti-microbial
  - o Adjunct to pharmaceutical tuberculosis treatment
  - o Potentiates
  - o Pathogenic fungi
  - o HIV
  - o Herpes virus
  - o Western equine encephalitis

- Cancer
  - Gastric
  - Breast
  - Lung
  - Liver
  - Melanoma
  - Adjunct to chemotherapy
- Immunomodulation
  - Colitis

Results of Studies in Veterinary Species for this Mushroom

- No studies *yet* on veterinary species. Multiple published studies in humans and laboratory animals. These published studies support the value of the mushroom and some of its isolated components, such as the lentinan for various types of cancer (gastric, breast, lung, liver, and melanoma), and viral infections like HIV, hepatitis B, C, and tuberculosis.

Synergistic Mushroom Pairings

- w/oyster, maitake, and/or agaricus for digestive and metabolic support
- w/turkey tail for cancer and viral infections
- w/cordyceps for improved stamina and energy

SNOW MUSHROOM (*TREMELLA FUCIFORMIS*, HYDRATING AND SUPPORTIVE)

This mushroom is a type of mushroom called a "jelly fungus" or "jelly mushroom." Its appearance is gelatinous or jelly-like. It has an unusual lifecycle in that it is a parasite to another fungus, a yeast. The yeast must be growing on dead and dying hardwoods, like oak. When it infects the yeast, that triggers its transformation into its mycelial vegetative stage, which then grows into the wood, proliferates, and when conditions are right, it mushrooms into its fruiting body, commonly called the snow mushroom.

It is a prized edible mushroom in Asia and is served fresh or reconstituted from the dried mushroom, a form in which it stores for long periods of time very well. Look for this mushroom in formulas for cognitive impairment, atopic dermatitis, gastritis, and chronic lung issues. It also offers properties that protect against ionizing radiation, cancer, and infectious diseases.

Mushroom Scientific Name: *Tremella fuciformis*

Mushroom Common Names
- Snow fungus
- White jelly mushroom
- White cloud ears
- Snow ear
- Silver ear fungus
- White wood ear
- White tree jellyfish

Where This Mushroom Grows

- Southeastern U.S. and warmer parts of the world, including Asia
- More commonly foraged and a related species that is both edible and medicinal is the *Tremella mesenterica*, also known as "witch's butter." It is distributed widely globally.
- *Auricularia auricula*, wood ear, or tree ear, is a very delicious and sought-after edible jelly mushroom in Asia, and it is distributed widely, globally.

Type of Mushroom: Basidiomycete: atypical spore-bearing structures; some can be teethed and others pore-like.

Traditional & Historical Uses

- Moistens, especially the lungs and stomach
- Upper respiratory inflammation and cough
- Tonic for longevity and energy
- Reduces cholesterol and atherosclerosis
- Supports healthy neurological repair from trauma
- Improves impaired cognitive function
- Supports a healthy immune response to challenges like cancer and infection
- Anti-diabetic
- Anti-aging
- Radiation protection
- Hepatoprotective
- Anti-allergenic
- Enhances beauty; used in cosmetics

Active Ingredients
- Mannan polysaccharides
- Beta-glucans
- Ergosterol
- Ergothioneine
- Phenols
- Chitin

Key Power: Rejuvenating, hydrating, moisturizing, and mental clarity

Traditional Chinese Veterinary Medicine Characteristics
- Organ Affinity
  - Lung
  - Stomach
  - Kidney
- Taste
  - Sweet
  - Bland
- Energetics
  - Neutral
- Actions
  - Nourishes Lung Yin and Stomach Yin
    - Asthma
    - COPD
  - Treats cough due to Lung deficiency
  - Hepatoprotective
  - Stimulates the Heart
  - Nourishes the Brain
  - Enriches the Kidneys, including Kidney Jing

Potential Applications for Veterinary Species

- Immune modulation
  - Cancers
  - Infectious agents
- Hydrates
  - Skin
  - Lungs
  - Kidneys
- Neurological support and protection
  - Especially post-trauma
- Benefits learning and memory
- GI Support
  - Gastritis
  - Ulcers
  - Constipation due to its hydrating effects
- Counteracts toxicity of radiation therapy
- Anti-aging and Longevity
- Supports the integrity of blood vessels
- Dermatologic support
  - Hydrates dry skin
  - Support for atopic dermatitis
- Strong anti-clotting effect, so use with caution if taking blood thinners

Results of Studies in Veterinary Species for this Mushroom

- A 2012 study in mice found that the unique polysaccharides found in tremella protected the subjects from radiation damage and side effects from the toxic radiation.[43]

- There are quite a few published studies on humans and laboratory animals. These studies have supported its value when being used for cholesterol reduction, certain types of cancer, normalizing blood sugar levels, circulatory disorders, memory impairment, and neurological damage. Based on a recent study, it may also be helpful as an adjunctive therapy for atopic dermatitis, commonly known as allergic dermatitis.[44]

Synergistic Mushroom Pairings
- w/lion's mane and reishi for calming, neurological support, and cognitive impairment and memory
- w/turkey tail for cancer
- w/chaga and reishi for allergies
- w/cordyceps for chronic cough and lung issues

TURKEY TAIL (STRONG MEDICINE)

Turkey tail mushrooms have centuries of use by humans for a variety of health complaints. Based on modern research and human studies, we have a greater understanding of the benefits of the many individual bioactive constituents in the turkey tail mushroom.

While there are few studies using the turkey tail mushroom in dogs to objectively suggest its benefits, many veterinarians believe that the same historical benefits and safety for humans will also translate to our pets' health and wellness.

The turkey tail mushroom contains multiple different types of molecules of beta-glucans. Beta-glucans are a type of indigestible fiber found in the cell walls of certain plants and fungi. These structural molecules for fungi and seaweed have been studied extensively for their capacity to help regulate the immune system, lower cholesterol levels, allow for healthy inflammatory responses, and help keep blood sugar levels within normal ranges.

There are many different variations of the beta-glucan molecule in turkey tail. It is this multitude of similar but different beta-glucan molecules that give turkey tail such robust immune enhancement properties.

Terpenes, both triterpenes and sesquiterpenes, are a second source of the strong immune-enhancing compounds found in the extracts of the turkey tail mushroom. Terpenes have many beneficial effects, including antioxidant and anti-inflammatory activity. Triterpenes in the turkey tail mushroom are, like the beta-glucans, found in a variety of molecular variations, all of which have potent bioactivity against infectious agents and neoplastic cells.

Turkey tail's cocktail of terpenes and beta-glucan molecules combine to provide the amazing therapeutic profile of immune effectiveness for which it is so well known.

Mushroom Scientific Name(s)

- *Trametes versicolor*
- Formerly known as *Coriolus versicolor*

Mushroom Common Names

- Turkey tail
- Yun Zhi
- Kawaratake

Where This Mushroom Grows

- Worldwide

Type of Mushroom: Polypore; Basidiomycota

Traditional & Historical Uses

- Endurance and longevity
- Anti-cancer
- Night sweats and coughs from tuberculosis (TB) and other pulmonary diseases
- Topical for ringworm, acne, eczema
- Rheumatism
- Fevers
- Leprosy
- Hemostatic (can be used to stop bleeding when used topically)
- Treats bacterial infections
- Abscesses
- Upper Respiratory Infections (URI)
- Urinary Tract Infections (UTI)
- GI
- Hepatitis B
- Chronic active hepatitis
- Immune weakness

Active Ingredients

- Beta-glucans (many variations)
- Polysaccharide Krestin (PSK)
- Polysaccharopeptide (PSP)
- Triterpenoids (many variations)
- Ergosterol
- Beta-sitosterol

Key Power: Defensive support, the mushroom to use for cancer and immune defense

Traditional Chinese Veterinary Medicine Characteristics

- Organ Affinity
  - Lung
  - Liver
  - Spleen
  - Heart
- Taste
  - Sweet
  - Slightly bitter
- Energetics
  - Slightly warming
- Actions
  - Increases circulation
  - Dispels Damp
  - Clear Wind and Heat

Potential Applications for Veterinary Species

- Cancer
- Viral infections
- Immune deficiency
- Microbiome support
- Helps reduce obesity
- Diabetes
- Arthritis/Analgesia
- Hepatoprotective
- Cardioprotective
- Inflammatory Bowel Disease (IBD)

NOTE: A safety study in rats showed safety for doses up to 7,500 mg/kg by mouth when given for 90 days.[45]

Results of Studies in Veterinary Species for this Mushroom

There are two studies published in dogs with splenic cancer (hemangiosarcoma). These studies used a pharmaceutical extract extracted from the turkey tail mycelium growing in a liquid nutrient broth. This polysaccharide peptide (PSP) is a single ingredient versus the multiple anti-cancer and immune-modulating ingredients found in the whole turkey tail mushroom.

The first study, published in 2012, was conducted at the University of Pennsylvania Veterinary School. The results were surprisingly good. The high-dosage group of five dogs survived this toxic and aggressive, and nearly always fatal, cancer of the spleen longer than dogs that had received chemotherapy.[46]

These study results caused a lot of pet parents to become really excited that PSP turkey tail extract could help their own dogs or cats with cancer. It is a very expensive extract, provided only by the Chinese company that owns the patent on its production. The product name is "I'mYunity™." Due to the high cost of this product, many pet parents have chosen to use the whole turkey tail mushroom extract and have, anecdotally, been finding some benefits to its use for a number of different cancer types.

The second published study of this PSP turkey tail extract in dogs with hemangiosarcoma took 10 years to complete and publish. In this study, they used groups of 50 and 25 dogs, with 100 dogs total in the study. The larger the study, the more likely those results indicate a true finding.

In this second study, published in 2022, also conducted at the University of Pennsylvania, one group of dogs received the PSP extract only. There were 50 dogs in this group. The second group of dogs received chemotherapy and the PSP extract. There were 25 dogs in this group. The third group received chemotherapy but also received a PSP placebo.[47]

The results of this second, larger study that was randomized, blinded, and placebo-controlled did not reflect the same findings as the first, smaller, pilot study. In fact, it found no benefit at all to the use of the PSP turkey tail product I'mYunity™ in these dogs, especially when combined with chemotherapy.

It was disappointing to see these negative results, and it was interesting in that there was a slight advantage for the male dogs over the female dogs in all three groups. The dogs on PSP alone did better than historical controls that did not receive chemotherapy or any other treatment other than the removal of the diseased spleen. It may be that the dosage wasn't high enough for this study.

In the first study, the group of five dogs that did so well comprised four males and one female, which would have skewed the results toward thinking that was a good dose to use. I would like to see this study repeated using the whole turkey tail extract at very high dosages. I suspect we would see better results than with an isolated single pharmaceutical extract of the mycelium.

What this second, larger study did reveal is that the degree of anemia of the dog with hemangiosarcoma is a prognosticator (predictor) of its length of survival from this cancer. For instance, if a male dog had a hematocrit (index of anemia) greater than 30%, they were in better shape than a male dog with a hematocrit lower than 30%. If it's a female dog, then its chances are much lower, even with a higher hematocrit than was found in male dogs. As the cancer spreads through the body by means of metastasis, the chances of lengthy survival become even more reduced.

Synergistic Mushroom Pairings
- w/lion's mane for cancer of the nervous system or stomach
- w/reishi for antiviral activity
- w/cordyceps for cancer of the kidneys or lungs
- w/chaga and/or maitake/shiitake for cancer in general

CHAPTER FOUR SUMMARY

Each of the important mushrooms presented in this chapter are complex organisms with many active ingredients. All mushrooms contain beta-glucans and triterpenes, which give them many similar properties. However, each mushroom species has variations of these common active constituents that give each mushroom its unique properties.

Since all mushrooms contain beta-glucans, all mushrooms have a very positive benefit to increasing immune system vigilance and function. This is why nearly *any* mushroom, given in appropriate amounts, could help address cancer, chronic infections, or cholesterol levels.

As another example, all mushrooms contain compounds called "terpenes," and each mushroom manufactures a variety of different terpenes. Terpenes can have very specific effects. Some address pain, others address anxiety, and others have anti-cancer effects. Terpenes generally reduce inflammation and exert a calming influence through serotonin receptors. Some terpenes are very specific, like the antihistaminic effects of certain terpenes in only chaga and reishi.

This is why learning more about what each individual mushroom contains, as I have detailed in this chapter, can help you better decide which mushroom(s) to choose for your pet's health, or for your own.

In Chapter Five, you will learn about how to give mushrooms to your pet. It will cover how mushrooms are provided in the marketplace, what would be best for a pet to use, and how to figure out the amount to give to your pet based on size and condition that way you can see first-hand how well a mushroom can improve your pet's quality of life.

HOW TO GIVE MUSHROOMS TO YOUR PET

Mushrooms can be fresh, they can be dried, or they can be processed into a supplement. **Fresh mushrooms** need to be cooked for at least 15-30 minutes to help release their active components that have been bound up in, or are part of, the fiber make-up of the fungal cell wall. Do not give raw mushrooms to your pet; they may not have any effectiveness in helping your pet's condition.

Dried mushrooms will keep for a long time at room temperature and are still the most common means of preserving mushrooms. Dried mushrooms can be found in Asian markets at local farmers' markets or can be ordered online. Before using a dried mushroom, you must first soak it in water for a number of hours to rehydrate it. The rehydrated mushroom must be cooked for at least 30 minutes, but it is even better if it is cooked for 120 minutes. The dried mushroom can also be powdered and consumed as a powder, which will have better absorption than a raw mushroom but not as good of a release of its fiber-based active components after heating for several hours at near boiling temperatures.

Mushroom extracts are the best way to get more of the active components of mushrooms into your pet—or yourself. Mushroom extracts come as powders, which can be added to your pet's food if they will accept the taste. Powders can fill capsules or be pressed into tablets. Powders can also be blended into soft chews or hard biscuits. Due to their being highly concentrated, some of the potential mushroom extracts that might be increased in the extract powder may exceed many pets' comfort zone of palatability. This is especially true with the bitter reishi, chaga, and turkey tail triterpenes. Of these three mushroom species, reishi is the most bitter.

Regardless of which form of mushroom you choose to use for your pet, it is easiest to mix it with some food in order to facilitate administration. It is important that you use the appropriate amount of mushroom or mushroom extract in order for your pet's condition and size to be accounted for. Too little mushroom will have a lesser effect. Too much mushroom is not a "thing." Mushrooms are extremely safe to give to your pet. Giving more won't hurt your pet and may ensure it gets enough to help.

Read the next section to better understand how to achieve an effective dose in your critter...

ESTABLISHING AN EFFECTIVE AMOUNT TO GIVE YOUR PET

When deciding how much of a mushroom extract to give your four-legged friend, the best way to come up with an effective "dosage" is to take your pet's weight and use that number of pounds or kilograms in combination with the type of condition your pet is experiencing, to arrive at an effective amount of mushroom extract or powdered dried mushroom to begin with.

All mushrooms have in common their beta-glucan content as their most studied active ingredient. As described earlier in the text, mushrooms have multiple components, all of which are biologically potent. The beta-glucan is produced by the plant in a proportional amount to the other active ingredients in the mushroom. When we use the beta-glucan percentage measured in a mushroom extract, we also give the other active ingredients in a fixed amount relative to that beta-glucan content in the mushroom extract.

Many mushroom products are analyzed for their beta-glucan content. Very few, if any, are analyzed for their triterpene or ergosterol content. When you are looking for a mushroom extract product, look for an extract from a company that also measures the beta-glucan percentage of that extract. By dosing for this beta-glucan amount, you will be giving a proportionate amount of the other active ingredients.

Here are the **three administration levels** I recommend considering when establishing an effective amount to give to your pet. Dried mushroom powder needs to be hot-water extracted for the best bioavailability of the mushroom active ingredients. To use these administrations by powder weight and pet weight, you will need to know the weight of your animal and the weight of the powder; a kitchen scale would be very useful here. You can estimate the weight of the mushroom powder as ½ teaspoon being equal to about 1 gram.

For people, we give the powder as follows:

Human Administration Guide

Wellness & minor problems:	1-3 grams once or twice daily
Moderate problems:	3-6 grams once or twice daily
Serious problems:	6-9 grams once or twice daily

Since there are so many different sizes of dogs (e.g., Chihuahua and giant mastiff) as compared to adult human sizes, I've adopted the above administration guidelines to be calculated based on your pet's body weight. This administration chart is below. You will need a kitchen scale that measures in grams to measure out the appropriate amount for your pet. This can be given once daily or twice daily for a more enhanced effect.

For pets, we give the powder as follows:
Critter Administration Guide

A simple place to start as a guide for administration is to simply use kitchen measuring spoon amounts per body weight of your pet. The powders all have very similar densities, which means that their volume measurement, which is easy to do without a scale, is a fairly accurate means of measurement.

Wellness & minor problems:	⅛ teaspoon/10 pounds of pet body weight daily
Moderate problems:	⅛ - ¼ teaspoon/10 pounds of pet body weight twice daily
Serious problems:	¼ - ½ teaspoon/10 pounds of pet body weight twice daily

These are the medical conditions that match each of these three administration levels:

Wellness & minor problems:	Daily wellness; mild stress relief
Moderate problems:	Chronic infections, vaccine titers, calming, significant stress relief, anti-histamine effect
Significant problems:	Cancer, bone marrow suppression from chemotherapy and radiation, serious acute infections, increased anti-histamine effect

NOTE: These are just estimates of good places to start on amounts to administer; you can modify these amounts, up or down, based on your pet's response and upon the advice of your veterinarian.

HOW TO SELECT AN EFFECTIVE MUSHROOM

Mushrooms are extremely effective in creating balance and harmony in your pet's life as a superfood and functional medicine. It is important for you to select a product that is clean and free of contamination, that meets its label claims for potency, and that does not contain myceliated grain.

Short of analyzing the mushroom extract yourself to check its potency claims, you should be able to find everything you need just on the bottle label. The label will tell you what mushroom species are in the product, how much of each mushroom is in each serving, and what the potency is of that mushroom species in terms of its beta-glucan content.

I have devised a method of determining how much to give your animal based on the type of condition being addressed. This method is based on:

1. Your pet's weight

2. The type of condition

3. The measured beta-glucan content of the product

It's a bit more complicated but is adapted to your pet's specific issues and its body weight and the beta-glucan content of the product.

You will need to source a mushroom product that has its beta-glucan content measured. Not many companies provide this information, but Real Mushrooms does measure and print the percentage of beta-glucan content of each of their mushroom products. They also maintain the same standardization of beta-glucan content, so you can give the same amount of that mushroom extract each time you purchase another bottle, as you will get the same potency from one product to the next.

If the label of the product you are considering giving to your pet does not contain the analysis of beta-glucans on it, call the company to ask them if they can share that data with you to help you establish an effective dose.

Chinese herbal formulas are commonly "decocted" or boiled for at least an hour before serving the liquid herbal (and mushroom) soup. Remember that the dried unprocessed mushroom powder has not released its fiber-bound medicinal compounds, so it will be less potent than an extracted mushroom powder.

Companies that manufacture and sell dietary supplements, like mushrooms or CBD, are forbidden to make "medical claims" about their products. According to the U.S. Food and Drug Administration (FDA), if a dietary supplement makes claims that it cures, prevents, or mitigates a disease, then it needs to be approved by the FDA as a drug, which is a long, complicated, and expensive process. The FDA reserves the right to stop the sales of a supplement, confiscate the inventory of that supplement, and fine the company if the claims are truly egregious.

In 1994, the U.S. Congress passed the Dietary Supplement Health and Education Act (DSHEA), which allowed the sale and marketing of human dietary health supplements as long as medical claims were not made in the marketing of the supplements. The FDA does allow companies to make "structure and function" claims. These types of claims describe what an ingredient or blend of ingredients does in the body in terms of the science that supports the use of these ingredients to benefit the structure or function of the body, but not about treating any specific disease.

For instance, when we use glucosamine in a product, we say that the glucosamine is in the formula to provide lubrication of the joint. A mushroom, for instance, may have evidence that it can help support healthy kidney function, as with the mushroom *Cordyceps militaris*. One could also say that a mushroom supports a healthy immune response to occasional inflammation or seasonal allergies in that the occasional use of a supplement for an acute symptom, like sneezing with allergies, is acceptable, but using it to treat a serious case of allergic dermatitis becomes a health claim.

This is why many of the labels on supplements and the marketing language used for that product do not tell you what it really is *for*. Instead, the label language would tell you what it *does*: what systems it supports or what structure of the body it helps maintain. The FDA frowns upon making medical claims for a product that has not undergone the extensive drug trials the FDA requires for something to be approved as a drug.

An educational book such as this is so very helpful in that there are no constraints by any agency, state or federal, to my First Amendment right of freedom of speech to write about what mushrooms do and what diseases they treat. It's just the label language and marketing of commercial products that are regulated by the government and subsequently need to follow these strict guidelines.

CHAPTER FIVE SUMMARY

Edible mushrooms contain so many functional ingredients that they have often been called "superfoods." Health benefits can be obtained by adding cooked mushrooms to one's daily diet in sufficient amounts.

However, for more substantial health benefits for more serious conditions, better results can be achieved using dried mushrooms, and even better results than ingesting them dried can be achieved with hot water extraction, as described in Chapter Five.

Although people refer to "doses" of mushrooms, they really aren't drug-like in how they work. The addition of mushrooms to your medicinal arsenal usually takes a few weeks of ingestion before benefits begin to occur. When used regularly over weeks and months, and even years, their benefits are more substantial.

This chapter has helped you understand better how to give mushrooms to your pet, and most importantly, how much mushroom you need to give to benefit the health of your pet. With this knowledge you will be better able address your pet's needs, especially with complex health issues.

This wraps up **"Section One: Our Marvelous Mushrooms."** In this section, we have focused on the history, scientific explanation, and active compounds of the most important mushrooms for a healthy pet. In Section Two, we will explore more specific conditions, along with case studies and specific recommendations, to help put this information into practical use.

In **"Section Two: Your Healthy Pet Guide—There's a Mushroom for That!"** we learn how to use mushrooms for specific problems that are common to dogs and cats. We explore more specific conditions by the use of eight stories I tell about pets I've helped or tried to help with integrative medicine, mushrooms, and cannabis. You will find this section to be the most useful for you if you are looking for some new tools and new tricks to help your pet stay healthy.

SECTION TWO

YOUR HEALTHY PET GUIDE
There's A Mushroom for That!

The pet problems covered in *Your Healthy Pet Guide* are examples of the conditions most commonly responsive to the use of cannabis, CBD, medical mushrooms, supplements, and diet. Every dog or cat's problem, although similar to other pets with similar problems, is actually very special and very unique to that critter. I'm sure you feel that your pet is a very special and unique individual.

The unique and special programs I have developed for this book address the individuality of your pet's genetic and acquired traits. The examples presented in this book are there to help you better understand the use of cannabis, mushrooms, and integrative medicine in the treatment of common problems we often see in our pets.

The information in this book is based on the scientific literature, and I've included references throughout this book so you can read these for yourself as well. The integrative programs I am recommending may help your pet's specific problem(s), but I can't guarantee they will eliminate it. Each pet's problem is similar to other pets with similar problems but also unique based on its biochemical individuality.

Please remember that this book cannot substitute for a thorough examination and advice by a licensed veterinarian. Your veterinarian will learn a lot from your pet's medical appointment by physically examining them in their office. They will listen to their heart and lungs, take their temperature, and look closely at them. There is only so much a book can do for your pet, but in partnership with your veterinarian, this book can help guide you in the use of supplements supportive of the conventional treatments your vet has recommended. This is the definition of integrative medicine, blending the best of conventional medicine with complementary and alternative therapies.

In this book, I am sharing my 40-plus years of experience as an integrative and holistic veterinarian with you. This way, even though I've retired from day-to-day clinical practice, I can still help the critters and leave this world a better place for our beloved pets.

ALLERGIES AND INFLAMMATORY DERMATITIS

ALLERGIES IN A DOG:
"POOCHIE" SMITH'S ALLERGIC DERMATITIS

"*My dog is scratching herself so much she is keeping me awake at night, causing sores and bleeding on her skin. She is also making disgusting licking sounds when she isn't scratching herself!*"

"*Her greasy skin and haircoat are so smelly, I can smell it the moment I open the front door!*"

"*Can you help me help my poor, miserable pet without using steroids, which make her fat, aggressive, and pee in the house? That's all my vets have ever offered to treat her, and although they stop the scratching, the side effects just get to be too much for me to handle.*"

I hear this type of thing so often from my clients who have allergic dogs. Although not life-threatening, gaining control over these types of allergies is really challenging and sometimes seems impossible without the use of strong drugs like steroids.

Fortunately, modern medicine has created some unique pharmaceuticals to address this issue that aren't as toxic as the steroids prednisone, prednisolone, triamcinolone, and dexamethasone.

These new medications, such as Apoquel™ and Cytopoint™,

are not as problematic as the long-term use of steroids but certainly can have their own side effects that still may be a problem. The feedback from a number of pet parents who have tried Apoquel™ and/or Cytopoint™ in their dogs is that it works well at first but its effectiveness seems to taper off over time.

The use of "allergy shots" can also be given orally. This hyposensitization approach is traditionally considered the best way to treat allergies, but these take quite a bit of time to become effective. These hyposensitization strategies don't always do a perfect job in terms of stopping that incessant scratching, licking, and the trauma to their skin that comes from scratching and licking. Still, these can help make life a little easier for you and your pet.

When "Poochie" walked into my exam room, she was wearing a t-shirt wrapped around her waist, with her front legs through the arm holes and her head through the neck hole. I could smell the foul odor of her skin when she walked into my veterinary hospital; it was so strong in my exam room that it was almost overwhelming. Vets learn to "mouth breathe" to be able to be close to that kind of smell for long periods of time and not "die" from it. If the odor doesn't come up through the nose, the smell is much less bad!

Before I examined Poochie, I spent considerable time learning the history and background of her problem. Poochie is a six-year-old, spayed, female, black, standard poodle weighing 65 pounds. Carol, Poochie's mom, said that she started scratching herself at about 18 months of age, and it had only worsened over the years. She had seen a dermatology specialist who suggested allergy testing and hyposensitization (allergy) shots. Carol tried the shots but hadn't seen much in the way of results after a year. She tried the new allergy medication, Apoquel™, and that seemed to work for a while, but now it wasn't so effective. She had tried steroids and antihistamines, but the steroids made Poochie too aggressive to other dogs, and she started peeing in the house. The antihistamines just made Poochie sleepy all the time. Carol tried supplements, fish oil, homeopathy, and even acupuncture, all to no avail.

So, when all else fails, they come to see me in their eleventh hour!!!

I'm used to seeing the most difficult cases that aren't responding well to conventional medicines. Many times, my suggestions make a difference, and they improve. Sometimes, I fail, too, and my suggestions don't make a difference. I prefer seeing these patients with difficult-to-treat conditions when they are just starting with the early symptoms. If I can see them before they start the use of medications, especially immune-suppressive medications, such as cyclosporin, prednisolone, prednisone, triamcinolone, dexamethasone, Cytopoint™, or Apoquel™, I feel I can make more progress early in the case than if they have been on the drugs already, especially for a very long time.

I don't hesitate to use these strong medications if my patient is suffering. In the short term, these medications are manageable. However, in the long term (months and years), their continued use makes it more difficult for the immune-supportive therapies I use to work as well as they can due to the pre-existing suppression of immune function from these medications.

For Poochie's care, I wanted to run a food allergy/sensitivity saliva test that Carol could purchase herself and conduct in her own home. The testing company would share the results with me, and I would then advise her on which foods to avoid that might be complicating the allergy picture. The results would take a few weeks to arrive, so in the meantime, I wanted to start Poochie on a few important supplements for her allergies and healthy skin that are discussed, in-depth in the following pages.

POOCHIE'S ALLERGY SUPPLEMENTS

1. PEA
(*palmitoylethanolamide*)[48]

A number of well-conducted, placebo-controlled, clinical trials in allergic dogs and cats found that PEA (palmitoylethanolamide), a tasteless fatty molecule found in all animals, can help to reduce the symptoms of allergies—the itching and red skin, especially. It needed to be given for a month before results were seen, but overall, many animals in the studies received comfort from their incessant scratching.[49]

PEA is a type of fat molecule naturally occurring in humans and all animals, as well as in common foods, such as eggs.

When the body experiences the immune dysfunction of an allergic response, it begins to produce more PEA. But if that PEA is added orally in addition to what the body produces, it has a much more substantial effect. This beneficial effect may take as long as a month (or longer for more severe cases) to develop, so be patient and give this supplement regularly.

Dog Dose: 10 mg/kg/d = 4.5 mg/pound/day for dogs
- 10 pounds: 45 mg/d
- 25 pounds: 112 mg/d
- 50 pounds: 225 mg/d
- 75 pounds: 336 mg/d
- 100 pounds: 450 mg/d

Cat Dose: 15 mg/kg/d = 7 mg/pound/day for cats

- 5 pounds: 35 mg/d
- 10 pounds: 70 mg/d
- 15 pounds: 105 mg/d
- 20 pounds: 140 mg/d
- 25 pounds: 175 mg/d

2. CBD
(30 mg twice daily for her 65-pound weight)

A recent Japanese study found that allergic dogs would scratch themselves less when given doses of CBD by mouth.[50] CBD reduces inflammation and the pruritus caused by inflammation of the skin.

3. CBDA
(30 mg twice daily for her 65-pound weight)

A second study, published in 2022, used a combination of both CBD and CBDA given to dogs with allergies. This study confirmed what the first study found, that CBD and other cannabinoids can help with the symptoms of allergies, mainly the itching, to some degree.[51]

4. CBG
(15 mg twice daily for her 65-pound weight)

This novel and emerging cannabinoid has good evidence that it can reduce inflammation in the skin and has been measured to have increased anti-inflammatory effects over CBD. CBG also inhibits an enzyme that breaks down PEA, thus contributing to higher blood levels of this important cannabinoid-like molecule for a longer period of time. CBG has been found in studies to help with autoimmune skin conditions like psoriasis. No study has been published yet about the value of CBG for allergic skin disease in dogs or cats. The evidence does support that it plays a positive role in managing allergic skin disease, according to reports by pet owners and a few veterinarians.[52]

5. Mushrooms

(reishi, chaga, tremella; ⅛ teaspoon of powder/10 pounds of body weight once or twice daily of each single mushroom)

Poochie was given ¾ teaspoon once daily of each mushroom.

Mushrooms and the many beneficial bioactive compounds they contain benefit the health of the skin and haircoat in a number of ways:

Microbiome Support[53,54]

The fiber in mushrooms consists of beta-glucans and chitin, which provides food to the many beneficial microorganisms that make up the population of the microbiome. We are learning that a healthy microbiome will improve the health of the skin and support a more balanced immune response to potential allergens.

Immuno-Modulation[55]

The beta-glucans and other immune-active molecules found in mushrooms, such as the triterpenes, nucleosides, flavonoids, and phenols, all contribute to a better-balanced immune system in those who take mushrooms regularly for long periods of time. With allergies, it is the immune system that "goes out of whack" and responds to harmless substances, like pollen or dust, with an exaggerated reaction. Supporting the immune system can help to reduce its reactivity to allergens.

Antihistamine Action[56]

Mast cells of the immune system are the allergy cells that cause many symptoms of allergies by releasing the chemical histamine that it stores in little intracellular sacks or "vacuoles." An allergic reaction triggers these cells to release their histamine, which causes the symptoms of an allergic reaction, which includes itching, local swelling, and redness.

Two mushrooms, reishi and chaga, contain special molecules called triterpenes that counteract the effect of the histamine release. I recommend that either or both be given. You might find that one works better than the other for the antihistamine reaction or that both together work better than any one of them alone.

Moistening and Hydrating Effect on the Skin[57]

The snow fungus, *Tremella fuciformis*, is used in Asia in cosmetics due to its hydrating effect when used topically in cosmetics or in topical medication. When ingested, the Tremella will also hydrate the skin. Benefits to the skin are often seen in two to three weeks, but some pets can benefit sooner.

6. Fish Oil (EPA+DHA)[58]

Of all the supplements available, fish oil is the most versatile, affecting nearly every system in the body, including the skin. Its value is not so much for the condition of the skin moisture; we look to linoleic acid (LA) for that and find the LA in flax seed meal. EPA and DHA are potent anti-inflammatory agents, although they require consistent daily use for two to three months for their full effect to be felt or observed.

7. Borage Seed Oil
(24% gamma-linolenic acid [GLA]: 240 mg twice daily)

This is another seed oil that contains a different fatty acid than fish oil and flax seed meal. This fatty acid is technically an omega-6 fatty acid oil but acts as an anti-inflammatory fatty acid like fish oil and flax seed oil. When all of these oils are given together, they have an additive effect in reducing inflammation of the skin and improving the allergy symptoms of scratching, licking, and chewing the skin.

8. Flax Seed Meal
(1 tablespoon per meal)

It is best to keep this in the refrigerator. Flax seed, once it's been milled, only has a three-month shelf life. Flax seed is a rich "superfood," containing omega-6 and omega-3 fatty acid oils, soluble and insoluble fiber, and something called "lignans," which have been found to help balance the body's hormones, provide antioxidant benefits, and can help with certain conditions such as Cushing's disease when combined with melatonin.

9. Quercetin
(5 mg/kg twice daily)[59]

This flavonoid has been found to reduce the release of histamine by mast cells, which is one of the most important mechanisms that create the symptoms of itching also known as pruritus. When combined with the PEA, its effects are amplified by their synergistic relationship.

Why have I chosen so many supplements for Poochie's skin problem?

I explained to Carol why I thought so many of these supplements together could benefit Poochie. After listening for a bit, she agreed that it was worth a try. I advised her to take it slowly and to introduce one new thing at a time to be sure it was not causing her a problem. I suggested a gradual introduction over four weeks. I knew that if Poochie had an unexpectedly bad reaction to a supplement or two, it would be difficult to convince Carol that we needed to keep at it for success.

Carol gradually introduced all of these supplements to Poochie's daily regimen, who accepted them in her food or with a little bit of "bribe food" with no problems or side effects. It's always good to introduce new things to your pet gradually to avoid adverse reactions like diarrhea, vomiting, or hives. I suggest starting with 25% of the final dosage and gradually increasing that over a period of two to three weeks to be safe.

Once we got the results of the food allergy/sensitivity saliva test from Nutriscan, Carol and I discussed the results and looked at foods she could feed that were not on the reactive food list.

Eating foods that the immune system is reactive to can create "whole body" inflammation. You can draw a direct line between excessive inflammation in the body and the itching symptoms of the skin. If an ingredient is not defined as having a food allergy-positive reaction, it can still contribute to increasing or decreasing inflammation.

This is why it is important to find a non-inflammatory diet. Better yet, it would be an anti-inflammatory diet. These kinds of diets are always a good idea for pets with allergic dermatitis like Poochie. Using a very detailed and unique test, such as with Nutriscan.org, increases your ability to create a true anti-inflammatory diet individualized for your pet. Individualization means it is targeted to your pet and will work better in reducing inflammation.

ABOUT SKIN ALLERGIES IN PETS

One of the more common problems seen in pets is the skin allergies that dogs, cats, and horses can be afflicted with. Allergies usually manifest on the skin but can also have digestive system manifestations, as well as upper respiratory symptoms.

Allergies occur when the immune system reacts to something that is not a threat to the health of the animal but which, due to the reactivity and hypersensitivity of the immune system, causes symptoms of itching, redness, and inflammation of the skin, digestive system, or respiratory system. Often, allergies will progress to become ulcerated sores that are worsened by the scratching, biting, and chewing that dogs and cats often do when their skin is irritated and inflamed.

Most often, dogs and cats are sensitive to pollen, dust, and mold they inhale, but they can also be sensitive to food ingredients and things they come into contact with, such as insect bites, plants, and chemicals in the environment.

The most common symptom of an allergy is the incessant scratching or licking of the skin due to an itching sensation, also called "pruritus," which is secondary to the inflammation and histamine release from specialized immune cells called "mast cells."

Excessive scratching and licking can be damaging to the skin and can easily turn an area of inflammation into an ulceration of the skin, creating what is commonly called a "hot spot." Another term for hot spot is "acute moist dermatitis." This is an area of the skin that your dog has been licking and/or scratching so much that the hair has come off and the naked skin is red, thickened, and inflamed.

The use of CBDA is the best topical treatment for a hot spot, in my opinion. The traditional treatment for hot spots is to wash it with an antiseptic soap and apply a topical steroid and antibiotic. It is important to keep the animal from scratching and licking the hot spot.

Often, an "Elizabethan collar" is used to prevent the dog from its self- destructive behavior. With the application of a CBDA salve or salve made from other cannabinoids, such as CBD and/or CBG, for instance, it is also important to keep your pet from licking and scratching. So, using a collar could be helpful, or using a t-shirt or some other means to cover the area so they can't get to it will also help.

Cannabis contains CBD and other compounds that are potent anti-inflammatories. Two studies have been published recently, one from Japan[60] and the other from the U.S.[61] (We further discuss these two studies later in this chapter.) Interestingly, both studies found that CBD and other cannabinoids like CBDA can help to reduce the itching (called "pruritis"), which drives the incessant scratching and licking that causes self-destructive sores on the skin. These two studies also found that CBD wasn't able to improve the redness around skin sores. This may be because the appropriate dosage has not yet been determined. It may be, however, that allergies are so complicated that simply giving the animal an anti-inflammatory drug or supplement, such as CBD (or a steroid), is not strong enough to counter its all of the symptoms.

There might still be some hope for allergy sufferers. Another compound, similar to cannabinoids, is found in common foods like eggs and is also found in the cells of all mammals, like dogs and us. I am referring to the tongue twister "palmitoylethanolamide," abbreviated as "PEA," which we discussed as part of Poochie's treatment earlier in this chapter.

CONVENTIONAL APPROACHES TO ALLERGIES IN PETS

Allergies are complicated diseases with a potential number of caus-es that are not the same from one allergic pet to another. There are three types of therapeutics currently being used to treat allergies in pets using conventional medications that are worth looking at:

1. Immune Suppressive Remedies

Immune-suppressive remedies give the quickest and strongest response over time. However, they are associated with adverse side effects when used for long periods of time at the high doses needed to control the symptoms of allergies.

Examples of immune suppressive therapies include:
- Corticosteroids like prednisone
- Transplant rejection drugs like Atopica™ (cyclosporin)

2. Symptom Modifying Treatments

Symptom-modifying treatments interfere with the chemicals our immune system creates that are the cause of the symptoms of al-lergies.

Examples of symptom-modifying therapies include:

A. Antihistamines counter the effects of the histamine released from mast cells of the immune system when an allergic response is activated.

Dosages of Common OTC
Antihistamines for Dogs and Cats

- **Benadryl™ (diphenhydramine)**
  - o Dogs: 1 mg/pound 2-3 times daily or as needed in a single dose
  - o Cats: not used in cats
- **Claritin™**
  - o Dogs: 0.5 mg/pound 1-2 times daily
  - o Cats: 5 mg 1-2 times daily
- **Zyrtec™**
  - o Dogs: 0.5 mg/pound 1-2 times daily
  - o Cats: 5 mg 1-2 times daily
- **Chlorpheniramine**
  - o Dogs: 0.2 mg/pound 2-3 times daily or as needed in a single dose
  - o Cats: 2 mg 1-2 times daily

B. Monoclonal antibodies use genetically engineered antibodies specific to the pro-inflammatory compounds produced during allergies. These compounds are produced by the allergy-activated immune cells and are responsible for creating the annoying symptoms of allergies. These monoclonal antibodies (MAB) will only bind to a specific cytokine. Cytokines are molecules produced by immune cells that are responsible for increasing or decreasing inflammation. These immune-based therapies do not cure the allergies but can provide a better quality of life than long-term steroid use by reducing or eliminating the symptoms without the steroid side effects.

For many dogs, these monoclonal antibody treatments are a godsend. Severe allergies can be very difficult to treat or manage. They can be costly without any successful outcome. Some pet parents get so frustrated with their inability to help their beloved dogs who are suffering in their own skin that they consider euthanasia.

Monoclonal antibody treatments can really help, especially with those patients with severe disease when nothing else but high, toxic levels of steroids are needed to control their run-away symptoms. I've heard of some adverse reactions, some that were actually allergic reactions to the anti-allergy drug! These are a new type of therapy and are non-toxic in comparison to corticosteroids, but still have a few issues.

Monoclonal antibody treatments are administered by injection and will last two to four weeks before another injection is needed. They are effective for atopic dermatitis in dogs.

Currently, the only MAB available for atopic dermatitis in dogs is a Cytopoint™ (Lokivetmab) injection, manufactured by Zoetis Animal Health. A single injection can reduce itching within 24 hours and can be effective for up to a full month. It is a monoclonal antibody treatment that binds the IL-31 cytokine, which is a major chemical mediator of itching in allergic dogs.

C. Immuno-modulatory therapies are similar to monoclonal antibody therapies in that they interfere with the cascade of chemical signals in atopic dermatitis that cause itching. Apoquel™ (Oclacitinib maleate), manufactured by Zoetis Animal Health, inhibits the chemical mediators that are "upstream" from the pro-inflammatory, pro-itch cytokines. These chemical messengers, when activated, will stimulate the production of IL-31 and other similarly-acting cytokines from immune cells. These cytokines create the itching and other symptoms commonly seen with allergies. Apoquel™ is a tablet that needs to be taken daily. It has been found to be effective for atopic dermatitis, food allergy dermatitis, flea allergy dermatitis, contact dermatitis, sarcoptic mange, or unspecified allergic dermatitis. It can be effective for a number of allergic-type conditions that affect cats, as well.

Contact and food allergies are best treated by avoidance of the offending foods and environmental causes, but the use of this immunomodulatory drug will address those allergic symptoms from foods and contact with environmental materials.

It is important to note that if you are thinking about performing the Nutriscan.org saliva test to find out which food ingredients are allergenic for your dog, you will have to stop the Apoquel™ treatment.

3. Disease Modifying Treatments

Disease-modifying treatments will actually treat the disease through hyposensitization treatments. Examples of disease-modifying therapies include:

A. Hyposensitization therapy: These are traditionally what have been called "allergy shots." These injections consist of the specific antigens that your pet is allergic to, determined through intradermal skin testing (most accurate) or blood tests.

The injections are given on a regular basis, daily, weekly, or monthly, depending on the specific needs of your pet. The injections start with an extremely diluted solution of the antigens, and over time, the concentration of the antigens gradually increases, which allows your pet's immune system to stop being so reactive to these antigens. As a result, your pet will have fewer symptoms.

These shots will need to be given regularly by you to your pet over a period of months and probably years, with gradually increasing concentrations of antigens and longer intervals between shots until they are one month apart.

They now have oral hyposensitization treatments available, as well. These oral treatments need to be given more frequently than the injection therapy.

Hyposensitization has been considered the "gold standard" in allergy treatments and still is the best and least toxic way to treat allergies in pets and in people.

B. Elimination diets: Allergies can be caused not just by environmental antigens that are inhaled but can also be caused by contact with allergens and from food ingredients or food chemicals, such as preservatives, additives, etc. Hyposensitization is specifically for inhalant allergies.

The elimination diet is the most accurate means of determining which food ingredients your pet is allergic to, sensitive to, or intolerant of. This is a hands-on, empirical approach to directly testing your pet with individual foods to observe a reaction or no reaction.

You have to start with a very bland diet that has limited ingredients that you have observed have not been reactive to your pet. Some people advocate for a pure diet of just tofu or potatoes and nothing else. I like to start with a saliva test and use that to guide my creation of the very bland, hypoallergenic diet. This is best done in partnership with your veterinarian or with a veterinary dermatologist.

After you feed this bland diet for four weeks, you should see the symptoms that are characteristic of food allergies get less or go away. Often, these symptoms are smelly, goopy ears, licking between their toes, licking their anus, or anal gland problems.

Next, you introduce one food ingredient, say chicken or beef, and observe your pet for developing food allergy symptoms again in two weeks. If they do not develop symptoms, then that ingredient is probably okay to feed. Put that ingredient on your "good" list and try the next ingredient. This is the most accurate means of food allergy testing but extremely time-consuming and tedious.

Pets who have allergies to food ingredients, when fed a food ingredient they are not allergic to, may, over time, develop allergies to that previously non-reactive ingredient. The amount of time it takes for a pet to become allergic to a food ingredient to which it was not previously allergic is different for each pet, and it is impossible to predict.

My recommendation is to "sacrifice" one set of hypoallergenic ingredients in order to determine how long it takes to develop allergies to an originally non-allergenic food material. Once you determine how long it takes, you then change the one hypoallergenic diet for another hypoallergenic diet so it doesn't become allergenic. That way, you can rotate back and forth between the hypoallergenic diets and not worry about them becoming allergenic.

Whew! It's a lot of work to have an allergic pet!

C. Contact allergies: identify the cause of the allergy and avoid contact with it, which is a logical approach.

D. Food allergies: identify the allergenic ingredients and materials in the foods we are feeding and then feed a diet that does not contain these allergens.

Identifying the allergenic ingredients in your pet's diet is not that easy a problem to solve. Often, pets are fed a variety of different pet foods, may also be given treats, and not uncommonly are fed table scraps and people food at random.

Two types of tests can help identify these allergens:

1. A blood test for food allergies can identify one type of allergic reaction to food materials, but the experts tell us that these blood tests are not very accurate over time. The blood test measures the IgE antibody, which traditionally has been the antibody involved with allergies.

2. A saliva test is now available that tests for several other categories of immune reactions to food ingredients. The saliva test determines if there are food intolerances or food sensitivities, which are also immune-mediate

The antibodies tested with the saliva test are the IgG and IgM antibodies, which are more involved with immune reactions to food ingredients that classically have not been defined as "allergies" since IgE is not involved. Nonetheless, the reactions we see in pets to food ingredients are very commonly orchestrated through the IgG and IgM antibodies more than the IgE antibodies.

I've used this test many times and have found it more useful than the IgE blood tests, which are the standard testing for food allergies.

You can administer the saliva test yourself at home, but the blood test will have to be performed at your vet's, where they can draw the blood and submit it for testing.

The site where you can order this test is:
www.nutriscan.org

You can add the name of your veterinarian on the test request form so they will also receive the test results.

INTEGRATIVE/HOLISTIC TREATMENTS

CBD and cannabis: two studies were published in 2022 reporting the results of treating allergic dogs with cannabinoids. One study used CBD in eight client-owned dogs without any placebo controls.[62] The second study recruited 32 client-owned dogs that used a product with a 1:1 ratio of CBD:CBDA, with a placebo control group.[63]

Both of these studies found, with the use of these cannabinoid formulations, that itching, called "pruritus" in medical terminology, was significantly less with the use of the cannabinoid products. The other symptoms of skin allergies in dogs, such as redness of the skin and skin sores, were significantly less in the group of eight allergic dogs receiving the cannabis extracts in the CBD only study. The dogs in the second study were not observed to receive any benefits to these skin lesions with the use of the CBD/CBDA product.

The doses used in the CBD-only study were within the same range of dosing that I have been recommending throughout this book. This study used the same process of starting with a lower dose of 0.25 mg CBD/pound of body weight twice daily, taken with a small amount of fatty food before each meal. The dosage was increased if, after two weeks, no changes were observed. Some dogs found relief with this lower starting dosage, but others needed a higher dosage, which in some cases was as high as 1 mg/pound twice daily with food.

In the CBD-only study, some of the dogs improved enough on the CBD to be able to reduce their steroid medication. Itching was less, as were skin lesions. They used a broad-spectrum CBD product containing no detectable THC.

The CBD/CBDA study used a dosage of 0.5 mg/pound twice daily of each of its two cannabinoids, CBD and CBDA. This study used the fixed dosage of 0.5 mg/pound each of CBD and CBDA but only found a reduction in itching, with no observed benefit to the skin, with this higher dose. Whether this is due to the CBDA in the product can't be determined from the evidence, but future studies may help to clarify whether CBDA is able to help improve skin lesions in addition to itching.

Both of these studies support the use of cannabinoids in the treatment of allergies in dogs. Using a dosing approach, as has been recommended throughout *Your Healthy Pet Guide*, to start with a low dose of 0.25 mg/pound twice daily with food and increasing it as needed for improved response, is an empirical approach that will determine the most effective dosing for your dog with allergies.

PEA (palmitoylethanolamide) PEA is a cannabinoid-like molecule with objective evidence that it can help with skin allergies in dogs, cats, horses, and humans.[64,65,66]

PEA was discovered in the 1950s during a rheumatic fever outbreak. It was found that populations of children for whom eggs were a major part of their daily food intake were more resistant to this infection than children who did not eat eggs as much.

Detailed laboratory analysis of eggs found this mouthful of a molecule that we simplify the polysyllabic name down to three letters: PEA. This material is found in all mammals and is part of the molecules in the body that are involved in the "entourage effect" of cannabis. In fact, when we take in some CBD, or your pet does, it causes this molecule, PEA, to stimulate cell membrane receptors that are involved in the immune system to have this anti-infective activity.

Further study into PEA found that it also had a good influence on relieving pain. Furthermore, it was found to be an anti-allergic and neuroprotective molecule. When it was given to dogs with allergic dermatitis, or "atopy," it was able to significantly reduce itching and redness of the skin. In cats who have a type of severe dermatitis called an "eosinophilic granuloma complex," commonly called "rodent ulcer," they would go into remission when fed relatively small amounts of this tasteless and odorless fatty molecule.[67,68]

There are a number of studies in dogs and cats that show PEA to be able to modulate skin allergies in both dogs and cats with twice-daily oral doses. It may take four to eight weeks for the PEA to have its maximal effect. PEA is considered to be GRAS by the U.S. FDA, which means it is "generally recognized as safe" and means just what it says: PEA is as safe as food.

PEA is what we call an "entourage compound," which means it is part of the body's endocannabinoid system and that it works together with a number of other naturally occurring molecules in our cells to reduce the allergic immune response.

There are studies in cats and dogs that showed PEA to be safe and effective to use for canine and feline atopic dermatitis (skin allergies usually from allergens that are inhaled). PEA was also found to be helpful for cats who have a chronic inflammatory granulomatous condition commonly called "rodent ulcer," but which has the medical name "Feline Eosinophilic Granuloma complex."[69]

In the study of 160 dogs with atopic dermatitis, otherwise known as "inhalant allergic dermatitis," PEA was given at 10 mg/kg of body weight (~5 mg/pound) once daily for eight weeks. The amount of itching (pruritus) and the types of sores that resulted from atopic dermatitis and the overall quality of life of the canine participants were measured. A total of 146 dogs completed the eight-week study. It was determined at the conclusion of this study that the PEA significantly improved the pruritus and sores, and the overall quality of life was improved, as well, in these dogs. After the first month, 80% of the dogs had improved on the daily PEA dosage.[70]

There is a similar study in cats diagnosed with "non-flea hypersensitivity dermatitis," which is how feline atopic/allergic dermatitis is described by veterinary dermatologists. Our understanding of feline allergic/atopic dermatitis lags behind that of canine allergic/atopic dermatitis, hence the differing terminology describing very similar problems in these two species.

A total of 25 cats completed this study. They were given 15 mg/kg, or 6.8 mg/pound, of PEA daily. It was determined that, compared to the group of cats that received a placebo treatment, the cats that received the PEA remained symptom-free for a significantly longer period of time.

Some of the cats in this study also were dosed with a corticosteroid for a short period of time, and these cats who received the steroid and that also received the PEA had significantly less pruritus than the control group. This means, if your cat cannot be taken off of a steroid without disturbing its quality of life, that the concurrent use of PEA with that steroid might allow you to use a lower dose of steroid and still get the same benefits without the potential toxicity that steroids can have on the liver.[71]

Supplements for allergies are many, but their effectiveness varies. Some pets will respond very well to these herbs and nutraceuticals, others not so well. Dosage is important, as well as the duration of therapy. It can take two to four months of therapy for diet and supplements to make a significant difference in your dog's response to allergies.

Listed below are the supplements for which there is the best evidence in the literature for them to work for allergies.

EPA/DHA fatty acids are most commonly found in fish oil but may also be found in other marine lipid sources, such as green-lipped mussel oil, Hoka fish roe oil, or high DHA oil from algal sources.[72]

When used at sufficiently high doses for at least three months, EPA and DHA can reduce inflammation in the body as a whole. Inflammation drives the pathology we see with skin allergies: the itching, the redness, and the skin sores.

We give a therapeutic amount of EPA/DHA by using the sum of the amount of each fatty acid (EPA+DHA) in each milliliter (mL) of oil and dose it at 50 mg/pound of body weight daily of EPA+DHA. It can take 90-120 days for fish oil to have a full effect in your pet.

GLA (*gamma linoleic acid*) is found in borage oil, black currant seed oil, and evening primrose oils. It is a slightly different fatty acid than EPA and DHA structurally, but it works together with EPA and DHA to help reduce the inflammation associated with skin allergies. The dosage for GLA hasn't been worked out as well as for EPA and DHA, but one paper used 12.5 mg of GLA for each pound of body weight daily successfully. Using these three fatty acids together is the best.[73]

Quercetin is a flavonoid, derived from fruits and vegetables. It is a powerful antioxidant that also has the ability to inhibit the release of histamine from mast cells. Histamine is a chemical produced by the mast cells, which are immune cells involved in the allergic process. It is one of the main driving forces that create allergy symptoms.[74]

There are different forms of quercetin, with differing amounts of bioavailability. Quercetin is not well absorbed, except when found in foods. The phosphatidylcholine-bound quercetin is the best-absorbed form of quercetin. Generally, we give our cats and dogs 50-250 mg of quercetin twice daily with food.

Probiotics – Microbiome Support

Beneficial bowel bacteria help to improve immune system function by providing the bowel with the appropriate strains of healthy bacteria and microorganisms. There are a number of available probiotic products available. I suggest finding a product with multiple strains and a very high bacterial count in the billions for each dose. There is no single "best" probiotic in the marketplace. Each pet defines for itself which probiotic formula works best for them.

Spore-forming probiotics and fungal-based probiotics are more heat stable than lactic acid bacteria probiotics. They do not need refrigeration and have copious research supporting their value for digestive health. The microbiome of the gut plays an important role in all of the functions of the body, including the immune system's response to allergens. The skin has its own local microbiome, and its health is directly related to the health of the microbiome of the bowel. Keeping the microbiome "happy" by inoculating your pet daily with probiotic cultures is essential for healthy skin and a healthy response to allergens.[75]

Prebiotics are food for the microbiome. Healthy fiber supplies this nourishment. This is another good reason to ensure adequate fiber in your pet's diet. Not only is fiber good for healthy stool formation, but it also feeds the microbiome. Mushrooms have some of the best insoluble fiber of all foods. Not only does mushroom fiber feed the microbiome, but the mushroom fiber that contains chitin will help to moisturize and reduce the inflammation of the lining of the bowel, which can help with bowel problems like colitis, inflammatory bowel disease, and leaky gut. Recently, a study from Japan was published in which they fed lion's mane mushroom powder with a dry pet food product and were able to measure improvements in the microbiome ratio of "good" bacteria to "bad" bacteria.[76]

Postbiotics are fermentation by-products of bacteria, yeast, and fungi that contain constituents that support a healthy microbiome and immune system. Foods like fermented vegetables (think sauerkraut), yogurt, tempeh, soy sauce, and miso contain these valuable nutrients, which are good additions to your pet's diet, whether you are making a home-prepared meal or just feeding them dry food. As an aside, mycelium grown on grain (MOG) is also a post-biotic, not a mushroom.

Herbs for Allergies

Traditionally, over the years, herbs have been used to address the symptoms of allergies in humans. We can use the same herbs for our pets with allergies. It is best to consult with a veterinarian skilled in the art and science of veterinary herbal medicine. The Veterinary Botanical Medical Association (www.VBMA.org), of which I was president a number of years ago, has a directory on its website that can help you find a holistic veterinary herbalist for your pet's allergies. The American College of Veterinary Botanical Medicine, of which I was president for a few years, and Charter Fellow of this College (FACVBM) also has a directory of veterinary clinical herbalists on their website: www.ACVBM.org.

Some Supportive Herbs to Consider
Giving Your Pet with Allergies:

- Nettle leaf
- Dandelion
- Red clover
- Yellow dock
- Licorice root
- Detoxifying herbs
    - Burdock root
    - Milk thistle seed
    - Turmeric

CHAPTER SIX SUMMARY

In Chapter Six, we learned that pet allergies are complex and not uniform between animals. As such, each pet needs to be approached as a unique individual. Allergies can be reactionary to things that are ingested, inhaled, or you and your pet come into contact with.

For a number of possible reasons, the immune system overreacts to innocuous substances that pose no threat to your pet, but because of this exaggerated response, the immune system causes the symptoms commonly associated with pet allergies.

These symptoms include sneezing, scratching, reddened skin, weeping skin, hair loss, edema of skin, wheals and urticaria, and running nose.

The most successful approach to pet allergies is multi-pronged, starting with testing to determine what are the allergens, and then a concentrated program of avoidance or hyposensitization with micro-exposures to the allergens over a long period of time.

Mushrooms and probiotics, as well as healthy oils can be very healthy for the skin, creating a lusterful hair coat, and moist, healthy skin.

ANXIETY AND BEHAVIORAL PROBLEMS IN DOGS AND CATS

CAT ANXIETY

Cat Fights! Two Male Cats Literally Pissed Off with Each Other!

Jessica (not her real name) brought her new young, purebred ragdoll, male cat into my office for fighting with her other male cat and urinating in her house.

She was a cat lover and had five in her household when she added little "Johnny" to the mix. She bred these cats to make a little extra cash to help pay for their food and medical care. She did not have Johnny neutered, as she wanted him to breed her youngest female, Sasha. If their offspring was as she had hoped, she was going to keep him to replace her existing aging male stud cat, Sebastian.

Unfortunately, the introduction of Johnny didn't go over so well with Sebastian. He hissed and spit at poor little Johnny, and as a result, he cowered and hid whenever Sebastian came into the room.

They would fight occasionally by the food bowls or when Johnny wasn't submissive enough to Sebastian. Johnny grew older, larger, and stronger as he matured into an adult cat. One time, their fighting was so bad that Johnny (who lost) developed a catfight abscess that needed to be treated at my office. I lanced it and put Johnny on antibiotics to get over the bacterial infection that resulted from the puncture wounds of Sebastian's sharp claws.

At that time, Jessica and I discussed her "social" problem with these two males, and I suggested trying some CBD for both of them in hopes that its calming nature would allow them to get along better. I sent her home with a CBD:CBG product which has superior calming properties to CBD alone due to the additional CBG it contains. I also sent her home with some powdered lion's mane mushroom extract to blend in with their wet food for its calming properties. I advised her to give each cat two to four drops of this formula in their food, twice daily, along with ¼ teaspoon daily, also mixed in the food, of the lion's mane mushroom extract, and to call me in a couple weeks with a progress report.

Jessica called a couple weeks later to say that the CBD:CBG tincture had settled them down some, but the household wasn't perfectly calm all the time. I explained that the testosterone both cats had as a result of them not being neutered was driving this behavior problem, and if she had them neutered, which she was NOT considering since they were breeding males, the problem had a 70% chance of being solved based on historical statistics tracking male behavior before and after neutering.

I offered a few integrative approaches that didn't involve neutering her males to help with her problem. Cats are very territorial, and part of the issues happening between Sebastian and Johnny was "turf wars." Cats express their "ownership" of a territory by marking it with their scent. They have scent glands on the bottoms of their paws, around the chin and jowls, and on top of their head in front of their ears. If you thought that your cat was rubbing up against you just because it loves you, think again.

Your cat, I am sure, loves you, but he or she also "owns" you by rubbing up against you or scratching your furniture or carpet.

When they scratch, it's not to sharpen their claws as many believe, but to mark it with the scent glands on the pads of their paws. This tells other cats that they "own" you, much like they own territory in your house. There is probably no stronger scent than that of cat urine. So, urinating in the house is also a means of owning it by marking it with their scent.

You can use this scent marking to your advantage with the use of commercially available feline pheromones to mark your household with that generic feline scent. All cats "own" this scent, so if you mark your household with the pheromone, it will help to reduce this inter-cat conflict. It helps, but it is not always 100% effective, so using the pheromones in combination with a CBD type of formulation will work even better than using either technique alone.

Now, Jessica's problem is not easily solved since she needs to keep these cats intact for her breeding program. However, for most cat owners, neutering your male just before the time it reaches sexual maturity and begins the "bad" behavior of urine marking or inter-cat aggression, will solve this problem very well.

EXAMPLE OF DOG ANXIETY: OLLIE'S PTSD AND ANXIETY AS A RESCUE DOG

Ollie's story is a very personal one for me. I'm a "Labaholic," a serial Labrador retriever lover and keeper. In my life I've had three labs so far. Beanie was my first lab, a black lab from a hunting dog line. He came to us as a young puppy from a breeder. He was our "baby" and we mourned his loss at 11 years young to dilated cardiomyopathy (DCM). He went into cardiac arrest while having surgery to remove a tumor in his groin.

Trigger was my chocolate lab, who came to us after having been chained up outside for years, with only one eye, having lost the other to glaucoma. He lost his other eye playing ball with me a year later. He misjudged the distance of the ball I was throwing, having only that single eye. It hit his good eye, which then developed glaucoma, and he became totally blind. I was his seeing-eye person!

I learned a lot about living with a blind dog through Trigger, who also had bad knees and hips and was 90 pounds and pretty overweight. I hurt my back a few times lifting him into my pickup! He later developed lung cancer, and in spite of all the good care and supplements I gave him for that, he did finally cross that "rainbow bridge" to the next world. Trigger was the sweetest dog I'd ever had. He was so grateful to not be tied up and neglected anymore.

Both Trigger and Ollie were found through a Labrador retriever rescue group in Golden, Colorado. Safe Harbor Lab Rescue is an organization I highly recommend if you are looking for a sweet Labrador to come join your family. This group sends out a monthly newsletter, and one month I saw this incredibly cute light yellow, almost white, puppy that had just come up for adoption. I shared that photo with my family, and they all agreed that we had mourned the loss of Trigger long enough, and we were all ready to bring another lab into our lives!

Ollie was found as a stray three-month-old puppy in a small town south of Houston, Texas. He was rescued with a broken leg (femur) and dislocated hip. He had been an injured stray for so long that the broken bones had already healed. I can only imagine what terror he experienced with the pain and abandonment and having to forage for food and shelter from the elements with a broken leg bone.

The animal control officers put him in a "kill" shelter, which meant that there was no vet at the shelter to give him pain meds, and he was slated for execution in a week. But, lucky for him (and for me!), a good Samaritan visited the shelter and saw Ollie, who is a very sweet and friendly little guy. They called Safe Harbor Lab

Rescue to come and get him if they could. Safe Harbor sent a pilot who was a member of this rescue group down to pick Ollie up with his private plane. They also brought a few other labs that were in that kill shelter in Texas back to Golden, Colorado.

Safe Harbor took him to their vet orthopedic specialist, who did surgery on his hip to relieve his pain and then fostered him out to a family until he found his forever home. That was when I saw his cute little picture in the *Lab Gab* Newsletter from this rescue group.

Ollie fit in right away with my family. He was really happy that we had a second dog, an older female, Violet, and the two of them were inseparable. I started him on a homemade raw diet and adaptogens and other supplements to help strengthen him from his experience as a stray and from his post-surgical stress. The way he felt and was behaving was very understandable, given the awful situation from which he had just been rescued.

I hoped that with our family's love, and the "tincture of time," he would get over his fears and the obvious PTSD he was experiencing. Lab's tend be very "needy," always wanting be physically close to their primary human companion, which in Ollie's case, was me. Labs are always underfoot, and in the way, because they want so much to be near to their human.

Ollie loved it when I would lie down with him on his dog bed, but after about five minutes, he would start getting nervous, as he was aware of how physically close I was to him, and he would then get up and move away from me. He was very nervous about being too close to me at the same time that he needed to be close to me—quite a conflict for him.

When I was not in my bedroom, he would then get up onto my bed. But, if I was in the bed, he never would get up. When my wife was watching movies with me on the bed, he'd start whining and getting excited and jump up on the bed to be with us. I imagined that he was scared of me because I am a man and not scared of my wife because she is a woman. If one of the cats were on the counter eating some food that had been left out, I'd raise my voice to reprimand them, and Ollie would slink out of the room as though I was scolding him. Loud noises or shouting would really set him off.

This is PTSD; the loud voice must have triggered a "flashback," as it brought back to him the memory of the original trauma he had experienced. When first adopted, I had thought perhaps he had wandered off from the yard where he was a young puppy and had gotten hit by a car that had fractured his femur, and dislocated his hip on that same side.

He reacted to me, a male, and my loud voice. He was completely comfortable with the female members in my household. Even when other women would come visit our house, strangers to him, he would be very friendly to them, but not to the males who came to visit. For these reasons, I came to believe that maybe a man had yelled at him and had kicked him in his hind end. A kick like that from a big man could very easily cause that kind of injury to a small puppy's hip and leg. I've thought about talking to an animal communicator to get another perspective on his early history.

Watching Ollie lie on his doggie bed, his eyes always had this fearful/depressed look. When I'd call his name, he would cower a bit, like I was scolding him. These were consistent behaviors for poor little Ollie.

Once I saw that Ollie's PTSD was not going to go away on its own, I began a program of supplements and behavioral training in the hopes of freeing him up from the "prison" of his emotions.

Here's what I've been doing with Ollie to help him manage this fear and anxiety.

Anti-Anxiety Pharmaceuticals:
Prozac™ & Paxil™ Helped Ollie a Little Bit

As an integrative vet, I blend the best of conventional medicine with the best of alternative medicine. I'm not against the use of drugs, when appropriate and when there isn't a natural therapy that could work. I thought that Paxil™ (Paroxetine) might help Ollie. Paxil™ is a pharmaceutical drug, similar to Prozac™ (Fluoxetine), but with a strong anti-anxiety effect. It normally takes one to two months for the Paxil™ to have an observable anti-anxiety effect. I observed Ollie to be friendlier than usual, and to wag his tail more at about six weeks into the Paxil treatment. I was happy with these changes, but they were only minor changes, and he was still unhappy a lot.

I wanted to improve upon Ollie's fearful behavior, better than just the Paxil™ alone, so I tried a mushroom and CBD:CBG product I had recently designed and had manufactured for my website, The Well-Pet Dispensary.

CBD and CBG are found in all of my Doc Silver Naturals™ pet CBD products. Studies have shown that lower doses of cannabinoids work better for anxiety than higher doses, which work better for pain. Ollie weighed 60 pounds at that time, and I dosed him with 0.25 mg of CBD for each pound of body weight. That would mean giving him about 14 mg of the tincture twice daily, given with a little bit of fatty food, just before his meal. The Silver Bullet™ tincture contains 60 mg of CBD per milliliter of volume. 14 mg is about 0.25 mL. There are measurements on the dropper pipette to make it easier to draw up a precise amount.

The Relax Mushroom Chews™ are a formula I designed for the Real Mushrooms™ company. It contains two calming mushrooms, reishi and lion's mane, along with the calming amino acids, tryptophan, and theanine, the latter of which gives green tea its "zen," even with its caffeine content. I also included in the formula some calming herbs like valerian, catnip, lemon balm, and passion flower for an added calming effect. What's really cool is that when you give both of these two formulas together, the tinctures and the mushroom chews, they work even better than either one of them alone.

I found that Ollie didn't like it when I gave him the liquid tinctures. Even though it was in his food, it still made him suspicious of me and his food. So, for Ollie's sake, I designed a soft chew especially for him, a tasty treat with hard-to-resist savory flavors from salmon and pork.

I added CBD and CBG, but also added organic lion's mane and cordyceps mushroom extracts in substantial amounts. Ollie loves these! So now I can give him the supplements in these chews. He looks forward to them; he thinks they are just treats. (I don't tell him they are "functional" treats.)

I call these new tasty soft chews "SilverDog Chews™." I give him both the SilverDog Chews™ and the Mushroom Relax Chews™ at the same time. I gave both of these chews to him regularly, twice daily for six weeks.

After a week of giving Ollie these two products, he started to act less nervous and more willing to let me lie down with him for longer periods of time. After several months of giving him the two types of soft chews twice daily, I noticed that he started to wag his tail when I'd call his name. This was definitely a positive change. His eyes had a fearful and depressed look much less frequently. He also would just spontaneously get up on my bed when I was reading or watching TV.

I was hopeful because I knew that these new behaviors were a sign that he was becoming less anxious and less under the influence of his PTSD.

Behavioral Training, Training Aids, and Hands-On Therapies

When I first adopted Ollie, I spent a lot of time with a professional trainer. Training is essential for a healthy relationship with your dog. Training creates a language of communication between you and your pet, in addition to teaching your puppy to follow commands that can provide a safety net. For instance, if they run out into the street in front of a car, and you "command" them to "COME" or "STOP," hopefully that will keep them from being hit by that car and avoid suffering a huge injury or even death.

I tried a Thundershirt™ on Ollie, but in trying to get it onto him, he felt stressed by that. I've seen Thundershirts™ or equivalent products work pretty well with some dogs. In fact, our other dog, Violet, really took to wearing one, which lowered her anxiety considerably. But for Ollie, there was no way I could get one of those on him.

In order for Ollie to become more comfortable with physical contact, I started to use my hands to rub him in ways that would feel really good to him. I pet him as much as he would allow me and massaged him, especially his damaged leg and hip. Once he relaxed into the good feelings from my hands, he started to really love my massages, especially of his sore hips and back. As he became even more comfortable with my massages, I would make them last longer and longer. Pretty soon, when I would stop the massage, he'd look back up at me and, with his eyes, implore me to continue or go deeper!

Interestingly, after Ollie had been taking the SilverDog Chews and the Mushroom Relax Chews regularly for two weeks, he was much more receptive to my petting and massages. Before the chews, he would tolerate only five minutes of massage before he would get nervous and get up to leave. By the time he had six weeks getting these chews regularly, he would complain when I stopped! He loved it so much, and his fearfulness was so much better.

When I think of all the things I was doing for his anxiety and PTSD fears, this hands-on contact worked the best, made him feel loved, and less fearful. I know that this was a very important factor in his progress. I could not have gotten that physically close to him for that long of a period of time without the benefits of the cannabinoids and mushrooms!

ANXIETY AND BEHAVIORAL PROBLEMS EXPLAINED

Behavioral problems are one of the main reasons dogs and cats are relinquished to animal shelters and are the main reason that they are euthanized, as well. Behavioral problems can reflect fears, phobias, anxiety, or aggressiveness on the part of your pet.

You can recognize a behavioral problem in your pet when it displays unwanted responses—urinating, destructive behavior, or aggressiveness—to environmental stimuli, such as loud noises, encountering new persons or animals, new and unfamiliar environments that are not the familiar home environment, and separation from their primary person.

When a dog or cat experiences fear or anxiety, they exhibit specific body language that can tell you they are stressed. They may lay their ears back on their heads, their tail carriage may change from a happy wagging to a more stressed position, they may pant, or they may be reclusive, among other stress-related behaviors.

Unwanted dog behaviors include destructive behavior, inappropriate urination or dribbling of urine out of fear, or if left alone, they may be destructive to their environment.

Dogs who have "separation anxiety" when their pet parent leaves them alone at home, can destroy the home environment by clawing at the doors and walls and have even been known to jump through windows and run away in search of their pet parents; they are *soooo* freaked out by being left alone.

CONVENTIONAL APPROACHES TO ANXIETY

There is no **"magic pill"** for pet behavioral problems, but there are a few pharmaceutical drugs that are used to help manage this difficult-to-fix problem. Sometimes, these drugs, like clomipramine, gabapentin, or trazodone, have sedating activity and thus will slow down a pet expressing its anxious behavior by causing the pet to become "groggy" as a side effect to their anxiety-reducing effect.

Other drugs, like Prozac™ or Paxil™, may alter behavior by modifying the same neurotransmitters that CBD and other calming nutraceuticals affect. Although behavioral training is preferred to the use of drugs, sometimes our pets are so freaked out by circumstances or their PTSD from traumas that have occurred, that they need to have their racing minds slowed down enough that they are receptive to behavioral training.

Pharmaceutical drugs may help, but better yet, CBD and CBG can also help do that. Other natural supplement options to help "settle" a pet's behavior are the mushroom extracts of lion's mane (*Hericium erinaceous*) and reishi (*Ganoderma lucidum*).

Behavioral training or modification is the best and most lasting approach to changing your pet's unwanted behavior. It's not an easy thing to do, and you may need a specialist pet trainer or veterinary behaviorist to help you with the specific process, but it is worth the time, effort, and cost. When you adopt a pet, it is for the life of the pet, which may be 10-20 years. To have an unruly pet who hasn't been properly trained, or who has behavioral problems for a life span of 10-20 years, is a lot for people to manage and live with on a day-to-day basis for that much time.

DOG ISSUES

Maybe your dog is constantly barking, or your pet can't be left alone without it destroying your house's inner walls by scratching at them incessantly. Whatever the problem, finding a solution through training is the best way to go and provides a long-term solution, as well as making your pet easier to live with.

It is a good idea, when you adopt a new pet, either a puppy or an adult rescue dog, that you immediately begin training them to understand commands like "stop," "come," etc. Training establishes a language and understanding between you and your pet.

Training also can help keep your dog safe, if for instance, they get out into the street accidentally. If they are trained to come when you call, they may avoid being hit by a car by obeying your command.

Dogs want to know how to please you. They want to know what they need to do to get another treat, a pat on the head, a scratch behind the ears, go on a w-a-l-k, or receive a kind word of encouragement.

When it comes to training, the main principle is to use **positive reinforcement** versus negative reinforcement. With positive reinforcement, you reward good behavior at the moment that it happens.

With **unwanted behavior** (*let's not call it "**bad**" behavior, as that puts a negative emotional spin on it*), you first distract them from the behavior so they will stop. Sometimes just calling their name or slapping your hands together loudly works. Some folks take an empty can of pop, fill it with rocks, and then rattle that to get their pet's attention so that they stop that particular behavior.

You only reward the desired behavior at the moment that they are doing it.

Dogs have a short attention span, and if you are rewarding them 10 minutes later for their behavior, they won't associate the reward with the behavior. It is that association of desired behavior with immediate reward that trains them to continue to do that desired behavior.

Punishing unwanted behavior is not effective at all, and it can create fears in the dog of being struck or reprimanded in an angry way and may make them shy away from being touched out of fear of being hit.

Anger has no place in training pets.

CAT ISSUES

The most common behavioral issue with cats stems from their social interactions, especially between two males or in multiple-cat households. Cats are very territorial, and most household problems with cats result from what I call "turf wars."

In order to "own" a household, a cat uses its own scent to mark its territorial boundaries. They do this by scratching, especially near entryways, as a "signpost" of their ownership. This can be very destructive to expensive furniture or rugs and can be a very challenging behavior to change. Even more challenging is when they mark their territory by urinating or defecating in your house.

Even after you clean up the urine, it has such a persistent scent that it will attract repeat urination in that same spot by the same cat or may attract another cat in the household to urinate on top of it to mark it with their own scent in competition. (Fun!)

Cleaning up the mess with enzymatic cleaners helps a lot. Locating the mess before it dries up, if possible, also really helps. If the urine is left to dry, and especially if over time there are repeat urination episodes in that spot, you may have to pull the carpet and the carpet pad and use a strong odor killer on the subfloor to remove the scent.

I know of a number of cases where, even with all of those efforts, enough scent remained to attract more urination. Very frustrating, for sure! In these cases, the only solution is to remove the subfloor that had been soaked through with cat urine over a long period of time.

From a holistic, integrative, preventative perspective, it's best to try to avoid having the cats in your household getting started with their urine marking.

The most effective way to prevent this household soiling is to neuter both your male and female cats around six months of age before they reach sexual maturity. Once past puberty, their increased levels of reproductive hormones will increase this territorial behavior, and without those hormones, this behavior will be reduced or eliminated.

The use of generic feline pheromones in your household can also help all of the cats in the house feel like it is their scent that they are smelling, hence they "own" the territory of your house and have no need to scratch or urinate to scent-mark.

INTEGRATIVE/HOLISTIC APPROACHES
TO ANXIETY AND BEHAVIORAL PROBLEMS IN PETS

CBD

One of CBD's highest callings is to reduce anxiety and fear-based behaviors. It does this by activating two different membrane receptors at the same time, thus stimulating the production of two of the compounds (serotonin and anandamide) that are produced by the body upon activation of those receptors. Each of these neurotransmitters has a calming effect on the nervous system and emotions.

CBD does not sedate at the dosages that we normally use for anxiety, but it will have a sedative effect at higher doses if using full-spectrum CBD products due to their THC content. Products with higher levels of THC than are legal for hemp (>0.3%) will also cause this, as well as in products that have higher amounts of myrcene and/or linalool, which are sedating terpenes, found in THC-dominant cannabis dispensary products, in hops and mangos for myrcene, and lavender for linalool.

CBD is known to "sharpen the mind" at lower doses.

For anxiety and other behavioral issues addressed by CBD, I have found that lower doses seem to actually work better, in general, than higher doses for most animals.

I recommend that you start with the lower dose range, which can be effective for anxiety and even for mild pain, and then gradually increase that dose over time (wait two weeks to determine if the lower dose is not working as desired).

There are a few animals I've treated that needed a higher dose for behavioral problems. Still, it is best to start dosing low and slowly increase the dose over time to achieve the desired effect.

Giving the CBD at an initial lower dose for 7 to 10 days to develop a "steady state" of CBD blood levels is a good idea. Once you reach that steady state, and if the results are not what you desired, then I suggest trying a higher dose (double the dose as a starting point for the change).

A good starting dose for anxiety is around 0.1 mg CBD/pound of body weight twice daily, given with a small amount of food before each meal

It might be that after starting at that low a dose, you see absolutely no change after 10 days. That means that:

1. CBD won't work for your pet's behavior issue at all, or

2. You need to give it longer, for a full month at least, or

3. Your dog needs a higher dose to affect its behavior

I give a range here because the dosage needed for a given individual can vary. It might be that the lower end of this dosage range works fine for behavioral issues in some dogs, and it might be that the higher end of this dose works better for behavioral issues in other dogs. this is the unusual thing about CBD and other cannabinoids: individuals respond to a given dosage differently for the same condition. Because of this, we have to start with lower doses and then increase them gradually over time after establishing steady-state blood levels to find that "sweet spot" of *perfect dosing.*

"Steady-state" blood levels occur after giving the cannabinoids for 10-14 days when the CBD (or THC) saturates the tissues and the bloodstream to maintain a stable level of cannabinoids in the tissues for the dosage given.

CBG

Cannabigerol (CBG) is a minor cannabinoid. CBG has been found to have some of the more profound anxiolytic effects of all of the cannabinoids. When combined with CBD, its anti-anxiety effect is amplified. CBG helps with anxious behaviors by activating two different receptors other than the two receptors that are activated by CBD. This means there are four unique pathways that reduce anxiety with the use of these two cannabinoids. When they are combined with other compatible anti-anxiety supplements, like lion's mane, as detailed below, the calming nature of these three extracts, when taken together, is very effective![77]

In a 2008 study, it was determined that when you measure the comparative anti-inflammatory effect of CBD with CBG or with the acidic cannabinoids—THCA, CBGA, and CBDA—CBD was 10 times less effective than these other cannabinoids in relieving inflammation due to the COX2 enzyme inhibition. This is the same mechanism of action that CBG and the acidic cannabinoids have, as do NSAIDs such as carprofen, meloxicam, or even ibuprofen. (It's not safe to give your dog ibuprofen, by the way.)[78]

LION'S MANE MUSHROOM EXTRACTS

Although the effects of lion's mane mushrooms on dogs or cats haven't been experimentally studied yet, it is reported anecdotally by both pet owners and vets that anxious dogs will relax more when they are given lion's mane mushroom extracts.

A published study in adult humans found that after four weeks of receiving a daily dose of lion's mane mushroom, scores for anxiety were statistically lower than those individuals in this group receiving a placebo treatment.[79]

EXAMPLE OF A PROPRIETARY PRODUCT
FORMULATION FOR BEHAVIORAL ISSUES

A start-up company making dog supplements asked me to formulate an effective formulation for calming and relaxation in dogs. They wanted me to use broad-spectrum hemp extracts and wanted them in the soft chew format that is so tasty to dogs and easy to administer.

CBD has been found to be quite calming and good for anxiety. I knew that it acts by attaching and "activating" cell membrane receptors that increase serotonin. Serotonin is known as the calming neurotransmitter. The free-form amino acid l-tryptophan is the precursor in mammals for the formation of serotonin. By giving tryptophan, you can naturally increase serotonin levels, thus leading to a calmer demeanor.

This is why many people with insomnia will take tryptophan to help them sleep. CBD can do that, too. It doesn't sedate; it just settles the mind to facilitate sleep.

Choline, which is similar to B vitamins, and phosphatidylcholine, a phospholipid containing choline, both have an influence on healthy cell membrane function and are precursors to the important neurotransmitter, acetylcholine, which has a positive influence on memory, mood, muscle control, and other nervous system functions.

Finally, I added the herb chamomile to this blend for its calming actions, but also because chamomile is good for digestion. It is commonly used as a tea for children with tummy aches.

In order to determine how well my calming formulation worked, we conducted a survey of pet owners and published the results online.[80]

We conducted a 20-question survey on 98 dogs in Chicago, Denver, Minneapolis-St. Paul, and Seattle. Pet parents filled out the survey about their pet's behavior traits before and after four weeks of giving these pet-calming treats.

The answers were based on a scale of 1-10 and scored accordingly. Pre-Pet Chew and post-Pet Chew scores were compared statistically.

Results from this study indicate that the use of this proprietary formulation was statistically significant in improving the negative behavior scores, including for the following negative behaviors:

- Thunderphobia and fireworks fears

- Panic in car rides

- Nervousness when at the groomer or vet

- Separation anxiety

- Excessive barking at strangers or doorbell ringing

- Fear or aggression when meeting other dogs

ALTERNATIVE THERAPY CALMING DEVICES

Thundershirts™

Thundershirts™ and similar intentioned products use the same physical, emotional comfort and security that "swaddling" an infant in blankets provides them from being held tightly in the wrappings.

PEMF (Pulsed Electromagnetic Force) Loops

This advanced technology using electromagnetic waves of a certain frequency has multiple influences on the body to reduce pain and inflammation and has also been shown to influence and improve behavior.

Currently, there are multiple brands available on the internet for pet-based PEMF units. The Assisi Loop™ is the first PEMF branded for use in dogs, and this company funded a study to show the benefits of using the PEMF loop over the head of the animal (they actually have a holder for the loop that looks like the pet has a halo like a doggie or kitty angel!).

CALMING SUPPLEMENTS

A number of herbs and nutraceuticals have been found to reduce anxious behavior, soothe, and calm. Some of these I included in the calming formula example above and repeat here, but others, also quite good at calming, are added as well.

Tryptophan

This amino acid is a precursor in the formation of the ultra-calming neurotransmitter serotonin. Many people take it to allow them to calm down and thus fall asleep more easily. It is a safe and very effective calming agent.

Theanine

This amino acid is commonly found in green tea and has been found to have a number of applications, including down-regulating cancer cell growth and for calming. Theanine is what gives green tea its "Zen" effect and helps to keep the caffeine effect of green tea mellower.

German Chamomile (*Matricaria* recutita)

The flowers of this plant and its essential oils contain terpenes and flavonoids that have a calming effect on the nervous system.

Phosphatidylcholine and Choline Chloride

These two forms of choline provide a wide variety of benefits to the nervous system and the body as a whole. Choline is an important structural component of the cell membrane, and since all health depends on the ability of cells to communicate with each other using cell signal molecules that attach to membrane receptor proteins, the health of the cellular membrane is crucial to the health of the entire body.

Choline is a precursor in the formation of the neurotransmitter acetylcholine and has a positive influence on memory, mood, muscle control, and other nervous system functions.

Other Herbs to Consider to Add to Your Four-legged Friends Calming Protocol

- Valerian root
- Passion flower
- Hops
- Skullcap
- Catnip
- California poppy

DIET: "YOU ARE WHAT YOU EAT"

Diet can have an influence on behavior in several different ways.

High protein: studies have found that feeding a very high protein diet can contribute to aggressive behavior. In the same way, tryptophan has been shown to reduce aggressive behavior, so foods that are tryptophan-rich can be fed to take advantage of this amino acid's calming effect.

Ketogenic diet: This is a variation of what has become known as the "Atkin's Diet" in humans. It uses a very high-fat content, moderate protein amount, and very low carbohydrates to convert your pet's metabolism from a carbohydrate-digesting metabolism to a fat-digesting metabolism. It has been found to be helpful to reduce or eliminate seizures in epileptic patients and has also been found to benefit issues in dogs, such as anxiety, ADHD-like behavior, mood, and cognition.

Foods Rich in Tryptophan

- Milk
- Canned tuna fish and fish in general
- Turkey, chicken, poultry
- Oats
- Cheese
- Nuts and seeds
- Tofu, beans, and lentils
- Eggs
- Other meat: pork and beef

Processed Foods versus Minimally Processed Foods

Just as with our children, the feeding of fast foods and ultra-processed foods, especially those with added carbohydrates, sweeteners, and fried fats, can also make our pets hyper and emotionally less stable than on a wholesome, minimally processed diet.

Pet parents who feed a raw or home-prepared diet often remark that their pets seem "better behaved" on these wholesome foods.

LIFESTYLE MODIFICATIONS

The single most important thing you can do for your pet to ensure good behavioral health is to see that they are trained as soon as they join your household. Training creates a language of communication between you and your pet and, when properly done, provides positive reinforcement to show your pet how you want it to behave. Negative reinforcement, as mentioned earlier, creates an adversarial relationship between you and your pet and is much less effective in getting them to do what you are training them to listen to you.

CHAPTER SEVEN SUMMARY

Pet anxiety is a growing problem in our stress-ridden world. Training your pet so it will listen to you is an important step toward managing its anxiety. Certain foods and diets can help to reduce stress, as can certain herbs and mushrooms. Combining the use of these foods and calming herbs with behavioral training to instruct your pet what is expected of them is often associated with behavioral success.

ARTHRITIS
(AND OTHER PAINFUL CONDITIONS)

ARTHRITIS IN A DOG: CHESTER
"WHEN IT HURTS TO JUST GET UP AND WALK..."

My favorite breed of dog is the Labrador retriever, and I've had three in the last 30 years. I still have Ollie; he's aging, about 10 years old now. Labs are bred from the sturdy Newfoundland breed and are built for the cold environment of that Canadian maritime province. As a result, they have big "keel bone" sternums and deep chests with an extra layer of fat to break through the ice in pursuit of a downed gamebird. They also have thick, short tails to use as a paddle and webbed toes on all four paws. Labs are water dogs but will never turn down the opportunity to run and play with their human companion.

Many runners keep labs and run with them on their long-distance training routes, over and over again. As a veterinarian in Boulder, Colorado, a very health-conscious and athletics-conscious town, I would see many dogs of these marathon, triathlon, and Ironman athletes, and many of them were labs with bad arthritis that were coming in for acupuncture. Acupuncture for pets was rather new at that time, and many pet parents went out of their way to schedule with me due to the good results.

One particular athlete and her black lab, "Chester," sticks in my mind as being remarkable, and I want to share that experience here.

Mandy strode into my office looking like she had just come from the gym, and her dog lagged a bit behind her, limping on his left rear leg. I noticed he was also having trouble with his right front leg. (I thought it looked like his shoulder was affected based on how he walked.)

"Doc," she said, "I don't know what's wrong with Chester these days. He used to run with me every day when I was training, but now he can't last more than 20 minutes before he lags behind and then lies down. At home, I don't see him limp much at all, but once he starts running with me, he starts to limp really badly."

We took some X-rays of Chester's hips and knees, and they showed a lot of bony arthritis, technically called "osteoarthritis," the most common form of arthritis we all get with injury, age, and post-infection. Another form of arthritis is "rheumatoid arthritis," which is what we call an "autoimmune" disease. This means that the body is attacking itself through its immune system. Typically, rheumatoid arthritis attacks the joint cartilage. It's relatively rare in dogs and cats, as compared to osteoarthritis, which is commonly called just "arthritis."

I sat Mandy down with the X-rays and also some blood tests we had taken. I explained to her what I thought was wrong with Chester that made him limp like that. I also shared with her what steps she could take, from an integrative medicine standpoint, to help him feel better.

Chester had developed, over a long period of time, arthritic changes in his joints with a lot of bone being deposited. These bony deposits around the joint are what we call "bone spurs," and they are where the pain is the worst. Every time he would run with Mandy, the bone spurs would act up and be very painful. Mandy's training schedule and her desire to take Chester with her never gave him enough time to rest and heal.

CHESTER'S ARTHRITIS PLAN

- Two weeks of leash walking only for 30 minutes twice daily; then increase to 45 minutes for two weeks

- Veterinary acupuncture weekly for three weeks, then every other week for three times and once monthly after that

- Cold laser every other day at home with a rental laser unit

- tPEMF loop (e.g., Assisi Loop™) over the affected joint(s) 15 minutes twice per day, every other day, alternating days with the laser administration

- Fish oil EPA+DHA = 50 mg/pound once a day

- CBD: 0.5 mg/pound twice daily with food, as directed

- CBG: 0.25 mg/pound twice daily with food, as directed

- Starting a glucosamine/chondroitin type of formula twice daily

- MSM high dose daily

- Turmeric/Boswellia in an anti-inflammatory dosage

After coming in weekly with Chester for treatments described in the bulleted list above, he started to perk up. By the time we had completed the eight treatments over 12 weeks, he was back to his old self again.

I warned Mandy to take it easy with him from now on. His spirit is willing, but his body, due to age, and the wear and tear of time, was weak.

Mandy was pleased that Chester's mobility had improved, and he seemed less pained to her, but as a competitive athlete, she expressed frustration at having lost her running partner. Dogs and runners are a match made in heaven. What dog would ever turn down a chance to run and run and run? Especially with their beloved human. And what athlete wouldn't want to have as a running partner a four-legged friend who could not only keep up with them but who could stay ahead of them enough to keep their daily run competitive?

Unfortunately, the toll that repetitive activities, such as long-distance running, take on joints, affects many dogs (and their pet parents). Usually not while they are young and vibrantly healthy, but over time, over the years, as the dog ages, so do the joints.

We can reduce the damage of repetitive activities, like running, on joints by the use of "joint lubricants," like glucosamine and chondroitin products and fish oil. We can keep our four-legged running partner's weight down to a lean body mass so there is less damaging impact on the joints. But there is no way to escape the inevitable stress and strain that gravity, activity, and time take on your pet's joints.

As much as their human companion hates to hear it, the solution is to reduce the distance and/or the time and/or the terrain to reduce the forces that stress the joint and cause it to develop inflammation, and ultimately, bony arthritis and bone spurs.

UNDERSTANDING AND DETECTING ARTHRITIS IN YOUR PET

The term "arthritis" literally means "inflammation of the joint." It's a general term that covers several diseases of the joint.

"Osteoarthritis" is a "bony" arthritis and is often associated with the formation of bone spurs and calcium deposits around the joint that can cause significant pain, even when the individual is not moving. Commonly, osteoarthritis is caused by trauma, repetitive motion of a joint, or a genetic malformation of the joint that leads to excessive wear and tear and, eventually, the formation of bone spurs. This is the most common form of arthritis in dogs and horses.

"**Rheumatoid arthritis,**" if present for a long time, will cause the joints and the bones around them to become misshapen. Rheumatoid is an autoimmune disease in which the body reacts to itself, in this case, the cartilage that is found in the joint itself. It causes long-term high-level inflammation of the joint cartilage, and over time it causes the joint to become misshapen and painful to move. With rheumatoid, it is common to see the skin around the joint become swollen with fluid, which is the excessive joint fluid and inflammatory molecules that build up with the immune system's reaction to tissues in the joint capsule. This is where the body attacks itself, which is the essence of autoimmune diseases.

"**Juvenile arthritis**" is the early onset of arthritis in younger people and animals. Generally, arthritis occurs in older individuals, as it usually takes quite a bit of time to develop, but in some unfortunate individuals, it can be genetically programmed to occur while the individual is still young. In humans, juvenile, or childhood, arthritis is similar to rheumatoid arthritis as a defect of the immune system.

Hip or elbow dysplasia in dogs can create early arthritis secondary to malformations of the hip and/or elbow joints that were present at birth. Another word for these types of diseases present at birth is "congenital." This malformation is present at birth due to genetic tendencies and other complicating factors. Some breeds of dogs are more likely to have this problem than others. Complicating factors include excessive activity or excessive weight, as well as diet. Unfortunately, the pain from this genetic condition can be extremely painful and disabling to a dog and can be the reason they are euthanized.

What to Look For *(Self-diagnosis)*

Dogs who have arthritis will have certain symptoms that are characteristic of this disease. Some dogs can have these arthritic bony changes in their joints and do not show arthritic symptoms. On the other hand, some dogs will show strong arthritic symptoms with very little obvious pathology in the joint. Other dogs may not have any arthritic symptoms with the same amount of joint pathology as the pained dog. Symptoms of arthritis could be confused with sprains or strains, or problems with muscles, tendons, or ligaments, as well.

Arthritis is commonly diagnosed with a variety of approaches. Sometimes, you have to use two or three of these techniques to confirm the diagnosis.

- Physical exam with deep palpation over joints, tendons, and ligaments

- Orthopedic manipulation of that joint

- Measuring range of motion

- Gait analysis

- Imaging

There now are blood tests that measure certain inflammatory molecules associated with arthritis to help with the diagnosis. There is also the orthopedic exam and gait analysis which are very thorough and specialized physical exams. For the gait exam, your vet will watch your dog as they move at several different paces. These observations of your dog's movement, and the orthopedic the physical exam, will help your vet figure out what is wrong, and how to treat it. They may suggest imaging such as X-rays to better understand the condition of the bones and joints.

Vets who specialize in orthopedics commonly follow this detailed examination protocol.

Symptoms of Arthritis in Dogs

- <u>Limping, lameness, and/or pain</u>
    - If your dog is walking on three legs, limping on one or more legs, or holding a paw up on the pained limb
    - Reluctance to get up on the furniture (this could be a good thing ☺)
    - Reduced stamina on walks, wants to stop and rest more frequently
    - Unable to perform tasks that were easy to perform before, like going upstairs, getting into the car, chasing a ball, and less play behavior in general
    - May cry out in pain if the joint is touched, even lightly
- <u>A swollen joint that is warm to the touch</u>
- <u>Bony swelling</u> of a joint or a puffy joint capsule filled with fluid

CONVENTIONAL APPROACHES TO TREAT ARTHRITIS

Pain-Relieving Pharmaceuticals

NSAIDs, Non-Steroidal Anti-Inflammatory Drugs, such as **carprofen** or **meloxicam,** have been in use for many years; newer NSAIDs that have more potency and potentially less toxicity to the liver or kidneys, such as **Galliprant**™ and **Onsior**™, which is specifically for cats.

As mentioned previously, NSAIDs reduce inflammation by inhibiting an enzyme that causes, pain, the COX2 enzyme. Cannabinoids have been shown to also reduce the COX2 enzyme's ability to cause pain, and some of the cannabinoids were as effective as NSAIDS in this study.[81]

NSAIDs are very effective for acute pain, as with post-surgical discomfort, and are also used for chronic pain without as good long-term benefits for some critters. Over time, the body may develop a tolerance to a given NSAID, and switching to a different one may improve response.

NSAIDs can be toxic to the liver and/or kidneys in some patients. Safe use requires pre-NSAID blood tests and testing two weeks after starting the drug to ensure their safety to your pet.

Some NSAIDs can also cause bleeding and ulcers of the lining of the stomach and intestines, which can cause vomiting and if prolonged, anemia.

NSAIDs can be used together with CBD and other cannabinoids. NSAIDs work in part by inhibiting the breakdown of anandamide, in the same way that CBD elevates levels of anandamide. This is also true for how acetaminophen (Tylenol™) works.

Opioids, narcotic drugs, work very well; if it weren't for their addictive nature, they are almost the perfect drug. They are safe, in terms of liver and kidney function, and don't cause hemorrhage of the lining of the gut.

Opioids, like NSAIDs, work best for acute, short-term needs. Over time, the body develops tolerance to the pain-relieving properties of opioids, and higher doses are needed to be taken for the same effect. This fact, combined with their addictive nature and the potential for pet owner diversion and abuse of their pets' narcotics, make them a prescription that is only given when absolutely necessary to manage a pet's pain.

Tramadol is a pre-narcotic, and a recent study indicates that it doesn't work that well in dogs for pain. Tramadol needs to be given at much higher doses than have been recommended in the past, and it needs to be given four times daily. Even at the right dosage, I've never seen it work as well as an actual narcotic or NSAID.

Gabapentin is a drug is indicated for neuropathic pain and to treat epileptic seizures. It is also used in dogs for non-neuropathic pain, although it's not that effective for those kinds of pain, such as a dog might experience with osteoarthritis.

Gabapentin is also sedating, and when combined with other sedating or calming drugs or herbs, can cause increased sedation.

My concern about gabapentin is that it is not working for the pain as much as we would want, but due to its sedating nature, your dog may not be complaining as much. We might be under-medicating their pain.

Pain management is the first thing you want to do for your pet. Pets are very "stoic" about their pain. It can be hard to tell easily that your pet is actually experiencing pain. It's better to assume they are painful and to treat them. Often, once they are treated, their behavior will often change for the better when their pain is relieved.

In the wild, if an animal were in pain and lagging behind their pack, not uncommonly, they would be left behind to be killed and eaten by predators. For this reason, instinctually, animals tend to not show their pain until it is really bad.

For many conditions for which patients come to visit me, I assume they are painful and make sure I treat them appropriately.

Surgery

With some types of arthritis, surgical procedures can be curative, or at least highly palliative. The success of a surgery really depends on the individual detail of that orthopedic problem in that individual pet. I've listed a few procedures below that often can permanently eliminate or significantly reduce their pain.

- Joint replacement surgery for hips and elbows

- Femoral head ostectomy for hip dysplasia in smaller animals

- Pelvic osteotomy for hip dysplasia

- Ununited anconeal process surgery of the elbow

INTEGRATIVE/HOLISTIC APPROACHES

CANNABINOID THERAPIES:
CANNABIS, CBD, AND OTHER CANNABINOIDS

CBD

Since the legalization of CBD in 2018, with the passage of the Hemp Farming Bill[82], its use by pet owners has "gone viral!" New pet products abound, and, fortunately, a number of good studies have been conducted to scientifically support their effectiveness for a few conditions.

The one condition studied the most since CBD became available to pet parents is arthritis. Observations from these studies and from pet parents are that the more severe the arthritis, the less well CBD works, except when it is given in larger amounts or more frequently. For some dogs, no matter how high the dosage, they have more pain than CBD's power to manage it.

The dosages used in these studies of CBD and arthritis have been pretty uniform, at 1 mg of CBD/pound of body weight twice daily (2 mg/kg twice daily).

A study that used a proprietary blend of 50% CBD and 50% CBDA, used 0.50 mg of CBD and 0.50 mg of CBDA/pound of body weight twice daily. This gives a combined dosage equal to 1 mg of cannabinoid/pound of body weight, which was also effective in helping with mobility.[83]

CBDA is the raw, acidic, and unprocessed CBD, and there are indications that for some things like inflammation and pain, it may actually be more effective than CBD.

I've used a dosage two to four times lower for osteoarthritis and found great success, so I normally recommend starting arthritic dogs at a lower dose: 0.25 mg/pound (0.5 mg/kg) twice daily.

Some dogs may respond *almost amazingly* immediately after the first day or two. Most dogs take longer, sometimes as much as 14 days or more. If after 14-28 days, the response of your pet to the CBD product is not what you were looking for, then I recommend doubling the dose ("doubling down," so to speak).

Remember to give the cannabinoids in a small amount of food or to at least offer food after administering the oil into their oral cavity (mouth).

Giving with food has been shown to increase blood levels at least four times higher than giving it sublingual or fasting. Giving with food will hasten the effect of the CBD. It has also been found a soft chew with CBD improves absorption and blood levels as much as if given with food.

"Ratio" Cannabis Products for Arthritis

Ratio products contain a blend of major and minor cannabinoids in a specific ratio, like CBD:THC, CBD:CBDA, or CBD:CBG, for instance.

The use of the "ratio" is intended to increase the potency of a full or broad-spectrum extract, or even an isolate, by the addition of another potent cannabinoid that was not naturally occurring in that extract.

Ratio products can be made either by adding isolates together to create a specific ratio, or the "ratio" cannabinoids can be added to a full spectrum or broad-spectrum hemp extract, creating a specific ratio of the desired cannabinoids.

There is a natural synergy called "the entourage effect" that happens when the many naturally occurring compounds found in hemp work together to improve the medical effectiveness of the hemp.

Full-spectrum hemp products may naturally contain small amounts of THC (<0.3%). Broad-spectrum hemp products will not have any detectable THC. Both types of hemp, though, can contain, naturally occurring minor cannabinoids like CBG or CBC.

If the hemp is processed without heat, it may contain acidic cannabinoids, like CBDA and CBGA. Raw, full-spectrum hemp will also contain THCA, which is the acidic form of THC.

THCA is non-intoxicating because the acid group on the molecule prevents it from activating the brain in an intoxicating way.

Ratio products with a THC amount greater than those found in hemp can only be sourced from dispensaries in the U.S. and provincial stores in Canada. They are combinations of CBD and THC in a specific ratio of CBD:THC, and they may be intoxicating.

A ratio product utilizes the fact that CBD and THC have similar but different effects on arthritic pain, and using them together creates a synergistic benefit that neither of them alone can provide.

CBD can temper the intoxicating effects of THC by using a ratio product with a high-starting CBD:THC ratio, like full spectrum hemp with its 30:1 CBD:THC ratio.

THC, at higher doses than in hemp, but at generally lower non-psychotropic doses, is a great pain medication, especially when combined with CBD. CBD reduces pain through its anti-inflammatory effects, and THC reduces pain by interfering with the function of the nerves that carry pain signals to the brain, as well as having an anti-inflammatory effect, which is less than CBD's anti-inflammatory potency.

I have designed two ratio tinctures (Sterling Silver™ & The Silver Bullet™) using broad-spectrum hemp blended to create a 2:1 ratio between its CBD content and CBG. The feedback about the benefits of this blend from my clients has been very rewarding. Some of my clients had been on the broad-spectrum hemp I had designed six years prior for a well-known veterinary nutraceutical company. In addition to this blend's benefits with arthritic pain, I was also hearing very good results with calming and even with some types of seizures.

This is an example of how you can increase, even more, the good benefits of naturally occurring cannabis extracts, with the addition of individual cannabinoids and terpenes.

Terpenes are discussed earlier in this book. Briefly, though, terpenes are small hydrocarbon molecules, naturally occurring in cannabis and other plants, such as hops, fruits, and vegetables, as well as mushrooms.

They provide the aroma for these plants and foods and have very strong biological effects, as well. If you've ever felt calmed by lavender, that is due to the terpene linalool. Terpenes can also be added to a cannabis extract to further increase its potency.

MEDICINAL MUSHROOMS AND ARTHRITIS: ANTI-INFLAMMATORY AND IMMUNE SUPPORT

Medicinal mushrooms, like cannabis, also contain terpenes, although typically, they are the larger and less volatile terpenes, such as triterpenes, diterpenes, and sesterpenes. These terpenes all have potent anti-inflammatory activity that can help your dog's arthritis.

Mushrooms also contain a number of other compounds that are beneficial in supporting a healthy response to inflammation. Some of these compounds are phenols, others flavonoids, and still others are unique fungal secondary metabolites, all of which are potent anti-oxidant and anti-inflammatory agents. Ergothioneine is one example of this kind of molecule that has strong effects.

The anti-inflammatory potency of mushrooms for arthritis is not as strong as CBD and other cannabinoids from cannabis. When medicinal mushrooms are used on a daily basis at moderate to high levels, they can be a very effective antioxidants, anti-inflammatories and analgesics (pain-relieving).

Mushrooms can contribute to improving your pet's discomfort from arthritis when used as part of a larger program of supplements, CBD, acupuncture, physical therapy exercises, lifestyle changes, including weight loss, and the appropriate use of pharmaceuticals.

The studies we have for mushrooms and arthritis have primarily focused on immune-mediated arthritis, like rheumatoid arthritis, not on the more common form of osteoarthritis, or "bony arthritis." Given the beneficial effect that mushrooms have on the immune system, this is no surprise.[84]

However, a few mushrooms are known for their ability to help with the inflammation and pain of osteoarthritis (bony arthritis due to bad joints, trauma, wear and tear, and age. Maitake, cordyceps, chaga, shiitake, and reishi are some of the better known to help with mobility issues. This study cited shows how mushrooms can signal the same receptors that cannabis does to relieve pain.

JOINT SUPPLEMENTS

Pet supplements can help with the discomfort of arthritis in dogs, cats, and horses, just as human supplements can help us. A number of supplements claim to be good for arthritis, but not all of them have the studies to support that they actually work. There are quite a few supplements that claim to help with arthritis. The following are the supplements that I've found to work in my own patients.

Typically, the most successful approaches to joint health are what we call "multi-modal," meaning that it takes several types of therapeutics to work together to help reduce the chronic pain and weakness we see with arthritis. This is why joint supplements, for instance, are made up of multiple nutraceuticals. The best joint supplements contain several different categories of nutraceuticals to address the different aspects of chronic joint pain.

<u>Three categories of joint supplements:</u>

1. Support for the structure and function of the joint by providing nutrients that are used in the repair and maintenance of healthy joint cartilage and joint fluid.

Examples:

- Glucosamine sulfate or hydrochloride

- Chondroitin sulfate

- Undenatured Type II cartilage

- Green-lipped mussel meat

- Sea cucumber extract

- MSM (methylsulfonomethane)

2. Anti-inflammatory effect: some of the same supplements that support joint structure and function are also anti-inflammatory.

Examples:

- Fish oil in high doses of EPA+DHA for at least 12 weeks for an effect
  - 50-150 mg/pound/day of EPA+DHA
- MSM
- Chondroitin sulfate
- Undenatured Type II collagen
- Green-lipped mussel oil and mussel meat
- Avocado/soybean unsaponifiables (ASU)
- Medicinal mushrooms such as reishi and cordyceps

3. Pain-relieving herbs have anti-inflammatory properties, which, in part, help them to reduce pain. They also commonly contain other constituents that reduce pain through other mechanisms.

Examples:

- Cannabis
- Boswellia
- Turmeric
- Devil's claw
- Yucca root
- White willow bark

Combination Joint Supplements

Most joint supplements for pets contain combinations of ingredients from these three categories listed above. These combinations are synergistic, which means they work better *together* than *alone* to improve painful joints.

Commonly, we find included in these formulations "joint lubricants," like chondroitin sulfate, which is commonly paired with glucosamine. Natural sources for chondroitin sulfates and glucosamines include green lipped mussels, sea cucumbers, and undenatured type II cartilage, which is often derived from chicken sternal bones, which are mainly this type of cartilage. Undenatured type II collagen has also been found effective for rheumatoid arthritis in humans.

These structural components are then combined with an anti-inflammatory agent, like MSM, for instance. MSM has dual functions in reducing inflammation but also providing nutritional support in the form of sulfur for the joint cartilage support.

In the more advanced formulations, we will also find one or more of the pain-relieving herbs listed above. CBD can be present in these formulas, and if it isn't, it can easily be added to your dog's program by sourcing it separately and dosing it appropriately according to the guidelines I offer in this book.

Usually, these products do not produce immediate results. The anti-inflammatory and pain-relieving herbs can take effect sooner, but the joint lubricants may take a month or two to have an effect. So, be patient and give it time. Fish oil at high doses can take up to 12 weeks for its full anti-inflammatory effect. Medicinal mushrooms can help reduce inflammation in the body, but they need to be given daily for extended periods of time, just like fish oil and other functional foods.

DIET – FEEDING THE ARTHRITIC DOG

Although we don't normally associate food with arthritis, there are a few connections worth mentioning.

Being obese or overweight causes increased weight-bearing on the painful limb(s), which will make any arthritis present even worse and can accelerate the progression of the degradation of the joint much more rapidly. This weight stress on the joints, over time, will make it much more painful for your dog to bear weight.

One study found that dogs (Labradors in this study) who are fed a 25% calorie-restricted diet lived, on average, *two years longer* than the control group that did not have any calorie restriction. The dogs fed more calories developed arthritis earlier in life than the calorie-restricted group. This was a major contribution to their reduced lifespans. Additionally, other weight-related conditions were less frequent in the calorie-restricted group, thus their longer lifespans.[85]

I know how hard it is to take the weight off a pet. I have a Labrador that loves his food, and it's so hard to look in those brown eyes and say, "No more." But it is something worth doing. It is a demonstration of your love for your dog that you would restrict calories to extend their longevity. Weight loss alone can be better than drugs, surgery, and even CBD, as demonstrated by this Labrador lifetime study.

There are commercial diets out there to help with weight loss. Portion control is crucial to limiting calorie intake to achieve successful weight loss. Nutrient profiles of commercial foods and home-prepared diets that have shown success for weight loss in dogs include: high protein diets, ketogenic diets, and high fiber-high protein diets. These all have studies supporting their ability to take weight off a pet.

It is most important for you to be consistent with the diet and the amount being fed. Slowly and gradually increase your pet's exercise to expend more calories. Over time this will gently reduce your pet's weight. Reducing the calories going in and increasing the calories going out is an equation that results in weight loss.

Weight loss = ↑ exercise reduces calories + ↓ calories being fed

HIGH CARBOHYDRATE DIETS ARE PRO-INFLAMMATORY AND ADD "EMPTY" CALORIES.

It is known that high carbohydrate diets and diets that are highly processed will increase inflammation in the body, which can have an adverse effect on joint function, joint inflammation, and pain. The best diet to feed your dog that is also anti-inflammatory is one that is home-prepared and contains the antioxidant benefits of brightly colored fruits and vegetables.

This diet contains higher protein and healthy fats, as well. Healthy fats include the right ratio of omega-3 oils to omega-6 oils (1:3). This ratio has been found to be anti-inflammatory. Fats are an important part of daily nutrition for a dog. They are more calorie-dense than protein and carbohydrates, so they need to be given based on how many calories they provide to your pet's daily needs. Overall, this is a good diet for dogs with arthritis, as long as you also pay attention to portion control to keep a handle on calories consumed.

There is an advantage to feeding home-prepared meals or commercially available raw or cooked diets because, as compared to commercial dry kibble, which only has 10% moisture content, wholesome food that is not processed contains 70% moisture. This allows your dog to eat more volume without consuming more calories. This moist food has more volume and thus can be more filling.

EXERCISE AND ACTIVITY CONSIDERATIONS

Activity will help burn fat off, but the catch-22 is that if they are overweight, it can be painful to increase their activity.

Getting some weight off first is a good idea, and if you have a swimming pool, a swimming hole, or a river, having them swim is the best because it's not weight-bearing but gets them moving and burns that fat. Be very careful with exercise. A flare-up will set you back a month in your progress as your dog recovers from its painful response to that excessive activity.

I was in veterinary practice in Colorado Springs, near the Olympic Training Center, and later, in Boulder, Colorado. Both towns are known for their bicycling and world-class athletes. These "career" athletes would bring their pets to me that were limping.

I mentioned earlier in this chapter about athletes and their dogs. It bears repeating again here:

Athletes are so competitive and driven that some train even when in pain. Training like this is inappropriate. It adds pain on top of pain and impedes healing.

When an athlete goes to run with their dog, it's rare for the dog to turn them down for the run even if they are pained. Dogs are such devoted companions and also competitive athletes in their own right. Dogs will ignore their pain for the joy of running with their human friend. Dogs are so stoic and won't clearly express their pain unless it is downright severe or disabling.

In conversations with my client athletes, they would say, "He limps, but when I take him running, he runs right along and follows me all the way for 5-10 miles. It isn't until the next day that he comes up sore again."

They were unable to associate their dog's pain with their excessive activity because of their dog's eagerness to run with them even if they were limping.

My instructions to them were that they needed to rest their dog sufficiently so its pain would reduce enough for that injury to heal. Not uncommonly, they would respond with, "How about if I just run him for half the distance?" ☹

For many runners, even half the distance was quite a few miles, and they would run that daily in their training for their Ironman or triathlon.

Be aware that activities in your life that your dog shares with you may actually be contributing to its painful arthritis. If you think that's the case, try to reduce or eliminate those activities completely (at least temporarily) until your dog heals.

MANUAL THERAPIES AND PHYSICAL REHABILITATION

Veterinary medicine now has a specialty called "physical rehabilitation." It is the same as "physical therapy," but the American Physical Therapy Association has that term trademarked, so vets can't say they are "veterinary physical therapists." Veterinarians are providing the physical therapy themselves. We call them "rehab" or "rehabilitation" vets now. There has been so much interest by veterinarians in this medical therapy that there is now a specialty in veterinary medicine for rehabilitation and sports medicine.

SIDEBAR

Sometimes, to me, a veterinarian, it seems like veterinary medicine isn't taken seriously by the human medical profession. We can't even call our nurses, "nurses." Due to trademarking by the human nursing profession, veterinary nurses must be called "technicians." They really aren't "technicians." They are "nurses," highly trained, compassionate, and competent, and in many cases able to perform procedures that in the past, only vets would do.

Veterinary nurses are the caregivers in our profession; they give pet parents emotional support when their pets are doing poorly. They truly are "nurses," but we are not allowed to call them that without trademark infringement! (It's a funny world we live in, isn't it?)

Acupuncture

Highly recommended

Animals seem to love the feeling they get from having those thin acupuncture needles inserted in specific "points" on the body. I've practiced it on animals since 1993 and am always amazed at how well they do after a few treatments and usually how calm they are while they have all those needles in them!

Chiropractic

Recommended

Many people prefer chiropractic, which doesn't involve the insertion of needles, which makes some folks nervous.

Combining the two (chiropractic and acupuncture) in the same treatment can be even more effective.

Massage

Recommended

My lab, Ollie, loves his massages! He was injured as a rescue puppy when I adopted him at five months. He had a fractured femur and dislocated hip when they found him as a stray at three months of age! So, he doesn't have a hip joint on his left side, just a hip muscle holding it together. That hip muscle will get sore after he and I are out playing. He loves it when I give him a deep massage of that sore hip muscle. I am careful not to press too hard, as I can tell that hip hurts him.

Underwater Treadmill

Recommended

These are great; they allow the dog to move and exercise but without as much weight bearing due to the buoyancy of the water in the treadmill. It significantly helps their rehabilitation back to normal movement.

Physical Therapy Exercises

Recommended

Weaving around posts or using a fit ball to balance their legs are just a couple of the many exercises that rehabilitation veterinarians use in dogs to help them recover from injury, surgery, or a painful joint.

Cold Laser

Highly recommended

I was an early adopter of the cold laser when it first emerged as a viable therapy for pained joints and other conditions. I found that its use improved everything else I was doing, such as acupuncture, herbal therapies, pharmaceuticals, and recovery from surgery.

Emerging Technologies

tPEMF (targeted pulsed electromagnetic field)

Recommended

This "Star Trek" medical technology is FDA-approved for treating pain in humans and animals. It uses the generation of these electromagnetic waveforms to reduce pain and improve healing. It has also been shown to be effective in helping with behavioral problems when worn around the head.

One brand is the Assisi Loop™, which is a loop that you can place over a joint or a painful area and run it for 15 minutes twice daily. It takes about a week of these treatments for it to start giving substantial relief from pain. I know all about this loop, because I use it for my aging knees and arthritic hands and it works.

There are other brands than the Loop, and more on the way, so shop around for the best deal.

May the "Force" be with you!

Shockwave Therapy

The microtrauma from the shock wave generated with this device stimulates healing. The use of the shock waves can be associated with discomfort.

CHAPTER EIGHT SUMMARY

Arthritis is a common condition that affects dogs and cats. It results from a number of factors and each dog or cat's arthritis is unique to them, and may take a different set of treatments to help than another dog with arthritis.

The best way to address the multifactorial causes of pet arthritis is with a "multi-modal" approach, using a variety of therapies, such as weight loss, anti-inflammatory diets, acupuncture, NSAIDS, herbs, mushrooms, nutraceuticals like glucosamine or Adequan™ injections, soft-laser, massage, and/or physical therapy.

CANCER AND CANCER THERAPY SIDE EFFECTS

CANCER IN A DOG: THE SUDDEN COLLAPSE OF GROVER, A 10-YEAR-OLD MALE LABRADOR RETRIEVER.

I called Mary as a favor for the friend of a friend. She was very concerned about her dog, Grover. I wasn't seeing patients then. I had stopped my clinical practice of medicine and begun teaching what I've learned in the practice of integrative medicine to veterinarians and veterinary students. I had also been sharing my knowledge online through webinars with pet parents and veterinarians about the science that underlies the veterinary uses for medical cannabis and medicinal mushrooms.

This case sounded really interesting. I was feeling the loss of no longer being in practice. It was only a few years since I had sold my practice and had moved on in my career to providing education to vets and pet parents. I was already missing "seeing" patients. It was only a few years since I had left the practice of veterinary medicine behind me.

And I did owe these friends that favor. So...

When I got to speak with Mary, she told me that Grover, an otherwise healthy, 10-year-old black lab, who lived to chase the ball, had collapsed last week while playing fetch with her husband. They took him to the vet, who performed an ultrasound and diagnosed him with hemangiosarcoma of the spleen. This is a blood-filled tumor on the blood-filled spleen. The mass on the spleen, when it ruptures, releases large amounts of blood into the abdomen. This causes immediate weakness, or even fainting, which she had seen with Grover.

I advised Mary that we needed to remove the spleen so it wouldn't continue to cause this blood loss. I was also concerned that the spleen, bleeding into his abdomen, will "seed" more tumors throughout the abdomen. Removing the spleen is the standard that veterinarians have always followed in treating hemangiosarcoma.

Mary informed me that Larry, her husband, had said he didn't want Grover to undergo surgery. If we couldn't fix his problem using diet, herbs, and mushrooms, then he would have Grover humanely euthanized (put to sleep).

Mary wanted to see if there were any holistic or natural options for treating Grover's hemangiosarcoma. She was adamant about no surgery or further diagnostics. It wasn't so much a money thing as it was a philosophy of end-of-life care thing. Larry's mother previously had chemotherapy and radiation for her lung cancer. He observed firsthand how toxic these therapies were to his mom. He watched his mom slowly fade away. He wasn't going to put Grover through all that only for him to probably die in less than a year!

Take a look at the statistics in the table below for how long a dog can live once hemangiosarcoma has been diagnosed. You will see that it is not uncommon for most dogs who do not have their spleens removed, and have no other treatment, to only live a month or two at the best. This table combines data from a published review of 208 dogs that were splenectomized and either received chemotherapy or did not.[86] I've added my own clinical experiences and those of my holistic veterinary colleagues for dogs that are not splenectomized and received no other treatment or received alternative therapies like Grover. It also includes estimated survival times for dogs that were splenectomized and who received alternative therapies, such as the results of the turkey tail hemangiosarcoma study published in 2022.[87]

The further progressed the cancer is at the time of diagnosis, the shorter the potential survival time. This means that if the splenic tumor is found before it ruptures, the dog will have a much better chance to live a longer life, which can be further extended with the use of chemotherapy. If the spleen has already ruptured at the time of diagnosis, it may have already spread to lymph nodes or other organs, and those more progressed cases have much shorter survival times.

There are no statistics available for survival times of dogs with hemangiosarcoma who did not have their spleens removed, as they are usually euthanized at the time of diagnosis (or shortly after) if no surgery or treatment is desired by the pet parent.

Additionally, there are no statistics available for dogs who weren't splenectomized but who received alternative therapies. Grover was the first patient in 30 years that I've not splenectomized but treated aggressively with alternative therapies.

There is no data published for dogs who are splenectomized, which is what I strongly recommend, but who do not receive chemotherapy and instead receive aggressive alternative cancer therapies such as Grover received, although he didn't have his spleen removed.

I've put values in this table based on my own clinical experiences and the shared clinical experiences of my integrative veterinary colleagues for this category of patient treatment without chemotherapy. If your dog is undergoing chemotherapy, the outcome of the chemotherapy can be improved, at the same time as the side effects are reduced, with complementary alternative therapies, such as are detailed in this chapter.

Survival Times for Canine Hemangiosarcoma
Based on Treatment Protocol[88,89]

Hemangiosarcoma Treatment(s)	Average Survival Time (months)
Dogs without splenectomy	1-2 months
Dogs without splenectomy **with alternative therapies (Grover)**	8+ months
Dogs with splenectomy **and no other treatment**	1-4+ months
Dogs with splenectomy **with alternative therapies (mushrooms/cannabis/Chinese herbs)**	2-8+ months
Dogs with splenectomy **and chemotherapy of any type**	2-4 months

Once the spleen is removed and the blood loss stops, the biggest problem is that the cancer has spread throughout the abdominal cavity, secondary to the tumor bleeding into the abdomen and seeding new tumor growth on other internal organs, like the liver. As the cancer progresses the tumor cells can spread by means of metastasis to the right atrium of the heart and the lungs. These metastatic tumors may also bleed.

It's not common for a dog to live nearly a full year after being treated by removing the spleen and performing strong chemotherapy.

Statistically, as we can see from the table above, dogs who are diagnosed with hemangiosarcoma and are splenectomized have very short survival times unless something aggressive is done. However, even in the face of aggressive chemotherapy, dogs with this cancer diagnosis may not live longer than six to eight months at best. It is not a good diagnosis in that the treatment options are few, and even with treatment, survival times are usually a year or less.

A short time before I spoke with Mary, I had read a study using mushrooms and Chinese herbs to treat hemangiosarcoma in dogs and wanted to give it a try with Grover. I had also been helping people whose pets had cancer with suggestions for dosing cannabis (for people who live in states with adult-use cannabis legislation). If they ask me about using cannabis to treat their pet's cancer, I usually suggest ratio products they can source from their local dispensary.

The legal issues with cannabis are still a bit grey, but for THC, which is a DEA Schedule I controlled substance, cannabis is still illegal at the United States federal level. It is federally legal in Canada, and a number of other countries are starting to legalize full-spectrum cannabis for medicinal and adult use.

Due to the grey legal issue with cannabis, I don't suggest its use unless the pet parent brings it up. In that context, I feel I am helping to reduce any harm to my patient that might come if the pet parent decided to try THC on their own without any veterinary supervision. Most veterinarians will not address this issue for fear of legal reprisals or action against their veterinary practice license.

I agreed to help Grover, as long as they were realistic about the potentially poor outcome that was possible. I understood and respected their wishes to avoid any aggressive, invasive cancer therapy, including a splenectomy. Given the very poor survival data for splenic cancer in dogs, I felt their instructions for his care were reasonable.

When cancer strikes a household pet, the entire family is affected. Often, the pet is elderly, has been in the family for years, grew up with the children, and emotionally supported their family through the good times and the rough times. Now that their beloved pet has been diagnosed with cancer, the treatments are often expensive, not to mention potentially toxic. Cancer treatments may cause the pet to become ill before it can become well. If surgery is involved, it is often expensive and disfiguring and/or disabling, as with an amputation. And…

There is no guarantee of any better outcome with these treatments. ☹

As an integrative veterinarian, cancer was one of the most common problems I would see in practice. Often, I found that the pet's "parents" were coming to see me **after** all of their other options had been exhausted. Often, they would come in just before they were going to make that difficult decision to put their beloved four-legged family member to sleep.

I was the "treatment of last resort."

I loved working with these patients! These cases are so challenging, and getting good results was never easy. When you have even small successes in treating these end-stage patients, the rewards are so amazing, and the emotional joy of their family is so wonderful to behold!

"Above all, do no harm" is the principle that all doctors follow, including veterinarians. When it comes to cancer therapies, you always have to balance the cost to the body of the therapy versus its benefits. Ultimately, the question your treatment approach has to answer is, "Will using this therapy improve my pet's quality of life?"

Quality of life (QoL) is determined by the following questions:

1. Is their pain able to be adequately managed?

2. Do they have an appetite, or can they be encouraged to eat?

3. Can they control their urination and defecation?

4. Are they ambulatory—can they move? If they can't control their urine or stool *and* they can't move, those two occurring together means that the pet is lying in its own excrement, which is a significant loss of quality of life.

I use a scale developed by a friend and colleague of mine, Dr. Alice Villalobos, who was the first woman to become a veterinary oncologist. She is a pioneer in the field of cancer care for companion animals and is a founding member of the Veterinary Cancer Society. She received the Leo Bustad Companion Animal Veterinarian of the Year Award in 1999, which is one of the highest honors in the veterinary profession.

Alice established the first pet hospice service, which she calls "Pawspice™," and she also published the first quality-of-life scale for veterinary oncology patients, which she calls the "HHHHHHMM Scale."

With her permission, I have included this scale here to help those pet parents reading this handbook who are faced with this difficult decision. This scale can be found in her book *Canine and Feline Geriatric Oncology: Honoring the Human-Animal Bond*.[90]

Pawspice™ HHHHHHMM Scale
Quality of Life for Veterinary Oncology Patients Scale

H:	0-10	**HURT:** Adequate pain control, including breathing ability, is first and foremost on the scale. Is your pet's pain successfully managed? Is oxygen necessary?
H:	0-10	**HUNGER:** Is your pet eating enough? Does hand feeding help? Does your pet require a feeding tube?
H:	0-10	**HYDRATION:** Is your pet dehydrated? For pets not drinking enough, the use of subcutaneous fluids once or twice daily will supplement fluid intake.
H:	0-10	**HYGIENE:** Your pet should be kept brushed and cleaned, especially after urination or defecation. Avoid pressure sores, and keep all wounds clean.
H:	0-10	**HAPPINESS:** Does your pet express joy and interest? Is she responsive to things around her (family, toys, etc.?) Is your pet depressed, lonely, anxious, bored, or afraid? Can your pet's bed be close to the family activities and not be isolated?
M:	0-10	**MOBILITY:** Can your pet get up without assistance? Does your pet need human or mechanical help (for example, a cart)? Does she feel like going for a walk? Is she having seizures or stumbling? (Some pet parents feel euthanasia is preferable to amputation, yet an animal who has limited mobility but is still alert and responsive can have a good quality of life as long as his parents are committed to helping him.)
M:	0-10	**MORE GOOD DAYS THAN BAD:** When there are too many bad days in a row, quality of life is too compromised. When a healthy human-animal bond is no longer possible, you need to be aware that the end may be near. The decision needs to be made, as difficult as it is, if your pet is suffering. If your pet's death comes peacefully and painlessly, that is OK, although very, very sad. ☹

Over 5 is acceptable in each category.

A total of 35 points or greater is acceptable for a good Pawspice™.

BUT: If the total is less than 35 points, it is time to prepare yourself for helping your pet make the transition over the rainbow bridge to end her suffering, as the greatest act of love you can give her. It takes courage to make that decision—be guided by your love for your pet. (This was added by Doc Rob.)

My recommendations, after discussing this condition and the options available to Mary, were based on her desire to not do surgery or chemotherapy. She stated she would like to try some of the better-documented alternative cancer treatments that might give Grover adequate QoL for as long as possible

GROVER'S PLAN FOR HIS HEMANGIOSARCOMA

1. Homemade diet, ketogenic nutrient profile, with moderately high protein, low to no carbohydrates, high medium chain triglycerides (MCT), and fish oil content.

The concept of the ketogenic diet is to switch your pet's metabolism from deriving its calories from carbohydrates and protein to deriving its energy from the metabolism of fats, which produces these "ketone bodies."

It is well known that cancers feed off of carbohydrates, simple sugars, and to a lesser extent, protein. They do not feed off of fats, though. Ketone bodies arise from the metabolism of fats. So, by feeding mostly fats, you are still nourishing your pet but not feeding the cancer. Ketone bodies can be used by the body for energy instead of metabolizing carbohydrates and simple sugars, but cancer cells cannot use these ketones for their own energy and growth.

2. Fish or algal oil = dose by its DHA content: 30 mg/kg/day (15 mg/pound/day).

3. Cannabis specially designed for your pet's needs. Start with broad-spectrum CBD at 1 mg/pound twice daily with food and then add THC gradually. After a week on the CBD, start with 0.05 mg/pound twice daily of THC, and then escalate that dose at a rate that depends on Grover's tolerance of the higher THC doses.

If he is tolerating the additional THC OK, you can gradually increase the THC content and reduce the CBD content to achieve a 1:1 ratio product. This is given twice daily at a dose just below the dose that makes him "loopy."

4. Chinese herbs for hemangiosarcoma (HSA):

Yunnan Pai Yao (also spelled "Yunnan Bai Yao") is a Chinese herbal product that contains pseudoginseng and helps to stop bleeding. It has been noted by veterinarians recommending this herb that the HSA stays in remission for a longer period of time with the use of this patented Chinese herbal combination than if not used.

Yunnan Bai Yao also can reduce the amount of bleeding if the spleen is not removed and it ruptures again, or if removed, bleeding of the metastatic tumors that may be on the surface of the liver or intestines. This herb can help reduce the amount of bleeding by promoting blood clotting more quickly in a safe manner.

Xue Fu Zhu Yu Tan (XFZYT) is a classical traditional Chinese formula originally designed for congestive heart failure and "blood stagnation" in the chest (Traditional Chinese Medicine terminology), but with modification, which is made by adding two additional Chinese herbs (*E Zhu & San Leng*) to the classical formula, this custom blend has the potency to slow down or stop the HSA cancer cells.

Prolonged survival times in dogs have been observed by vets and pet parents who have used these two herbal formulas.

Alternate TCVM Herbal Formulas include **Stasis Breaker**™ **& Wei Qi Booster**™ by Jing Tang Herbal, formulated by Huisheng Xie, DVM, Ph.D., and available only through veterinarians.

5. Medicinal mushroom extracts, such as the **PSP and PSK extracts**, are not naturally occurring in the mushroom in amounts as high as in the mycelium that is grown in super-nutrient broth.

The use of the whole mushroom versus the isolated extract for cancer is an approach that has been used by humans with cancer for hundreds of years with good success. This use of mushrooms for cancer has primarily been in Asia and Eastern Europe, where the cultures historically have been engaged for thousands of years in mushroom foraging and consumption.

Medicinal mushroom fragments were found in the clothing of Otzie, the ice-age man found perfectly preserved in the ice where he had died millennia ago. It is believed he used these to treat himself for various medical problems.

There are multiple healing ingredients in a mushroom other than the PSP or PSK extracts. These individual extracts from the mycelium grown in liquid culture may be potent enough to help with some pet cancers. They demonstrated their ability to help with hemangiosarcoma, even if they aren't as effective as chemotherapy, they still can help. This is based on the results of the most recent 2022 study of I'mYunity™ and hemangiosarcoma.[91] The success of its use in other cancer types is unknown, as is the appropriate dosage to use for those other types of cancer but anecdotal reports from veterinarians and pet parents whose animals had other cancers than the hemangiosarcoma.

I believe that the whole mushroom contains many more active ingredients than the individual extracts of PSP or PSK, and, if dosed sufficiently high, should help as much as the PSP or PSK. We just don't have any studies with the whole mushrooms since these two extracts were patented.

I suggest for your pet with cancer to use the **whole turkey tail mushroom extract** at a high dose (four to five times the recommended starting dose). Other anti-cancer mushrooms such as reishi, chaga, maitake, and/or shiitake can be added to the turkey tail for increased potency. I recommend dosing by the beta-glucan content of the mushrooms based on your pet's weight.

My recommendation is to use the whole hot water extracted turkey tail mushroom and use my dosing recommendation of 5-15 mg of turkey tail beta-glucans per pound of your dog's body weight daily.

6. Turmeric extracts that have been modified to be more bioavailable, are also highly recommended for Grover's cancer.

I suggest **10 mg of curcuminoids per pound of body weight daily**, preferably with fatty foods, which can be given at the same time as the cannabis with the same food to enhance blood levels.

NOTE: Immune-enhancing and cytotoxic herbal remedies work synergistically together. I suggest utilizing as many therapies as you can afford and which your pet will accept as the best approach. Higher doses of these herbs, mushrooms, and nutraceuticals will usually have a better chance of slowing down the cancer growth than lower doses and have been found to be non-toxic to our pets at these higher dosages.

NOTE: Some pets may develop reactions to the supplements, like diarrhea, vomiting, or a loss of appetite. For this reason, even if the "clock is ticking" in terms of the progression of their cancer, it's important to go slowly. If you create an adverse side effect due to increasing the dosage too rapidly and causing side effects, you may be reluctant to "get back up on that horse again" and give your pet those supplements again.

HOW DID GROVER DO ON THIS PROGRAM?

Hemangiosarcoma is an aggressive and nearly always rapidly fatal disease. I try not to get my hopes up too much in terms of the success of my treatment protocols to increase survival times substantially. My goal is QoL (quality of life) and giving my patient the chance to overcome this nasty disease. It happens; I've seen it a few times in my many years working to treat this cancer. The standard treatment, first, is to surgically remove the diseased spleen. This prevents further blood loss. If the tumor has not yet ruptured, it can reduce the spread of the cancer to other organs in the abdomen.

What was different about this hemangiosarcoma case for me was that Grover's family was very definite that they didn't want any surgery for him, which meant no removal of the spleen.

His family's thinking was that if he wasn't going to live much longer with this disease, and if removing the spleen wouldn't contribute substantially to his survival time, then why subject him to this stress?

Each dog who suffers from a diagnosis of hemangiosarcoma has their own, individual response to the cancer. For some, the cancer takes over very quickly, and their survival time is quite short, maybe a month, maybe two months. But for others, even without chemotherapy or supplement intervention, survival can be many more months.

The published statistics for survival times, with or without removing the spleen, are fairly grim, as can be seen from the data I shared with you earlier in this chapter. The use of chemotherapy following the removal of the spleen may provide minimal rewards in terms of **substantial** median survival times, but for many pet parents, those few extra months are precious.

When Grover's family had such a strong negative reaction to any invasive cancer therapy, I have to admit that I could not deny the logic of their thinking. The survival statistics for hemangiosarcoma are very grim. I was very curious to see how he would do, over time, with the spleen NOT removed.

If I had insisted that Mary's family subject Grover to the risks and stressors of the surgery to remove the spleen, and they had reluctantly gone along with my advice and something bad had happened, that would be the memory that they would have of his final days, suffering unnecessarily because of my advice. I didn't want to see that happen for Mary, her family, or Grover and was hopeful we could help him with my treatment plan for his hemangiosarcoma.

With another type of aggressive cancer, bone cancer, known as "osteosarcoma," it has been observed that when you don't amputate the diseased leg with the incredibly painful tumor on it, the dog is less likely to develop metastatic tumors in the lungs. I wondered if this might be a similar situation with hemangiosarcoma and "amputating" the spleen.

Mary was one of my best clients. She did everything I recommended, exactly as I recommended it. She and I spoke weekly, and I helped her with whatever issues she was dealing with in terms of fixing the ketogenic diet and sourcing supplements, mushrooms, and Chinese herbs. Grover seemed to be thriving on the new diet and the mushrooms, cannabis, and Chinese herbal formulas.

One night, on a hot night early in July, Mary called me upset and frantic. Grover had been feeling great this week when both of her daughters had returned home for the Fourth of July holiday. They had played ball with Grover like they hadn't for years since he was younger and spryer. But that evening, Grover just lay around the house. He wasn't interested in eating or being part of the family's dinner time. His belly looked a little bloated, according to Mary. This was about a month into his anti-cancer program, and I was unsure how he was doing.

Mary wanted to know if it was time to put Grover to sleep. I replied, "Maybe, but he doesn't seem to be in pain or suffering right now, so let's give him 24-48 hours to recover, and if he doesn't bounce back, then the 'writing is on the wall,' and we will know it's time to say goodbye.

That next night, Mary called me to say he was like Lazarus, returned from the dead! He bounced back, literally, the next morning and was in the kitchen demanding to be fed. (Grover was a lab, so we excuse his "rude" food behavior—food is *existential* to a Labrador retriever!) I breathed a sigh of relief and told Mary to stay the course, continue with all of the supplements as before, but to avoid excessive activity. It's likely that the jostling of movement from chasing the ball was too much and it jostled his mass to start another bleed into his belly.

In the weeks that followed, Grover continued to thrive, but his improvement was punctuated by these down episodes, usually following some sort of increase in activity. It seemed like they were occurring every month or two. Although Mary tried to keep him less active, when he was feeling good, he had a lot of energy, which made it harder to keep him quiet, and which continued to cause problems for this tumor.

Grover broke all of my previous records for post-hemangio-sarcoma survival times. And he was the only patient I followed for this long who did not have their spleen removed. Finally, after eight months and a number of episodes of weakness happening about once monthly, he had another episode that he only partially recovered from. Mary had to travel out of the country. She was his primary support person for administering his supplements. She made sure he was fed his ketogenic diet. Most importantly, she was also his "emotional support person." I wondered before she left, if, with being away for 10 days, Grover might decline even more.

And he did decline.

I received a text from Mary that he had continued to decline in her absence. His family watched him become weaker and "out of it" with each passing day. Finally, even though Mary was returning home in a few days, they called the in-home euthanasia service to come and humanely and painlessly relieve his pain and suffering and help him "pass over."

Understandably, Mary was disappointed she couldn't be with Grover for his final day. But she understood that it wasn't kind to

Grover to keep him going just for her sake, and she was glad that he was able to be euthanized at home, surrounded by his entire family, and could feel their love tangibly.

There is a certain kind of relief when your pet dies if you've been involved in giving a lot of time and labor-intensive care to them during their time in hospice. Often, pet parents, when mentioning to me that they felt this relief, feel very guilty to have such a positive feeling like that associated with their pet's death.

I let pet parents know that it is completely normal to feel that relief when an intensive period of caregiving ends with the death of your beloved four-legged family member. Most people will feel guilt over their feelings of relief. It's a normal response to this situation, and there is no need for guilt.

WHY DID GROVER DO SO WELL SURVIVING WITH THIS AGGRESSIVELY TERMINAL CANCER DIAGNOSIS?

He did so well due to a combination of:

1. All of these treatments working together synergistically against this cancer's growth.

2. His own inner strength. There is a small percentage of dogs stricken with cancer who have such strong immune function that they can survive much longer than most dogs with the same cancer diagnosis.

3. The incredible amount of time, energy, and money spent by Mary and her family in the hospice care of Grover. Without their attention to the details and sacrificing their time and energy in order to provide him with 24/7 care, his successful journey with this nasty cancer would have ended up entirely differently.

I've had patients like this in the past, who defied the statistics to survive longer and better than most of my patients with the same cancer diagnosis. It has been tempting, in the past, to ascribe the success of these patients to the strength of the anti-cancer properties of the supplement program I am using.

Certainly, both the cancer supplements and the cancer diet are critical to clinical success with cancer. However, it's most likely that our success was more due to a combination of the supplements we gave, the patient's immune system's vigilance against the cancer, and the motivation and energy of their families in helping fulfill these complicated cancer programs that worked so well against their cancers.

SUPPLEMENTS THAT MADE A DIFFERENCE WITH GROVER'S CANCER

I suggested to Mary that we use a **high dose of the whole turkey tail mushroom** extract instead of the I'mYunity™ product. Mary had asked about using that patented product based on an article she had read in a popular pet magazine.

Based on the success of the first study of the PSP Coriolus in the I'mYunity™ in canine hemangiosarcoma, I was very hopeful we might have found a new tool to use to treat this nasty disease. But with the publication of the larger failed study, I knew that using the I'mYunity™ for Grover was out of the question. This recent clinical trial demonstrated objectively (statistically at least) that there was no clear clinical advantage for Grover to use this single-molecule pharmaceutical extract (PSP Coriolus) from the liquid mycelial culture of turkey tail, especially given we didn't remove his spleen.

Historically, the turkey tail mushroom has been used successfully for millennia by humans for cancer. The whole turkey tail mushroom is found growing wild and naturally in our forests and is distributed worldwide. The PSP extract of turkey tail was only discovered less than 50 years ago and contains a single fraction of the turkey tail mycelium.

For this reason, I wanted to give Grover the *whole* turkey tail mushroom extract at a very high dosage. I had hoped that this would have a better effect on his hemangiosarcoma than using the PSP Coriolus individual beta-glucan as found in the I'mYunity™ product. The whole turkey tail mushroom extract contains a wide multitude of bioactive anti-cancer molecules, whereas the PSP Coriolus is a single polysaccharopeptide molecule. There is potency in diversity, as can be seen here.

The other therapeutics: the **CBD:THC ratio product,** the **Chinese herbs,** and the **ketogenic diet** all contributed to the success of this approach to Grover's cancer.

Mary lived in one of the 22 states in the U.S. that allow adult-use cannabis. This meant that she could walk into a dispensary in her state, show her driver's license to verify that she was 21 years of age or older, and pick up the correct dispensary product containing CBD and THC in the proper ratios to give to Grover to try and slow down this nasty cancer.

THC and CBD have been found, for certain types of cancer, to be able to slow down or stop the growth of that cancer. There are many stories of people, and now pets, who used a THC and CBD combo product that substantially helped to stop the growth of their cancer, and in some cases, actually caused the cancer to go into remission and be undetectable!

This is important: We have found, while **THC and CBD are helpful to reduce the growth of cancer,** that, if you stop taking them, the cancer will come back. It comes back with a passion, growing faster than before, and not affected by CBD:THC the second time around. This is not unlike the drug resistance we see that cancers can develop with chemotherapy drugs.

Yunnan Pai Yao, the Chinese patent formula for bleeding, is particularly effective in stopping the bleeding into the abdomen, and, it will also slow down the growth of the hemangiosarcoma.

Chinese herbs for cancer: Wei Qi Booster™, Stasis Breaker™, and Modified Xue Fu Zhu Yu Tang, improved immune function and had anti-cancer herbs to slow down the cancer's growth.

It is well known that cancer cells utilize an inefficient way to generate cellular energy that doesn't use much oxygen. In fact, oxygen is toxic to cancer cells. This is one reason that medical ozone can be used to treat cancer, by exposing cancer cells to ozone, which is like "super-oxygen," or oxygen on steroids.

I explained all of this to Mary. She promised to follow my instructions and make a custom formula containing both THC and CBD for Grover. I suggested she start with a very low dose and then very slowly increase that dose over time. Of all the animals, including the human animal, dogs are extremely sensitive to the adverse neurological effects of THC. We have to start slowly with very low doses over several weeks to get a dog used to higher amounts of THC without adverse side effects.

Mary told me the next time we spoke, that Grover tolerated the THC well, with no obvious episodes of "loopiness" from the THC.

The story of Grover illustrates how well a dog can do who has a nasty cancer and who follows a healthy diet and supplement protocol designed to reduce and eliminate cancer cell growth. We may not have been able to extend this 10-year-old dog's life much, but this was a success story for Grover, who didn't suffer, and who actually thrived, able to share those eight months with his family in a very happy way

HOW DO YOU KNOW WHEN IT'S TIME?
(to say goodbye to your elderly and/or terminally ill pet)

Probably the single hardest thing I have to do as a veterinarian is to advise a client to euthanize their beloved pet and then to actually administer that lethal dose in a way that is kind and loving, with the owner present. I've developed a technique for this procedure to minimize any adverse reactions our patients may have to the medications we are administering.

I take as much time as the pet parent needs to be ready for the inevitable. I encourage the pet parent to put out pictures and items of significance to them and their pet—kind of like a little tribute. I like to have them talk about their critter and find out what made it such a special member of their family. I encourage them to express their emotions, whether tears or laughter, as a sign of their love for their pet.

Most of all, we just take our time and treat this procedure with the importance that it deserves. When a pet, especially a geriatric, has been with their family for a decade or more, it is never easy to say goodbye, even if the pet's condition is causing it intractable suffering.

When I first meet the pet parent and their critter for a cancer consult, I always ask what their goals are in seeing me. Of course, they usually say to help their dog live forever! But then we discuss reality and what could be the predicted outcome of their pet's illness based on historical statistics. I then discuss with them objective criteria they can use to help with the difficult decision to put to sleep or euthanize their furry friend.

I share with them the Pawspice™ Quality of Life survey[92] as a way for them to have an objective means to evaluate whether it is time, yet, for them to "say goodbye" to their beloved pet. I talk with them as much as they need, to help them reach that decision they can remember was based on the facts and not just on emotions or their reluctance to let their pet go, no matter how much it is suffering.

It is not an easy decision to put a pet to sleep (never an easy decision), and I never feel comfortable insisting the pet parent euthanize their animal. I've seen a few pets that died naturally. In fact, two of my cats passed that way without my needing to make that decision.

Most of the pets I see clinically, though, will be suffering at the end with intractable pain, lack of appetite, an inability to move, or are even semi-comatose. I try to lead the pet parent to make that decision on their own, with a little help from me, discussing what the pet must be experiencing and the possibility that it would get better (usually no possibility if we are at this point in the process), and I encourage them to think of their pet's needs, versus their own emotions regarding the loss of their pet. I tell them the greatest act of love they can express toward their pet is to find the courage to let them go.

I had an experience many years ago when I was in clinical practice at Boulder's Natural Animal in Boulder, the clinic I founded in 1994, with a pet parent whose cat I had been called in to euthanize. My associate had seen this pet; I never had. He was on vacation that week when they called to bring the cat in to put it to sleep. They said it had diabetes that wasn't under control and the cat was destroying the house with its urination everywhere.

I am always an advocate for my patients and am forthright in expressing to the pet parent, my client, what I think is in the best interest of their pet. When I walked into the exam room and introduced myself, I saw a beautiful little butterscotch tabby cat, meowing and rubbing up against his owner, who was feeding him treats. He walked over to me and rubbed his temples against my hand in friendship.

I discussed with his mom his diabetes and urination in their house. I do not like to euthanize animals that can be treated. If it wasn't responding to the insulin and other medication, I am always looking for ways to improve patient response. So, I said to his mom, "You know diabetes is a treatable condition." I said that because I didn't want to euthanize him, because he was so bright and alert and apparently hungry and happy. The owner said they just couldn't get the diabetes treatment to work for them and they couldn't tolerate the household soiling.

So, I assembled the euthanasia medications and catheters, and returned to the room. What I didn't realize was that his owner was feeling very guilty about this, and my saying that to her made her upset with the situation. As a result, she started to act angry with me. It turned into an uncomfortable experience, and I really had upset this owner to the extent that she started to post bad reviews of me everywhere she could.

In retrospect, I could have handled it differently, especially if I had known the pet parent or the patient beforehand, which I didn't. I learned one important lesson from this experience. This lesson is to not participate in the euthanasia if I am not comfortable doing that. They will be able to find another vet willing to euthanize their pet if I am reluctant to do so.

The loss of a beloved pet is a very sad event. I give pet parents the advice, after euthanizing their pet, to allow themselves as much time as they need to grieve. I always like to quote the saying, "The body weeps the tears the eyes do not shed." I tell them that grieving is their way of honoring their pet's life and their life together, the love they have shared, and the wonderful times they spent together. I recommend that they speak with their pastor or therapist or look to pet-loss support groups if they think that they may need some help to make it through the grieving process.

WHAT IS CANCER?
WHAT CAUSES IT?
HOW IS IT TREATED?

Cancer is defined as the uncontrolled growth of cells that have had their genetic code altered through mutation, so they never mature and die as normal cells do; they just keep multiplying and spreading. It is by means of this growth and this spread that cancer does its damage, which ultimately may take the patient's life. Even if not terminal, cancer can cause a lot of distress and loss of quality of life for your pet and your entire family.

Not all cancers are the same. Each cancer has properties unique to itself and its tissue of origin. Cancer cells arise from mutations of non-cancerous cells. These cells can come from any tissue, and the tissue type they come from defines the type of cancer, and that definition also, in part, determines the optimal treatment(s) for that cancer cell type if, in fact, there is a standard treatment available.

For instance, malignant cancers that are called "carcinomas" are derived from epithelial cell lines. This type of cancer has been found to be more sensitive to certain chemotherapy agents and less sensitive to others. When the epithelial cell lines are forming ducts or glands, they are called "adenocarcinomas." CBD and THC have been found to be more effective with carcinoma-type cancers than with other types of cancers, *in general.*

"Sarcomas" are cancers that are derived from mesenchymal tissue, which typically includes connective tissue, bone, cartilage, the circulatory system, and the lymphatic system. Sarcomas are *generally* not as sensitive to cannabinoids as are carcinomas or adenocarcinomas.

Malignant tumors are usually destructive of tissue and are often terminal unless treated. There are exceptions to this rule. Benign tumors don't generally spread but can occupy space that healthy tissue would normally occupy. This can cause serious problems, especially in an enclosed space, as with brain tumors inside the rigid shell of the skull.

When cancer occurs in an individual, it often is the result of a series of slow processes. These events occur over a considerable amount of time. Cancer cells arise, possibly through mutation, and a weak immune system allows those cancer cells to escape immune system vigilance and destruction. Without control by the immune system, these cancerous cells will thrive and multiply to become a tumor, and in doing so, will disrupt the health of the animal.

Most cancer cells that arise in the body are destroyed by an active and effective immune system. When cancer finally emerges, it means that your pet's immune system has not been working up to snuff for quite a while in order for cancer to be able to develop, or, that your pet has been exposed to powerful carcinogens or dangerous ionizing radiation.

CONVENTIONAL APPROACHES

Veterinary oncology is the science of diagnosing and treating cancer in veterinary species such as dogs, cats, and horses. It has become a specialty college in veterinary medicine only in the past ~35 years. It is a relatively new specialty that has been growing in number of members but also in terms of the new and emerging cancer therapies it embraces.

DIAGNOSTICS FOR CANCER

Until recently, cancer needed to be diagnosed by locating the tumor, staging its progression in the body by observing whether it is in one location (stage 1) or has spread to regional lymph nodes (stage 2), then onto the organs (stage 3), and finally to the lungs (stage 4). The final absolute diagnosis is from looking at the cells of the tumor to identify its exact origin.

In the past few years some newer, non-invasive tests have been developed to screen for cancer. These can be done through blood (or urine) tests. The value of these non-invasive tests is that they can tell you pretty accurately whether your pet has some form of cancer. The best defense against cancer, other than living clean, and taking immune modulating and antioxidant supplements, is early detection. If you can detect that cancer when it is just in its early stages as a single mass that hasn't spread even to the regional lymph node, you have a much better chance of treating and curing your pet of that cancer.

When the veterinary oncology specialty college was first formed, the only treatments we had for veterinary cancer patients were surgery or **chemotherapy**. The use of chemotherapy agents in pets was modeled after the use of chemotherapy in humans. These agents are toxic to cancer cells but are not selective in their toxicity, so they are also toxic to healthy cells. Chemotherapeutic agents are given at the "MTD," which is the "**maximum tolerated dosage.**" MTD dosing may make the patient ill, which is the experience of many people with cancer who have had chemotherapy.

Over the years that chemotherapy has been used in dogs, cats, and horses, veterinary oncologists have learned to adjust and lower the dosages originally derived from human patients to their four-legged patients. As a result, the side effects of chemotherapy for veterinary patients are usually not as toxic nor as sickening as the same chemotherapy given to people.

People who have had experience with chemotherapy themselves or who have observed it's sickening effects on family members or friends fear seeing similar symptoms of toxicity in their pets. As a result, some pet parents choose not to subject their pets to this potentially harsh but often successful treatment for veterinary cancer.

Folks who are worried about the harsh effects of chemotherapy will often come to my office looking for alternative therapies that work and that would not be as harsh as chemotherapy or which may reduce the difficult side-effects of chemotherapy.

Surgery as a treatment for cancer can be curative. "To cut is to cure" is the mantra of the surgeon, and in many cases, it can be true. When cutting out the cancer, it's important for the surgeon to take what we call "wide margins" around the tumor of an inch or more to remove ALL of the cancer cells so the tumor will not come back. Clean margins can be determined when the surgeon sends in the excised tumor for histopathology.

Histopathology is used to look microscopically at the tumor to diagnose it and to check around its edges to observe whether there are any tumor cells extending to the edge of the excised mass. If tumor cells are found at the margins of the excised mass, it means there are still some tumor cells that were left behind in your pet. These cells left behind can go on to grow back into another tumor if measures aren't taken. When that is the case, the conventional oncologist will follow up with radiation or chemotherapy depending on the circumstances specific to your pet.

A recent approach to chemotherapy for a given cancer is to take some living cancer cells from the tumor, grow them *in vitro* in tissue culture, and in petri dishes to test individual chemotherapy agents to find the agent or group of agents most toxic to the tumor in your pet.

Another recent advance uses those samples of the tumor removed from the patient to analyze its DNA to see which chemotherapy agents would be most effective.

There are some new and promising conventional cancer treatments that are just now coming into regular use. Cancer vaccines are being developed. There is one vaccine for malignant melanoma commercially available. Another vaccine that looks very promising is for osteosarcoma, a crippling and terminal form of bone cancer. Preliminary results look very promising for these vaccines. Vaccines may be a game-changer for this nasty and painful bone cancer.

Monoclonal antibody treatments are similar to vaccines in that they recruit the immune system to attack the cancer with antibodies and activated T cells. As we better understand the many biochemical steps involved in the creation and perpetuation of cancer, "small molecules" are being synthesized that can interfere with these biochemical processes and, in the process, slow down or stop cancer cell growth. These are advanced and emerging technologies that are looking very promising. The details of these new treatments are beyond the scope of this book.

I think that in the future, we will approach the treatment of cancer entirely differently than we now do. Some say our current approach to cut and poison the cancer is pretty heavy-handed. We can look forward to future treatments being very targeted to the biochemistry and genetics of the specific cancer that is growing in your pet.

We have also been learning from recent experiences since medical cannabis has been made legal in many states in the U.S. and throughout Canada. Many persons suffering from a variety of types of cancer have found that CBD and THC can help to stop or slow the growth and spread of their cancer.

Currently, there is quite a bit of active research underway to better understand the details of treating cancer with cannabinoids.

I think it's important if your pet has cancer to learn about all of your treatment options so you can make the best decision for your four-legged family member.

I suggest to my clients that they consult with an oncologist near them. I have some oncologists that I've worked with near me in the Denver area who are open to integrative medicine approaches in the treatment of cancer. I also have several board-certified veterinary oncologist colleagues who practice integrative oncology and who can do telehealth consults for pet parents who are not close to where they practice.

It must be a tough job to be an oncologist, always dealing with terminal diseases and outcomes for the patient that may not be so good. They must have compassion and thick skin at the same time to deal with the sorrow and loss that come with pet cancer. It takes a special person to be an oncologist, and in my opinion, they are pretty special folks!

IS CHEMOTHERAPY RIGHT FOR YOUR PET'S CANCER?

Many people have had "bad" experiences with pet cancer or with cancer in someone close to them. Having had these bad experiences, many people will outright reject the possibility of aggressive cancer therapies in their pets and prefer to treat their pets with alternative therapies alone. In my humble opinion, cancer can be such a difficult disease to treat that I think you should use every possible advantage to treat it with as many different approaches as you can for the most successful outcomes.

This is where the concept of "integrative medicine" comes in, blending the best treatments from conventional medicine that are specific and as least toxic as possible with the best treatments from published studies of alternative medicine therapeutics that are also as minimally toxic and as maximally effective as possible.

Natural and alternative therapies often are not as immediately effective as the strong chemotherapy or radiation therapy agents used to treat an aggressive cancer.

It's possible that your pet's cancer may be so aggressive and growing so rapidly that unless it is treated aggressively, your pet may die of the cancer before the natural therapies have a chance to make a difference. I've seen this again and again. It's so sad, but also so true.

Some studies in dogs have found a better way to treat them with chemotherapy. Instead of using the MTD (maximum tolerated dose), which may make an older, weaker patient sick, they give oral chemotherapy agents at lower doses daily instead of higher doses every three weeks, which has been the standard for MTD chemotherapy. This approach, which is better tolerated, with fewer adverse reactions and side effects, has been shown to slow down the cancer's growth and to reduce the growth of new blood vessels, also known as angiogenesis, which normally feeds the growth of the cancer.

This less toxic form of chemotherapy is called "metronomic chemotherapy." I want you to know about this approach, as it might be the right thing to do for your pet if their cancer diagnosis qualifies them.

Each patient is an individual, and each case needs to be treated individually in terms of whether chemo or radiation is used or not. This is a decision that is up to you but which should be made based on the facts and evidence about your pet's specific cancer and how it is progressing in their body.

Discussing whether chemotherapy in some form is right for your pet's cancer with your regular vet and with your oncologist can be helpful to your decision-making process. I also encourage you to speak with a veterinarian trained in integrative medicine about your approach to your pet's cancer diagnosis.

TURKEY TAIL STUDY OF HEMANGIOSARCOMA IN DOGS

In 2012, the University of Pennsylvania College of Veterinary Medicine published a landmark study of dogs who suffered from hemangiosarcoma. These dogs also had the standard of care: spleen removal (splenectomy). The owners did not want the dogs to undergo chemotherapy but were interested in trying a mushroom extract, the PSP Coriolus found in the I'mYunity™ product. The Chinese company that has a patent on this extract funded this study in the hopes of eventually gaining FDA approval for its use in humans. The PSP extract has been used extensively and successfully in China as a companion to chemotherapy and radiation in human cancer patients.

In this study, they divided these research-bred beagles into three groups of five dogs each. Not a very large sample for statistical significance. They gave each group a different dose of the patented PSP medicinal mushroom extract from the turkey tail mycelium grown in a liquid broth. Much to the surprise of the researchers in this study, the dogs who received the highest daily dose of the PSP extract lived even longer than dogs who had their spleens removed and had chemotherapy but did not get the mushroom extract.

When this study was published, it created quite a stir for pet parents who are faced with the awful reality of their dog being diagnosed with cancer. Pet parents, desperate to find something that will stop cancer from taking their dogs' lives earlier than they should die from natural causes, have been giving this mushroom extract to their dogs for other types of cancer than hemangiosarcoma.

A larger, follow-up clinical trial was finally published 10 years after that first study of the I'mYunity™ product. This study was conducted in 100 client-owned dogs who had naturally-occurring hemangiosarcoma.[93] This larger, placebo-controlled, randomized clinical trial did not find any *statistical* benefit to the use of this PSP turkey tail extract, either when used alone or when combined with chemotherapy, as compared to those dogs who received chemotherapy alone. All dogs were splenectomized, which is the minimum standard of care for this diagnosis. A total of 50 dogs received the PSP alone. At the same time, 25 dogs received chemotherapy and PSP, and 25 dogs received chemotherapy with a PSP placebo.

Several important facts about the treatment of hemangiosarcoma were learned from this study. This is in spite of the lack of statistical proof that PSP was equal to or superior to chemotherapy alone. Clinical outcomes for these dogs in this study were improved when the chemotherapy was combined with PSP, even though the results were not statistically significant. From this second study, we learned that male dogs fare better with hemangiosarcoma than female dogs.

Another thing learned from this second study, as alluded to in the previous paragraph, was that the amount of anemia at the time of diagnosis could predict how well the dog will do with treatment, either chemotherapy, PSP, or both. When the hematocrit (an estimate of anemia) is 30% or higher at presentation, the predicted outcome for that patient is significantly better than if your dog presented with a hematocrit of less than 30%. Normal hematocrit is usually around 45-50%.

The third important point this study made is one that can be helpful for those pet parents who do not want chemotherapy. For the dogs in the study that received only the PSP, the best median survival times were for male dogs with hematocrits that were 30% or higher.

These male dogs were also all in stage 1 of cancer progression, which means that the tumor hadn't ruptured or spread to regional lymph nodes (stage 2 cancer), or worse still, had spread to other internal organs like the liver (stage 3 cancer); or to the lungs (stage 4 cancer). These survival times can help you to make the right decision for your pet. I'm not against chemotherapy if it works and prolongs the length and quality of your pet's life. Not all dogs have serious problems with chemotherapy.

Veterinary oncologists have modified the chemotherapy protocols used for humans to be less toxic to dogs and cats and, therefore, this treatment will have fewer side effects. When you combine chemotherapy with the appropriate herbs and mushrooms you can significantly reduce the adverse effects of chemotherapy on the liver, bone marrow and nervous systems.

That is the value of an integrative approach to cancer, blending the best of both worlds into a safer and more effective treatment. Studies have shown that mushrooms can actually improve the outcomes from chemotherapy without causing anemia, or low white blood cell counts.

Mean Survival Times for Hemangiosarcoma Treatments
(Males; >30% hematocrit; stage 1 cancer)[94]

PSP alone	240 days
Chemotherapy alone	373 days
Chemotherapy with PSP	407 days

Turkey tail mushroom, dried or extracted with hot water, has been in use for millennia, successfully, for a number of different types of cancer in humans. Recently, with the discovery of PSP in the late 20th century, a number of papers describing its successful use in humans have been published. This 2022 veterinary publication was one of the first studies of this cancer in pets who are using turkey tail mushroom extracts.

As described in Chapter Four, where I discuss important medicinal mushrooms for pets, the I'mYunity™ PSP Coriolus extract comes from the turkey tail mycelium grown in a liquid nutrient broth and then pharmaceutically extracted from the mycelium to create the purified PSP extract. The PSP extract is thought to be more powerful than a simple beta-glucan because it is a combination of a beta-glucan with protein fragments attached to it. This makes it more potent as an immune system enhancing agent.

It is common knowledge that mushrooms often are helpful when used in a comprehensive program that strengthens a patient's immune system who has cancer. Mushrooms not only improve host immune system defenses against cancer, but they also can have a cytotoxic (killing) effect on the cancer cells.

My recommendations for Grover were very specific to his diagnosis. Other dogs with similar or different cancer diagnoses might need a different protocol, so I suggest you find a holistic vet or integrative oncologist who can help you figure out exactly what your pet with cancer needs, which will give your pet the best possible outcome for its cancer diagnosis.

INTEGRATIVE/HOLISTIC APPROACHES FOR CANCER

USING CANNABIS TO TREAT CANCER

Cannabis has a long history of successful use to treat cancer and to treat cancer side effects and cancer therapy side effects. Its use for animals is fairly recent, though, with the legalization of medical marijuana and pet CBD.

Many of the compounds found in the cannabis plant have anti-cancer effects. In the whole plant extract, these different constituents work together synergistically to slow down or stop cancer cell multiplication and spread. Both CBD and THC have anti-cancer effects, as well as some of the terpenes and flavonoids found in the plant.

Below, I discuss how to prepare a ratio product to use for your pet with cancer, and I've also discussed in great detail how to safely introduce THC to your pet so as to avoid adverse reactions.

Ratio products are the best bet to try and reduce cancer growth and spread by using the synergy between THC and CBD. There is still so much work needed to be done for us to know more precisely what ratio to use and what the optimal dosages of THC and CBD are to improve outcomes and reduce side effects.

This is why I recommend a staged approach to treating cancer with cannabis, starting with CBD, the "safer" ingredient in cannabis, and gradually escalating the dose over several weeks to months and observing for a response.

In several dogs with oral or lingual (tongue) tumors, we found that a low dose of CBD of 0.25 mg/pound twice daily was able to cause the growth on the tongue or in the oral cavity to go into remission after six weeks. We were able to see the beginnings of a positive effect from the CBD after only three weeks in these patients.

I suggest increasing the dose of CBD when used in the absence of THC to as high as 1 mg/pound twice daily. If, after using that dose for a month, you are still not seeing a reduction in cancer growth, then it's time to think about adding on THC.

Not everyone will be comfortable using THC for their pets. It can be associated with some side effects if not introduced slowly enough over time. Not everyone lives in a state where they can legally access products with THC that also have precise analyses of the THC content for accurate dosing of your pet. The mid-term election of 2022 increased the number of states with legal adult use of cannabis to 23 states and the District of Columbia. That's nearly half our country that now provides access to products containing substantial amounts of THC.

If you are in a "legal" state, or if you are in Canada, then trying THC when you've exhausted other options may be your only hope in slowing down the cancer in your pet.

I must caution you that not all cancers will respond to cannabis, but in the absence of other credible treatments for your pet's cancer, I think it's a good idea to try the staged approach I am suggesting. Start with CBD alone in a broad or full spectrum product, and then, if getting an inadequate response after three to six weeks, try adding a ratio product with THC in it, and, of course, introduce it gradually.

CBD

We have already learned quite a bit about how cannabinoids like CBD and THC can be used to reduce the growth and spread of cancer in humans. Information about using these cannabinoids in pets is something I've personally been working on since the passage of the first farm bill in 2014.

Although there are only a few controlled clinical studies in humans and none in pets about the use of cannabis for cancer, there are quite a few anecdotal reports and case reports.

I have personally seen several patients with different types of cancer go into remission when they were given a fairly low dose of broad-spectrum CBD (0.25 mg/pound twice daily). Other patients didn't respond as well to just CBD without adding substantial amounts of THC, more than are found in full-spectrum products. For these patients, a "ratio" product of CBD:THC has the potential to work better against cancer than a full-spectrum hemp product due to the synergy between the effects of CBD and higher levels of THC than are found in hemp.

THC use in dogs, when it is not introduced very gradually over a week or two, can cause significant neurological and cardiovascular side effects that can be prevented using a slow and gradual introduction of THC, which develops tolerance in your dog to its adverse neurological side effects.

Research has found that not only can cannabis stop the growth of cancer cells, but it also can prevent cancer from spreading to other sites within the body. This spread of cancer from the primary site is called "**metastasis,**" and it involves a number of steps, including:

1. Formation of new blood vessels from the tumor to support its growth

2. Movement of the cancer cell from the primary tumor into circulation

3. Invasion of the migrating tumor cell into the distant tissue site where it

4. Implants and starts a new growth of a metastatic tumor

Cannabis has been found to prevent each of these steps in the growth and spread of the cancer. We are still learning exactly how much cannabis extract is needed to effectively treat a specific cancer type.

Until we learn these treatment details from future research studies, we will need to use an empirical trial-and-error approach to find the right doses and which parts of the cannabis extract work the best for that specific tumor type.

In addition to the benefit that cannabis extracts can have in reducing the growth and spread of the cancer, cannabis has also been found to be helpful with the side effects of cancer therapy and from the cancer itself. Both THC and CBD can reduce nausea and vomiting and can improve your pet's appetite. Cannabis also can help with the pain associated with the cancer and cancer therapies.

A recent *in vitro* study looked at the effect of CBD, CBDA, and THC on the growth of several common tumor types affecting dogs.[95] They found that CBDA had much less effect on cancer cells than CBD and THC. They also determined that the amount of CBD needed in the cancer cell tissue culture to inhibit cancer cell growth would correspond to a very high oral dose of CBD if given to a dog. *In vitro* studies are done in a test tube or petri dish, whereas *in vivo* studies are done in the living animal or person.

Higher doses of CBD could cause diarrhea and other side effects. For this reason, I recommend trying higher doses of CBD alone only when lower doses aren't working well enough. Start first at a lower dose and increase only if more potency is needed.

Adding THC to the CBD is a good strategy when the high dose of CBD isn't working well enough. Ratio products have been found more effective when used to address cancer and cancer side effects than high doses of CBD due to the increased potency with higher levels of THC.

Paying a visit to your dispensary can help you source the proper ratio product for your pet with cancer.

COMMERCIALLY AVAILABLE
RATIO PRODUCTS WITH CBD:THC

Ratio products contain a specific ratio of CBD to THC. Hemp, being a 30:1 CBD:THC ratio, is the only ratio product that can be sourced online or from retail stores, legally.

Many dispensaries are now carrying ratio products, but you should call around first to see who has the precise product you need. We want to start with a lower CBD:THC ratio, such as a 20:1 or the stronger 10:1, to get your pet used to lower doses of the THC. Once tolerance is achieved, we "switch up" to a higher THC ratio product, like a 1:4 or a 1:1. This last *even* ratio product is the most commonly used ratio product for cancer patients, as well as for other serious medical problems, like severe pain, inflammation, and immune-mediated diseases.

It's possible that the dispensaries in your state don't carry the exact ratio product in their inventory that you need for your pet's cancer. In this book, I give you a guide to exactly how you can make a ratio product using a distillate with high THC you can get from your local dispensary and a broad-spectrum hemp product.

We start dosing ratio products with a high-CBD to low-THC ratio and dose according to the THC content. If your pet, like most, has not been exposed to THC, it can be excessively sensitive to the adverse effects of THC. It needs to develop tolerance to the adverse effects of THC by the introduction at first of very small doses of THC.

I recommend a dose of 0.05 mg/pound twice daily of THC and a dose of 0.5 mg/pound twice daily of CBD. This creates a ratio that is a good starting place to introduce THC to your pet for their cancer.

DIY RATIO PRODUCTS – WHEN RATIO PRODUCTS ARE NOT AVAILABLE LOCALLY

You may find that where you live there are no dispensaries close, they do not carry any ratio products, or they do not have the desired ratios you need for your four-legged friend. If you can find syringes of THC distillate at your dispensaries, which is a very common dispensary product, then you have the tools you need to make your own dispensary product.

Here's how you do that STEP by STEP:

Step One: Source a THC distillate that has been analyzed for THC content.

If it is 85% for instance, it will contain 850 mg of THC in the 1.0 mL or 1 gram contained in the syringe. The syringe you get may have a different concentration, so plug that in so you know how many milligrams of THC/mL you have to work with.

In order for this to work, the product you get at the dispensary needs to have an analysis of its THC content from a state-approved lab.

Keep that analysis on hand; we will need it soon.

Step Two: Source a 30 mL (1 fluid ounce) **"Boston Round" amber dropper bottle.** They can be found online and possibly locally in a specialty store near you that carries that stuff. I often will find mine at the hardware store here in Boulder or at an herb shop located in the downtown area that reminds me of what Boulder used to be like way back when in the olden days.

Step Three: Decide on a "carrier oil" to use. I recommend medium chain triglyceride oil (MCT), which is derived from coconut or palm oils and has a bland-sweet vanilla taste that seems to be acceptable to most dogs, cats, and horses I've worked with.

Other oils, even some off your kitchen shelves, like **olive oil or safflower oil,** have been used with great success. The main contribution that carrier oil selection has is for palatability. The few studies we have that have looked at carrier oil and absorption don't show any significant benefit of one type of oil over another in terms of bioavailability or absorption when you compare that to the improved effect on absorption of giving any cannabis infused oil with food.

Step Four: Measure 29 mL of the carrier oil of your choice and pour it into that amber glass Boston Round. Put the dropper top back on that filled bottle and tighten it.

Put that Boston Round bottle into a double boiler using a water level that won't cause the dropper bottle to fall over.

Warm it up for about 10 minutes to just below the boiling point of water.

Place that syringe with its cap tightly on into the very warm water of the double boiler for about two to three minutes, which will make it easier to squeeze out the distillate into the warmed-up Boston dropper bottle with the carrier oil in it.

Step Five: Syringe all of the THC distillate into the warmed and filled Boston Round.

Shake well to mix the distillate completely with the carrier oil.

You now have a diluted THC tincture that contains X = number of milligrams of THC in the distillate syringe divided by 30 mL = THC milligrams/mL.

This diluted THC can be used to create your own custom ratio product if you source a zero THC, broad-spectrum CBD tincture with a published analysis of its concentration of CBD per milliliter.

See the section below titled, "How to Create the Exact Ratio Your Pet Needs."

How to Calculate How Much THC/mL
is contained in your custom THC tincture:

%THC = X

X = # milligrams THC in 1 mL

X divided by 30 = # milligrams THC per mL = Y

Y divided by 30 = # milligrams THC per drop = Z

Dosing by the drop is an approximate but convenient measurement; however, it is more accurate to measure using volume = mL.

This calculation assumes approximately 30 drops per mL. I've seen it range from 20-40 drops per mL.

Starting dose to establish tolerance =
0.05 mg/pound twice daily of THC

Once tolerance has been established, you can gradually, over time, increase the amount of THC you give your pet for better effects without causing adverse neurological side effects, although your pet may still get sedated from the THC dose.

1. **Sample Calculation, assuming 85% THC distillate**

2. You now have a safe dilution of the THC content of the distillate in the carrier oil. So, if there were 850 mg of THC in that 1 mL you diluted into the carrier oil, there are now **850 mg/30 mL = 28.3 mg/mL** in your tincture.

3. If you **divide the 28.3 by 30 drops per mL**, you will have a little less than 1 mg of THC per drop, which should

make it easy to start with a very low, safe dose. I would round that number up to be on the safe side. That will have you dosing a little lower than the calculated dose, which is a little safer when getting started.

4. **Give that low dose for one or two weeks** to create **tolerance** in your pet to the adverse reactions from THC, so you can then, over time, administer higher dosages of THC to help treat more serious, deep-seated, and possibly terminal conditions.

HOW TO CREATE THE EXACT RATIO PRODUCT YOUR PET NEEDS

Once you have a solution of THC whose concentration you trust, either from a reliable dispensary or made by yourself, you then need to **source a broad-spectrum CBD-dominant tincture (hemp cultivar)** and combine it with your **DIY THC tincture** to create the precise ratio.

My suggestion is to keep each bottle of THC or CBD unaltered and create a ratio product specific to your pet's needs by **giving separately** each amount of **broad-spectrum CBD tincture and DIY THC tincture** to your pet.

The 1:1 ratio product is commonly recommended for cancer, severe pain, and treatment-resistant digestive diseases, such as inflammatory bowel disease.

The 1:1 is an equal ratio product, so you simply use equal concentrations of CBD and THC for this ratio.

With this DIY approach, you can gradually transition without a huge expense on your part by not needing to purchase multiple bottles from the dispensary to work your way up from a lower potency to a higher potency THC ratio product.

MEDICINAL MUSHROOMS FOR CANCER

One of the highest callings that medicinal mushrooms have had both traditionally and historically has been their use for people diagnosed with cancer. Mushrooms contain a number of powerful bioactive anti-cancer constituents.

Beta-glucans are long branching chains of simple sugars like glucose that serve as structural components of the fungal cell wall. In nature, beta-glucans can occur as triple helixes, a similar structure as found in DNA. Beta-glucans will activate immune cells to be more vigilant against cancer cells and microbial pathogens. Mushrooms contain many different types of beta-glucans, which increase their ability to better help the immune system deal with the cancer growth. The mushroom associated the most with treating cancer historically is the turkey tail mushroom. It contains over 17 different types of beta-glucan molecules and has the highest percentage of beta-glucans of any medicinal mushroom.

Terpenes are anti-cancer molecules, some of which can kill cancer cells. They play a large role in mushroom anti-cancer activity and also have an effect on the nervous and digestive systems. Turkey tail mushroom is known for its high numbers of these terpene molecules. In mushrooms, most terpenes are larger molecules and less aromatic than the smaller-sized terpenes, such as are found in cannabis, like limonene, but these larger terpenes are often bitter tasting.

Other molecules, nucleosides, such as adenosine and cordycepin, and flavonoids and phenols also play a huge role in mushroom anti-cancer effects.

Specific Mushrooms for Specific Cancers:

This is only a brief list. Most mushrooms will benefit most cancer types.

- Agaricus
  - Prostate
- Chaga
  - Prostate
- Cordyceps
  - Lung
  - Kidney
- Lion's Mane
  - Esophageal
  - Gastric
  - Pancreatic
  - Brain/nervous system
- Maitake
  - Lymphoma
  - Prostate
- Oyster
  - Lung
  - Liver
- Reishi
  - Liver
- Tremella
  - Liver
- Turkey Tail
  - Cancer (many types)

OTHER SUPPLEMENTS FOR CANCER PATIENTS

There are a number of supplements that have shown benefits for patients with cancer. There are reports of cancers going into remission or the growth of the tumors slowing with the use of supplements. Additionally, when the appropriate supplements are used, they are also good at managing and reducing the side effects of chemotherapy or radiation treatments. Supplements generally will not "cure" cancer, but they can help turn a potentially terminal disease into a long-term, chronic, manageable disease. Supplements work best when they are given early in the course of the cancer before it has a chance to grow and spread around the body.

It's important not to delay important vital life-saving treatments by trusting in your supplements to fix your pet's cancer. They may be helpful, but it's dangerous to be lulled into a false sense of security to think that the supplements will cure the cancer.

Unfortunately, it's unlikely that supplements will immediately stop your pet's cancer (especially if the cancer is way far progressed and your pet is in its eleventh hour). The earlier you detect a cancer, and the earlier you can begin providing interventions, the more likely it is that your pet's cancer can be controlled.

By delaying a treatment that might save your pet's life, you are making things worse. I'm not saying don't use supplements—they are great—but don't put so much trust in them that you waste precious time that could be better used in earlier intervention for your pet's cancer.

Some cancers are like ticking time bombs—they have a short fuse before they "explode" and kill their host. Other types of cancer take their time and can be better managed using diet and supplements. This is why I will often suggest considering chemotherapy just to keep my patient alive long enough so the natural therapies can have a better effect.

This section on pet cancer supplements includes those supplements that I have used the most and with which I have found the best results. There are quite a few other compounds with comparable anti-cancer benefits, and new anti-cancer supplements are being discovered regularly.

It's beyond the scope of *Your Healthy Pet Guide* to provide huge depth or detail on all supplements. I provide here a broad overview of some of the more effective cancer supplements for you to consider for your pet.

There are three basic classes of nutraceuticals (herbs and supplements) for pets with cancer:

1. Antioxidant compounds

2. Immune system modulators

3. Cancer cell cytotoxic compounds

ANTIOXIDANTS

Antioxidants have been found to help protect the body from the damaging effects of both chemotherapy and radiation therapies, but the question always arises whether they also reduce the effectiveness of these therapies. I've spoken with oncologists who recommend against them being used at the same time as chemotherapy and radiation treatments, and other oncologists who didn't think it mattered.

My suggestion is to follow your oncologists' instructions, and if they don't allow cannabis, antioxidants, or other supplements to be used during chemotherapy or radiation therapy, still follow their instructions for the duration of their cancer therapy. Once conventional oncologic therapies have been completed, then you can start adding the cannabis, mushrooms, and other natural therapies that were recommended.

There are different types of antioxidants, and studies show that antioxidants that are part of food or an herb, and most nutraceuticals, do not seem to pose a problem to the success of chemo or radiation therapy. This is especially true when these antioxidants are given at lower dosages. Pharmaceutically-isolated antioxidant compounds have been found to be more likely to cause a problem with chemotherapy or radiation therapy.

There are some oncologists who don't feel that the use of antioxidants with chemotherapy is a problem at all, but they recommend against their use with radiation therapy.

You need to discuss this with your oncologist so you understand their position. It's important to be in compliance with their recommendations if you want to work with them.

One example, *Silymarin marianum*, or milk thistle, contains some strong liver-protective compounds, and it also has very potent antioxidant properties. There are studies that show that milk thistle can be used at the same time as chemotherapy without affecting the cancer cytotoxicity of the chemotherapy agent. This has also been found to be true in studies of the herbal extract from the turmeric rhizome (*Curcuma longa*), curcumin, as well as the antioxidants present in green tea and green tea extracts.[96,97]

In one study, rats with experimentally-induced cancer were treated with chemotherapy combined with fish oil. It was determined that the addition of the fish oil increased the cytotoxicity of the chemotherapy. When high doses of vitamin E were added, that cytotoxic benefit of the fish oil on the cancer cells was lost.[98]

I recommend the use of food-bound or plant-bound antioxidants concurrent with cancer chemotherapy and/or radiation therapy.

Add foods to the diet that are rich in antioxidants, like blueberries or raspberries. Use antioxidant herbs like the ayurvedic herb amla (*Phyllanthus emblica*) or CBD. Home-prepared meals with brightly colored fruits and vegetables are another good way to provide antioxidants to your four-legged friend without disturbing their conventional cancer therapy. Be careful to not add too many fruits, which are high in simple sugars, to your pet's cancer diet. We know that simple sugars, as are found in fruits, can promote the growth of cancer cells.

You can add fish oil, MCTs, and antioxidant-rich foods to your pet's processed kibble diet to be sure they are getting the good stuff. Even though you may want to do a home-prepared diet, you may not have the time, energy, or resources to do that. So the next best thing, if all you can feed is kibble, is to add supplements, oils, mushrooms, Western and Chinese herbs, and vegetables or antioxidant extracts from fruits and vegetables to their commercial food.

Green tea is one of the least expensive and most widely consumed antioxidant drinks in the world. Green tea is consumed as a beverage by more people than any other beverage, including coffee. Even a tea bag of green tea has value for its antioxidant properties. The amount of caffeine in green tea is not very much, and the l-theanine, an antioxidant amino acid found in green tea, provides green tea with its "Zen." L-theanine helps to temper the edginess of the caffeine in the tea, much the same way that CBD tempers the edginess of THC.

I recommend steeping a green tea bag in 6 ounces of hot water for 15 minutes. You can then take that tea and place it on your pets' food as a way of providing them with their daily antioxidants.

**Each 6-ounce cup of green tea will contain, on average,
25 milligrams of Epigallocatechin gallate (EGCG),
a powerful antioxidant found in green tea.**

If your pet is sensitive to the caffeine in green tea, even with it being tempered by the theanine, there is a simple way you can de-caffeinate your tea, or, you can get *decaffeinated* green tea bags.

To remove 75% of the caffeine in the green tea you are providing to your pet, steep the tea bag in 6 ounces of hot water for 45 seconds, remove the tea bag from the cup of hot water, and discard that hot water. It will contain most of the caffeine, thus substantially reducing the amount of caffeine remaining in the tea bag. Then, steep the tea bag again in hot water, this time for 15 minutes. This will not substantially reduce the amount of **EGCG** in each cup.

EGCG has many beneficial properties and has been found to have some cytotoxic properties toward cancer cells, as well.

I highly recommend **EGCG** as a daily healthy antioxidant to support your pet.

IMMUNE SYSTEM MODIFIERS

Immune system modifiers can help improve your pet's immune system response to the cancer. Cancer cells are being created through mutations of healthy normal cells all the time. A healthy immune system usually will detect these cancer cells and destroy them. When cancer becomes a disease, it means that the immune system is not able to remove those mutant cancer cells. Without immune vigilance, cells grow into a tumor. Malignant tumors have the potential to metastasize and spread their cancer to remote locations in the body like the lungs or liver. The goal of giving immune-modulating herbs and mushrooms is to "train" the immune system to kill cancer cells.

Immune modulators are balancing agents that "normalize" immune function. If the immune system is underactive, a modulator will bring its function up to normal. If it is overactive, which can result in a hypersensitivity-type of disease, such as allergies or an auto-immune or immune-mediated disease, modulators can help settle down its activity.

Immune system "stimulators" or "enhancers" will increase immune system activity, and not in a balanced way. An immune "suppressive" supplement, on the other hand, can reduce immune system activity. A "modulator" responds to what the body needs most from its immune system and helps it adapt to create balance and homeostasis.

With an under-active or over-active immune system, the body is not as competent to be able to remove these "pre-cancerous" cells. Immune modulators have a better chance of effective vigilance and action to remove these early cancer cells.

Common Examples of Immune System Modulators:

- Beta-glucans, isolated from yeast or mushrooms

- Mushroom extracts

- Vitamin D

- Curcuminoids from turmeric

- Larch arabinogalactan

- Inositol hexaphosphate

- Astragalus root

- Ashwagandha

- Wei Qi Booster from Jing Tang Herbal™

- Cannabinoids and terpenes from cannabis

BETA-GLUCANS

Beta-glucans, mentioned earlier in this section when discussing the active molecules found in mushrooms, are chains, or "polymers" of molecules of simple sugars that are used by mushrooms, yeast, seaweed, and grain to provide structural support to their cell walls. Our own and our pets' immune systems have developed to respond to beta-glucans with improved immune cell function. Studies have shown that when given beta-glucans from any source, cancer growth can be reduced substantially for many types of cancer. Other studies have shown that beta-glucans increase the ability of the cells of the immune system to kill cancer cells and infectious disease agents.[99]

VITAMIN D

Vitamin D levels in the blood have been found in studies of **canine cancer patients to be excessively low for all types of cancer.**[100]

Dogs and cats do not convert cholesterol molecules in their skin by exposure to sunlight into vitamin D_3. Dogs and cats are more likely to have excessively low vitamin D_3 levels, which may make them more susceptible to developing cancer.

Vitamin D can be toxic when too much is given, and the only way to know how much vitamin D_3 your dog or cat needs is by testing its blood for vitamin D first and then treating with the appropriate amount of vitamin D daily.

Dogs and cats get their vitamin D strictly from diet, and there is no way to predict what their levels are until they have been measured in the blood.

VDI Laboratory (www.VDILAB.com) provides vitamin D blood test kits to your veterinarian.

Your veterinarian will need to draw your pet's blood, apply it to the test kit, and send it in for analysis for your pet's vitamin D status. They will provide you with a report that includes the recommended dosage of vitamin D_3 you need to give to your pet to bring their vitamin D levels up to normal.

There are two types of vitamin D. Vitamin D_3 is derived from animals. It can be metabolized from cholesterol molecules in the skin following activation with UV light. The commercial vitamin D_3 product is derived from sheep lanolin (grease) that has been irradiated with UV light. This molecule is called cholecalciferol and is converted in the liver to vitamin D_3, which is then activated in the tissues where it has its activity.

The other type of vitamin D is vitamin D_2, which is derived from mushrooms that have been exposed to UV light. In mushrooms, the pre-vitamin D_2 molecule is called "ergosterol," which is almost identical to cholesterol with only a few molecular differences. Once exposed to sufficient UVB light, it is converted to ergocalciferol, which the liver then converts into Vitamin D_2.

Mammals can utilize either vitamin D_2 or vitamin D_3. The vitamin D_3 form has been found to be about 30% more potent than the vitamin D_2 form. These higher doses of vitamin D_2 have comparable benefits to vitamin D_3. Vitamin D_2 is a vegetarian product. Vitamin D_2 can be organically grown and is less toxic than vitamin D_3.

CURCUMINOIDS (*CURCUMA LONGA*)

The root (technically, it's called a "rhizome") of the turmeric plant contains some very potent compounds that have strong anti-inflammatory activity and are also able to interfere with the growth of cancer cells.

Some studies show that curcuminoids can also help with cancer therapy side effects, such as nausea, and can have a good effect in addressing pain from the cancer or cancer therapies. Turmeric extracts are considered to be very safe, even at higher dosages. The big problem with curcuminoids from turmeric is that they are extremely poorly absorbed.

Some turmeric products have been modified to increase their bioavailability so they will produce higher blood levels, which will be more therapeutic. There are different absorption technologies for turmeric, and some claim to be more highly bioavailable than others. When you are looking for a turmeric supplement, see if they have done anything with the product to increase absorption, as that would be the product you should source to help your pet with cancer.

POLYSACCHARIDES

Arabinogalactans (*Larix occidentalis*) are derived from the bark of the western larch tree. They have been approved by the FDA as a source of dietary fiber. As a prebiotic, it will promote the growth of beneficial intestinal probiotic species. It contains non-digestible polysaccharides that have anti-inflammatory and anti-allergic activity. They stimulate natural killer T cells (NK T cells), which can attack cancer cells. Arabinogalactan is dosed by teaspoon upwards of a tablespoon, with smaller animals getting 1 teaspoon two or three times daily and larger animals receiving as much as a tablespoon two or three times daily.

Inositol hexaphosphate (IP-6: Inositol-1,2,3,4,5,6-hexaphosphate) can be found in almost all plant and animal cells and is vital for regulating cellular functions. IP-6 is a strong antioxidant. It has been found to:

1. Cause cancer cells to differentiate and mature into normal, non-cancerous cells

2. Reduce cellular growth and proliferation

3. Interfere with cancer cell to cancer cell communication signals

4. Stop the cycle of cancer cell growth

There have been no studies of IP-6 for cancer in dogs or cats, but there have been several studies published in humans and laboratory animals that have used a dose for humans of 3 grams twice daily of IP-6. That dosage translated to dogs and cats would be about 20 mg/pound of body weight daily.

ADAPTOGENS

Adaptogens help the body and the adrenal glands deal with stress. They are considered very safe and most effective when given on a daily basis for a long period of time. Many adaptogens can help the body deal with cancer. Adaptogens have the adrenal gland as their target, and they involve the hormones that are produced in the pituitary gland as well. True adaptogens will affect the "HPA-Adrenal Axis," which are the interrelated endocrine glands in the brain and the adrenal glands. The two adaptogenic mushrooms are cordyceps and reishi.

Ashwagandha

Ashwagandha (*Withania somnifera*) is sometimes called "Indian ginseng" and is also considered an adaptogen, like Astragalus root.

Ashwagandha has been found to be able to sensitize tumor tissue to the damaging radiation of radiation therapy but not to sensitize healthy cells.

Ashwagandha will stop cancer cells from multiplying by:

• Regulating the cell cycle, which stops multiplication and proliferation

- Increasing cancer cell death (apoptosis)

- Inhibiting angiogenesis, which is the growth of new blood vessels from a tumor that supplies nutrients in the blood to support increased growth

- Inhibit NF-kappa-beta, a cell-signaling molecule that reduces inflammation and cancer cell growth.

NF-kappa-beta is an important molecule that turmeric, cannabis, and medicinal mushrooms inhibit to reduce inflammation and cancer cell growth.

Although an exact dose for cancer in veterinary species has not yet been determined, published doses for ashwagandha suggest ~50 mg/pound of the dried herb two or three times daily. Alcohol extracts of ashwagandha are dosed at 1 ml/10 pounds of body weight two or three times daily.[101]

Astragulus Root

Herbal Immune Tonic: Astragalus root (*Astragalus membranaceous*) is a Chinese herb, known as a "Qi tonic" and is immune modulating. Astragalus root is considered to be very safe and effective in modulating immune system function. It has been found to induce cellular differentiation and cell death (cytotoxic).

CHINESE HERBAL FORMULATIONS FOR CANCER

Wei Qi Booster™

This is a Chinese herbal combination formulated by Huisheng Xie, DVM, Ph.D., founder of Chi University and Jing Tang herbal that helps to improve immune system vigilance against cancer cells. It is only available through a prescription from your veterinarian.

Stasis Breaker™

In the medical philosophy of Traditional Chinese Veterinary Medicine, tumors are considered to be a "stagnation" of blood or phlegm. The herbal strategy to treat tumors with Chinese herbs is to use herbs that will "break up" the stagnation. Stasis Breaker™ contains those herbs that break up the cancerous masses so the body can dispose of them.

This formula can be used for a variety of tumors, including hemangiosarcoma, osteosarcoma, mast cell tumors, melanomas, and others.

There are numerous anecdotal reports from pet parents and veterinarians about the successful use of the combination of Wei Qi Booster™ and Stasis Breaker™ to slow down or stop many types of cancer growth and spread.

Yunnan Baiyao™

This Chinese patent formula originates from the Yunnan province of China. Its "chief" herb is pseudoginseng (*radix notoginseng* or Tienchi ginseng in Chinese pinyin), which is not the same ginseng that is commonly used as an adaptogen and energy tonic. This form of ginseng improves blood clotting and is used to stop bleeding and improve wound healing.

Legend has it that this is the herb that won the war in Vietnam for the Viet Cong because they would carry it in their field kits, and when injured, would use it and be able to return to battle sooner.

This herb is used currently by veterinary specialists who are doing endoscopy procedures that have a lot of hemorrhage, for instance, in the nasal passages. When given for several days prior to the procedure, the amount of bleeding during the procedure is significantly less.

For dogs who have been diagnosed with cancer of the spleen, hemangiosarcoma, giving this herb can help reduce the amount of abdominal blood that accumulates when the splenic mass ruptures and bleeds. It can help stop that bleeding from starting and also appears to have an effect on slowing down the growth of the hemangiosarcoma cancer cells themselves.

Yunnan Baiyao™ comes in a 16-capsule blister pack with a little red pill in the middle. The little red pill is called the "emergency pill" and is the equivalent of the combined clotting benefit of all 16 capsules taken at once. You can also open a capsule and sprinkle it into a bleeding wound, apply pressure, and it will help stop that bleed.

Recommended amount to give for Yunnan Baiyao™ in veterinary species:

For Acute Bleeding in Dogs Use These Doses:
- Give 1 capsule 2-3 times daily for pets who are 10-30 pounds
- Give 2 capsules 2-3 times daily for pets who are 30-60 pounds
- Give 3 capsules 2-3 times daily for pets who are 60-100 pounds
- The little red pill is called the "emergency pill" and is very concentrated. It can help if bleeding is severe.

For Chronic Use:
(After the acute bleeding is under control)
- Wound healing, use the chronic dosages
- Hemangiosarcoma, use the *Acute Bleeding* dosages

Chronic Dosages:

- Small pets, < 30 pounds: 1 capsule twice daily

- Medium pets, 30-60 pounds: 2 capsules twice daily

- Large pets, 60+ pounds: 3 capsules twice daily

- Try to find the lowest dose that is effective for long-term use.

Note: The herbal contents of the capsules may not be very palatable to cats as they are fairly bitter. It's best to give the entire capsule if possible versus mixing the content of the capsule in food.

Modified Xue Fu Zhu Yu Tang (XFZYT)

This formula takes an existing formula that is commonly used to relieve blood stagnation in the chest, *Xue Fu Zhu Yu Tang*, which is used for pets with congestive heart failure, and modifies it by adding two additional herbs, *E Zhu*, which is from the *Curcuma zedoaria* plant, a first cousin of the turmeric plant, and *San Leng*, *Sparganium stoloniferum*, an herb from the rhizome (root) of a reed-like plant that grows in shallow water.

With the addition of these two herbs, the tumor will be further broken up. This formula is especially effective if the tumor is a "blood stagnation" tumor, like hemangiosarcoma, mast cell tumor, or malignant melanoma.

The modified XFZYT is comparable to Stasis Breaker™ in that it also breaks up stagnation, especially blood-stagnation types of tumors. My suggestion is to consider alternating these every three to six months to give a different and fresh set of herbs to perhaps have a more effective activity in your pet.

If the mast cell tumor or melanoma is located in the lower abdomen, then the use of a modified *Shao Fu Zhu Yu Tang* would be indicated. This formula is modified with the same herbs as the XFZYT, but the formula itself is better adapted to treat stagnation in the lower abdomen, such as mast cell tumors around the rectum, or prostatic or bladder cancer.

Xiao Chai Hu Tang, or Minor Bupleurum, is a Chinese herbal formula with a variety of applications, including supporting the patient's immune system and energetics who has cancer, immune-mediated problems, or hepatitis, to name a few. It can be used concurrently with the modified formulas or by itself for patients with cancer. It can be used for lymphoma patients combined with medicinal mushrooms and a healthy ketogenic diet.

ALTERNATIVE CANCER THERAPIES

Ozone

Cancer cells are not like healthy normal cells. For one, their metabolism is different. Normal cells derive energy from metabolizing food in the presence of oxygen. They are able to produce large amounts of energy in the form of ATP in the presence of oxygen. Oxygen is toxic to cancer cells. Cancer cells metabolize foods in the absence of much oxygen and do not produce a lot of energy from that low-oxygen reaction.

Ozone is "super-oxygen." Normally, oxygen comes as O_2. Ozone is O_3, containing 30% more oxygen, which makes it very toxic to cancer cells. Additionally, the use of medical ozone treatments will stimulate the body's immune system to reduce inflammation and attack the cancer cells damaged by the O_3. Ozone can be added to the blood, administered by rectal insufflation, bubbled through intravenous fluids, and given IV or subcutaneously, or injected directly into the tumor mass.

Mistletoe Injections

Mistletoe is a semi-parasitic plant that lives off of the sap from the trees (apple, oak, pine, and elm) it attacks. This therapy is widely used in Europe to treat cancer in humans. It is administered by injection, so you need to work with a veterinarian to be sure it is safely and effectively administered. Very few side effects have been noted with mistletoe injections. There is an oral form of this mistletoe, but it's not as potent as the injectable.

Mistletoe works by increasing immune system vigilance against cancer cells and the immune cells that are stimulated, like natural killer T cells, which can destroy cancer cells.

My colleague, Dr. Kendra Pope, an integrative, board-certified veterinary oncologist (www.prismvethealth.com), has been using mistletoe injections, as well as high-dose IV vitamin C therapy for her cancer patients with a great deal of success in controlling their cancers. She is available for telemedicine consults, and if you are in northern New Jersey, you can take your pet with cancer to see her in person.

High-dose IV Vitamin C

Dr. Pope also provides high-dose Vitamin C injections in the form of ascorbic acid or sodium ascorbate. This common antioxidant, when given by injection directly into the vein of a person or animal at pretty high dosages, has been found to be cytotoxic (kills!) to cancer cells.

Although vitamin C is an antioxidant, when it is given at very high dosages, it becomes a "pro-oxidant" and can oxidize and kill cancer cells. A common oxidant is hydrogen peroxide, or ozone, as discussed above. These compounds kill bacteria, viruses, and cancer cells using the oxidizing properties of oxygen, ozone, hydrogen peroxide, or super-high doses of vitamin C.

The vitamin C is diluted into a bag of intravenous fluids and "dripped" into the vein slowly over several hours to avoid any adverse reactions. This treatment is given weekly and, for optimal benefit, is alternated with weekly ozone treatments.

DIETS FOR CANCER PATIENTS

When I was in day-to-day clinical practice, I would schedule 90 minutes to meet with pet parents whose critters had cancer. This amount of time allowed me to better understand their problem and gave me time to teach and explain the many steps I recommend to help pets who have cancer.

The first question I asked my client, the pet parent, was to tell me what their goals are for coming to see me. I was surprised that almost every pet parent's first goal (other than having their pets live out their natural lifespan and not die from the cancer) was to learn how to prepare a healthy diet to address their cancer.

There are no definitive studies that show which diets cure or treat cancer in pets or humans. From what we know about the metabolism of the cancer cell being different from a healthy cell, there are several approaches to diet that can improve outcomes in cancer patients.

These "cancer" diets are based on the metabolic fact that cancer cells feed primarily on simple sugars, complex carbohydrates, and to a lesser extent on protein, but do not use fats for energy at all.

There are two basic diets that seem helpful for feeding cancer patients. Each of them is low in carbohydrates. The first diet is **high in protein and fats**, and the second diet contains **moderate protein and high fats**. The second diet is called the "**ketogenic diet**," and due to its high-fat content, will create "ketones" (also known as "ketone bodies"), which cancer cells cannot feed off.

When cancer cells metabolize simple sugars and carbohydrates for energy, they produce an excess of lactic acid as a by-product.

The "ketosis" we see from ketogenic diets is different than the ketoacidosis with diabetes mellitus, although both involve the production of ketones. With diabetes, the metabolism is so out of whack that the ketones and acid condition of the blood are very pathogenic. The ketones that result from the metabolism of fats in a pet who does not have diabetes are considered healthy for most. Some pets have problems with ketogenic diets, so be aware of that.

When healthy cells are provided with zero carbohydrates, they are forced to metabolize fats or protein. They produce the ketones from fat metabolism. Healthy cells can metabolize these ketones, but cancer cells cannot. The ketogenic diet produces ketones, which can help "starve" the cancer. Cancer cells are limited in what they can metabolize. They can only derive energy, and fairly inefficiently, from simple sugars, lactic acid, and carbohydrates.

The best and easiest way to formulate a diet specifically for your pet's needs is by engaging the services of a veterinary nutritionist. At the end of the book, I've listed some Resources for you to find a nutritionist if this is something you would like to do. I recommend that you connect with a veterinary nutritionist to ensure the diet is properly formulated.

The diet formulation process I've given here will work in the short term, but over a long period of time, there may be nutrient deficiencies that your pet develops with this diet template. Your pet will, in the long run, be better served with a personalized custom diet formulation from an experienced expert.

There are few commercially available diets that can provide these specific nutrient profiles. Hill's prescription diet **N/D™ is a canned diet that contains higher protein and very high oil content,** including the fatty acids from fish, EPA/DHA, which have a lot of research suggesting they can help manage cancer through their anti-inflammatory and pro-oxidant effects. This diet is based on published metabolic studies performed on canine cancer patients with high doses of fish oil and protein.[102,103]

Commercially available ketogenic diets are just starting to emerge in the marketplace. I have not had any direct experience with any of these commercial food diets, so it's difficult to make specific diet recommendations. I've made my own ketogenic diets in the absence of commercially available ketogenic diets. What I would like to see in a commercially available ketogenic diet is some scientific evidence—in other words, analytical tests—showing that dogs fed these commercial diets did, in fact, develop ketosis. The proof of ketosis is determined by the measurement of ketones in the blood, or to a lesser extent of accuracy, in the urine.

BUT, there is a "hybrid" option:

Purina™ has a diet called "NeuroCare™" that is a dry, kibble format of dog food that was developed to address epilepsy, especially refractory epilepsy. For many years, it has been known that a ketogenic diet can help with epilepsy. In fact, it was the finding that cancers would go into remission with the use of ketogenic diets in epileptic patients who also had cancer, which led researchers to extend the benefits of ketogenic diets to cancer patients.

NeuroCare™ is a commercially available ketogenic diet, but it doesn't follow the standard ratios of high fat, moderate protein, and low or no carbohydrates. Instead, this diet, being from kibble, is about 50% carbohydrates, as the hard extruded kibbles need carbohydrates to hold them together.

When I read the studies around the development of Neuro-Care™ as a ketogenic diet, I was surprised to find that the diet was made from 50% carbohydrates, a moderately high protein content (28%), and 15% fat, with a third of the fat calories coming from medium chain triglycerides. The dry food contained 373 kcal per 100 grams of food, so its calorie content wasn't very rich. Measurements of ketones in the blood of these dogs were determined to be significant after three months on this "ketogenic" dry food.

This study with NeuroCare™ was for epileptic seizures or behavioral issues, so it's impossible to say that this same diet would be good for cancer. But it might be a good starting point for a homemade-hybrid ketogenic diet.

A potential compromise, in terms of using a commercial food as a starting point for a ketogenic diet, would be to look at a canned, raw, or cooked diet with comparable protein and fat levels as the NeuroCare™, but which would be substantially lower in carbohydrate content (10% at the most).

The key to a successful ketogenic diet is not just the proportions of fat and protein and the normally lower, to non-existent, carbohydrates, but also the *large percentage of fat calories provided by the MCT*.

MCT contains 9 kilocalories per gram of oil. Each teaspoon of MCT oil contains about 40-45 kcal. If we are to give about 10% of total diet calories from MCT, we would calculate the number of calories in the moderate-protein and low-carbohydrate diet and then add 10% of the calories of the diet with medium-chain triglycerides to each meal.

CHAPTER NINE SUMMARY

When your pet is diagnosed with cancer, it's a very stressful experience. Some types of cancer are relatively easy to treat. Some, you can surgically remove and they never return. Others, no matter how aggressive your surgery is and how strong the chemotherapy agents, the cancer still prevails and you will lose your beloved four-legged family member.

With early detection of cancer, such as is now available with a urine screening test that is 80-90% accurate, we can detect bladder cancer (CADET™ BRAF testing), lymphoma, melanoma, mast cell tumor, and hemangiosarcoma (Oncotect™ In-Home Urine Screening test) early enough to make a significant difference in the outcome of these often terminal cancers.

This chapter on my treatment of hemangiosarcoma in a Labrador retriever guided you through the process that can lead to successful outcomes when cancer strikes, including the addition of medicinal mushrooms, cannabis, special cancer diets, and selected nutraceuticals, like fish oil, which can work together to "tip the scale" in favor of your dog winning and its cancer "losing."

DIGESTIVE DISORDERS: THE DIARRHEA JUST WON'T STOP AND THE HOUSE IS A MESS!

DIGESTIVE PROBLEMS IN A DOG: TAWNY'S UNRELENTING DIARRHEA

Mrs. Shoemaker entered my exam room with Tawny, her spayed female, six-year-old vizsla. This breed of dog is beautifully muscled and athletic-looking, but they are also very high-strung, and many of their problems stem from that. Tawny had been seen by the specialist at the veterinary teaching hospital up north for her chronic diarrhea, and Mrs. Shoemaker had followed everything exactly, according to this specialist's recommendations, including feeding an expensive prescription special diet.

Nothing had worked.

None of the drugs had stopped the dog from pooping wet loads consistently and constantly, with straining. Tawny's anal glands continued to fill and make her so uncomfortable that she would "scoot" to try to empty them herself. This left stinky brown "hash marks" on the new white carpets.

If left untreated, anal glands can become infected, abscess, and rupture, and that creates the problem of a draining, painful rectum.

When Tawny defecated, due to the pain and swelling of the rectum from this infection, stool would remain on the rectum until it was wiped by Tawny onto the carpet when she scooted.

The Shoemakers were at their wit's end, and that's when they came to me.

"We've heard from our next-door neighbor who brought their dog to you, Dr. Silver, that you have a few tricks up your sleeve when it comes to this sort of problem. At least you really helped their dog's poopy problem. We are so frustrated by this problem, and it's so messy. Please, please help us!" Mrs. Shoemaker said.

I performed a digital rectal exam to be sure there wasn't a growth in the rectal area and emptied the anal glands, which were full of a stinky yellow secretion and some pus. With my gloved finger, I then extracted a stool sample to send to the reference lab to analyze for parasites and bacterial growth.

After I completed my examination, I sent in some blood for testing and sat down with Mrs. Shoemaker. I suggested that to start, we send in a saliva test sample to find out if there are food sensitivities we need to know about when selecting his food.

Until those results came back, I suggested that we start by feeding 50/50 cooked chicken and wet-cooked white rice. I've found that most dogs are not allergic to this combination. It is very well-tolerated by most dogs, and the white rice often will help control the diarrhea. I suggest cooking the white rice with 1 cup of rice to 2 cups of water. This will make the rice very soft and easy to digest.

Additionally, I had them add montmorillonite clay, probiotics, digestive enzymes, and a combination Chinese herbal formula (*Huo Xiang Zheng Qi San*) that I commonly reach for with my patients with diarrhea. I had them start a CBD:CBG tincture for both mental calmness and because this cannabinoid blend can help calm the gut.

Mushrooms contain several types of non-digestible fiber that help support a healthy gut microbiome and, at the same time, benefit the immune system. We used a lion's mane 1:1 mushroom extract from a Canadian company for its fiber and calming effect on the digestive system. The 1:1 extract contains all of the fiber from the fresh mushroom, as well as the other immune and digestive-supporting active ingredients.

Mrs. Shoemaker called at the end of the next day to say the stools were almost looking normal. She was happy. I agreed to review the Nutriscan™ test results when they returned. From these results, we better learned which ingredients to include in Tawny's meals and which ingredients to avoid.

I have a lot of experience treating digestive problems in pets, and I've found that sometimes just one new ingredient in a diet can throw off the entire digestion. This is why I take a thorough diet history, as well as run tests of the dog's reaction to foods, like the Nutriscan™ saliva test that looks for food intolerances and sensitivities. This will help guide the pet parent in the selection of diets and ingredients that are better tolerated by their pet. I have had a lot of positive results using this testing method to adjust pet diets to create a healthier digestive process.

Restoring healthy function to your pet's digestive system is not always that easy. It would be great if you could just change one ingredient, and everything would go back to normal. Unfortunately, it can be much more complicated than that, with many other factors than diet playing important roles in creating and maintaining your pet's chronic diarrhea.

In this case, a few of the ingredients in the food she was feeding Tawny were high on the list of sensitive foods. When we switched to just the rice and chicken, which were not foods that the test results suggested to avoid, the stools improved.

Honestly, we got lucky that it was relatively easy to learn what dietary factors were contributing to the diarrhea.

When I am seeing a patient with acute or chronic diarrhea, I nearly always start by suggesting cooked chicken and white rice because it's so universally acceptable and palatable to most dogs. It is bland and generally not inflammatory. I've found that it settles the stomach, especially when prepared with ginger root.

White rice, especially when wet-cooked (1 cup rice to 2 cups water), is one of the best foods to firm up stools I've used in my 40+ years in practice. Chicken is commonly found in many commercial pet foods. For this reason, it is one of the more common food allergens in dogs. But, if your dog is NOT sensitive to chicken muscle meat, it is a great food and great for the digestive system. Chicken liver often is not allergenic, but the muscle meat often is.

Tawny's blood test came back indicating a slight deficiency of pancreatic enzymes. I had her increase the amount of digestive enzymes she was adding to the food. These enzymes helped a lot.

The pancreas is the body's natural source for many of the digestive enzymes that are needed to break down food into smaller, more digestible units. In the absence of these enzymes, as was found to be the case with Tawny, the food is only partially digested, which can lead to diarrhea, as well as malnutrition. The digestive enzymes we added to her diet helped augment the poor production of naturally occurring digestive enzymes from Tawny's pancreas.

When the pancreas is unable to manufacture sufficient digestive enzymes to break down the food ingested, we call this condition "exocrine pancreatic insufficiency," or "EPI." The best treatment for EPI is with pancreatic digestive enzymes from dried whole pancreas. Dogs with EPI can have different levels of digestive enzyme deficiency, and some will respond when given enzymes that are not from the pancreas. Some dog breeds, like the German shepherd, are genetically prone to this condition.

Most commercial digestive enzyme products are fungal-based. Fungal enzymes have a wider range of activity for digesting food than pancreatic enzymes. With EPI, I've found that pancreatic enzymes work the best to treat this condition, which is a cause of chronic diarrhea.

One other factor contributing to her chronic diarrhea was Tawny's high state of mental energy. Vizslas are hunting dogs with a lot of energy. A working dog like a vizsla needs to be exercised quite a bit each day. This gives her an outlet for this energy. Without adequate exercise, some of that undirected excess energy can "overflow" to her bowel and create soft stools or diarrhea.

The use of CBD:CBG allowed her excited state to wind down and also helped to reduce some of the muscle spasms in her gut, wrenched by her nervous energy but relaxed by the cannabinoids. Lion's mane mushroom extract worked together with the CBD:CBG to create a more relaxed state of mind and gut. Many gastroenterologists (people who specialize in diseases of the digestive system) say there is a connection between the mind, emotions, and gut. They term this "the brain-gut axis," and it is why calming supplements like cannabinoids and mushrooms can help with diarrhea in highly excitable dogs like Tawny.

In humans with irritable bowel syndrome (IBS), medical doctors and gastroenterologists recommend the use of peppermint tea or peppermint essential oil drops in water. Peppermint will relax smooth muscle spasms, as well. It's easy to administer and works together nicely with cannabinoids and mushrooms.

Diarrhea and chronic bowel problems often have multiple causes. This is a perfect example of the use of an integrative medicine approach for Tawny's chronic digestive problem.

This was a *multi-factorial* approach to a *multi-factorial* problem.

The digestive system, or "bowel," stretches from the mouth to the anus, and there are numerous problems and conditions that arise at each location in the bowel:

- Dental problems (although these are tended to by veterinary dentists)

- Oral problems

- Esophageal problems

- Stomach problems

- Liver, pancreas, and gallbladder problems

- Upper bowel and lower bowel problems

- And, finally, anal problems

I could easily devote this entire book to just bowel health alone!

UNDERSTANDING THE DIGESTIVE SYSTEM

There are three important functions of the GI tract for nutrition and protection:

1. Digest food into its nutrients

2. Allow nutrients and other beneficial molecules to be absorbed into the blood system

3. Prevent the entry of "dangerous" molecules like pathogens, toxins, and antigens

When these dangerous molecules remain in contact over an extended period of time with the wall of the bowel, a chronic inflammatory state will occur in certain areas of the digestive tract. These pro-inflammatory conditions create a "perfect storm," leading to conditions such as chronic diarrhea, irritable bowel syndrome (IBS), inflammatory bowel disease (IBD), or colitis.

We see these inflammatory diseases of the GI tract in both dogs and cats. In cats, IBD can look a lot like small cell lymphoma. There are diagnostics that can help your vet differentiate feline IBD from feline lymphoma.

Digestive problems are the most common and easily noticeable medical problems in pets. Many of the same digestive aids that are available for digestive problems in people, like digestive enzymes, prebiotics or probiotics, or certain herbs like licorice root, ginger root, or turmeric, can safely provide symptomatic relief for pets, too.

For most types of digestive problems in pets, herbs, supplements, digestive enzymes, and beneficial probiotic bacteria will provide almost immediate relief. If these gentle natural therapeutics aren't sufficiently strong to help, we always have the ability to use antibiotics or pharmaceuticals to help control diarrhea, nausea, and/or vomiting. Most of my cases of digestive problems that I've seen in my veterinary practice resolve fairly easily after a day or two of treatments.

CAUSES OF BOWEL PROBLEMS

This section will focus on describing four types of chronic diarrhea:

"Neurogenic" causes are derived from stress, and those signals come from the brain. One example of this is irritable bowel syndrome (IBS), which is caused by stress and anxiety. Colitis is another condition that can be neurogenic. The constant stresses your pet experiences can cause this condition, which involves the infiltration of pro-inflammatory immune cells and pro-inflammatory proteins into the bowel wall. This cellular and pro-inflammatory protein "infiltrate" interferes with the bowel's normal function, resulting in soft stools or diarrhea.

It is thought that in addition to the stressors that trigger this condition, there may also be a genetic component, and dietary and immune system factors, which increase the risks for the development of IBS, IBD, or colitis.

Increased inflammation is characteristic of a more complicated and severe inflammatory bowel condition than IBS. This condition is called "inflammatory bowel disease" (IBD). It is characterized by much more severe infiltration of pro-inflammatory cells and inflammatory protein molecules into the bowel wall. Often, IBD may be associated with chronic pathogenic bacterial overgrowth. Inflammatory infiltrates can be so widespread in the bowel wall that ulcerations of the mucous membrane lining the bowel occur, and GI bleeding will result. In humans, this is called "ulcerative colitis" (UC). Crohn's disease is another lower bowel inflammatory disease in humans similar to but different than UC.

For cats, inflammatory bowel disease (IBD) looks a lot like **small cell lymphoma.** It is difficult to tell them apart; the treatments are fairly similar, and they are both difficult to treat, but small cell lymphoma can progress to a terminal condition. There are blood tests that look for cancer markers that can help to differentiate between these two diseases, and a biopsy of the bowel wall will usually decide which of these two problems your cat has. From a conventional standpoint, a low-grade small cell intestinal lymphoma in the cat can look very much like IBD, and often, they are treated the same way if the lymphoma is well-contained and low-grade.

Dogs and cats can also get an **idiopathic chronic diarrhea** that isn't associated with either of these two inflammatory conditions. This can be a real problem for the lifespan of your pet if not properly addressed. The cause of this diarrhea isn't known, which is why we use the word *"idiopathic."* In some cases, this diarrhea may be due to hypersensitivity to ingredients in the diet, byproducts of diet manufacturing, treats that your dog gets, or possibly something in the environment that they are ingesting that is making their bowel more inflamed. Cannabinoids and mushrooms can help lower the level of inflammation, but so can diet changes, digestion boosters, and probiotics, as well as other herbs and drugs as detailed in this chapter.

INTEGRATIVE/HOLISTIC APPROACHES TO DIGESTIVE DISORDERS

Problems with the digestive system, causing diarrhea, vomiting, poor appetite, and/or weight gain or weight loss are the most common problems we see in our dog and cat populations.

To a large extent, these digestive problems result from pets' reactions to the mass-produced commercial foods, especially the dried kibble format, but there are problems with canned food and with raw foods as well, depending on the circumstance. Modern-day stressors play a role as well in the development of digestive problems, and often stress itself is a key element in the cause of diarrhea or vomiting.

Changes in the diet to a more acceptable and healthy format and recipe often times will solve digestive issues. However, in a number of cases diet changes alone are not enough, and a variety of different digestion boosters also need to be added to your pet's daily gut health program. This may include digestion boosters, such as prebiotics and probiotics, digestive enzymes, antioxidants, soothing herbs for an inflamed gut, and supplements specific to help with leaky gut and all that entails.

Emerging therapies, such as cannabis and medicinal mushrooms, are finding an important place in their use as digestion boosters, with cannabis helping with GI inflammation and appetite, and with mushrooms providing important fiber and immune modulation to create a healthy and balanced microbiome.

CANNABIS AND THE DIGESTIVE SYSTEM

There are cannabinoid receptors throughout the bowel. The body's naturally occurring cannabinoids, the endocannabinoids, play many vital roles in maintaining healthy digestion and bowel health. Cannabinoids will reduce bowel inflammation and bowel hyperpermeability; they can help treat "leaky gut syndrome" and play a role in bowel motility and digestive processes. There are a number of studies that show that the use of cannabinoids *and mushroom fiber* can help create a healthier microbiome.

Cannabis is well-known to increase appetite. The "munchies" are a well-known side-effect of ingesting THC. CBD can also contribute to improved appetite through other mechanisms of action. CBD doesn't cause the munchies like THC but can create a feeling of well-being and can reduce pain and anxiety. If your pet is in pain, anxious, or not feeling well, their appetite can be affected. It is in this way that CBD can improve appetite.

Cannabinoids such as THC and CBD and a few of the minor cannabinoids such as THCV and CBG can affect the nausea and vomit centers in the brain to reduce nausea and vomiting. If there is inflammation of the stomach, or elsewhere in the digestive tract that is influencing nausea or vomiting, cannabinoids can reduce that inflammation, which also can reduce nausea and vomiting.

CBD

CBD alone or in a full-spectrum or broad-spectrum extract will stimulate the receptors in the digestive tract to reduce inflammation. It also activates other receptors in the bowel, which increase motility—the contractions of the bowel that transport digested food through the bowel from mouth to anus.

One side effect that is commonly seen with CBD when given

at sufficiently high dosages or in sensitive individuals is diarrhea. This is hypothesized to be due to the effect that CBD has on increasing bowel motility. The faster the bowel moves, the less time there is to reabsorb the fluids to firm up the stool, so the stool remains soft to liquid in consistency.

When CBD is given initially in much smaller dosages it is less likely to cause this embarrassing (to your pet) side effect.

Dosages for CBD for bowel inflammation are typically in the higher ranges to help reduce the inflammation and pain associated with these chronic GI problems. If your pet has problems with soft or loose stools, or easily gets diarrhea from changes in diet, etc., I'd recommend starting with a lower dose, such as 0.1 mg/pound of body weight twice daily, with some food. Otherwise, you can start the dose at 0.25 mg/pound of body weight twice daily, and if after two to four weeks, no benefit is seen, then double that dose and see if another two to four weeks at this higher dosage will help.

Combining CBD with diet changes and with digestive supplements like enzymes, probiotics, and herbs like ginger or psyllium often works better than using CBD or digestive supplements alone.

Terpenes

Terpenes are the small hydrocarbon molecules found in fruits, vegetables, and herbs like hops or cannabis that give them their aroma, but which also have a biomedical benefit to your pet. Certain terpenes can also affect the bowel. Full-spectrum and broad-spectrum extracts will contain terpenes, whereas CBD isolate does not unless specific terpenes have been added back to the CBD.

Terpenes are very volatile molecules that evaporate from the hemp oil distillate when higher temperatures are used in the extraction and purification processes. Terpene analyses can be misleading if the analysis uses too much heat, as with gas chromatography. The heat used in the gas chromatograph can cause some of the smaller, more volatile terpene molecules to be lost and not recorded. A special analytical method called "headspace analysis" is needed for the most accurate measurement of the terpenes in an extract.

Four Terpenes Found in Cannabis with Benefits to the GI Tract:

1. Beta-caryophyllene (*also from cloves and pepper*)
   - Analgesic
     o Gastrointestinal relief from pain
   - Anti-bacterial, anti-fungal
   - Enhanced gastric cell protection with THC
   - Enhanced anti-inflammatory effect with CBD

2. Limonene (*also from citrus*)
   - Suppresses gastro-esophageal reflux disease (GERD)
   - This effect is enhanced when combined with THC

3. Humulene (*also from hops*)
   - Suppresses appetite

4. Terpinolene (*also from conifers, mangos, apples, and coriander*)
   - Gastrointestinal relief from pain

Ratio Products with THC

THC has been found to be very effective in reducing the inflammation and pain of inflammatory bowel disease and colitis and in helping control the diarrhea associated with it.

The amount of THC found in full-spectrum hemp products (<0.3%) may not be enough to provide adequate benefit in these cases, especially if it is a particularly severe case. The use of a dispensary or provincial store ratio product would be more effective than just full or broad-spectrum CBD from hemp.

Before going to THC, which can have its own set of problems and side effects, try CBD at higher doses to see if it will be able to control the straining and loose stools. I suggest starting at the ratio of 20:1, which would still have a relatively low amount of THC in it, so it would be safer to start with and less likely to cause problems but still potent enough to address the inflammation.

If the 20:1 is not effective, even at higher doses, then going to the next higher ratio, whether that be a 10:1 or 4:1 depends on local availability. If you have your pet on the 20:1 for two weeks, then that should be enough for it to develop tolerance to the adverse side effects of the THC if you scale up the dosage or go to a stronger ratio product.

In order to introduce this 20:1 ratio product (and it's the same principle if this were a 10:1 or a 4:1 product), you need to have an accurate analysis of the exact amount of CBD and THC/mL. Until your dog develops tolerance to the THC, you start these ratio products by dosing for the THC content. The dosage amount for the THC is the dosage-limiting factor due to its intoxicating nature.

Example of Calculations for
Safe Starting Dosage of THC for GI Problems:

Sample Ratio Product:
20:1 ratio = 10 mg/ml CBD:1.0 mg/mL THC.

This is an example of a 20:1 product with 20 mg of CBD and 1.0 mg of THC in each milliliter (mL).

NOTE: You will have to see what the actual ratio and amounts of CBD and THC in each milliliter are for your specific product. Usually, it is listed on the label somewhere or on the receipt given to you at the dispensary. Each state's dispensary can have different standards for listing potency and ingredients in a product. Dispensary products are NOT FDA approved since at the time of this writing, THC is still a Schedule I controlled substance according to the U.S. FDA.

Dog's weight = 25 pounds

Dose for THC = 0.05 mg/pound twice daily

25 X 0.05 = 1.25 mg twice daily of THC

There is 1.0 mg of THC/mL

1.25 mg THC = 2.5 mL of this ratio product

1.0 mg/mL X 1.25 mg = 2.5 mL, which contains the **1.25 mg of THC.**

This blend will contain 1.25 mg of THC and 25 mg of CBD in 1.25 mLs of volume

Give this amount to your dog (if it weighs 25 pounds and has IBS/IBD) twice daily for two weeks and observe its stool quality and for any straining when it defecates to see if that dose is sufficient to help.

Be sure to give the THC with a small amount of food just before feeding them their normal meal twice daily. This is known to increase the amount of THC and CBD that is absorbed into the body.

If, after two weeks, that dose doesn't seem to be helping, then I recommend doubling that dose and giving it for another two weeks.

Continue this process of increasing and observing your pet to see if the dose you are using is sufficient to help your pet. If you find with a dose escalation that the amount of THC you are giving makes your pooch a little "loopy," at that point, you will need to reduce that dose to the next lower dose you had used where your pooch was NOT getting loopy. Loopy symptoms include being glassy-eyed, wobbly, excessively sleepy, hard to arouse, and possibly bumping into things or falling over. When you see your pet acting like this, your pet is telling you that it has had too much THC. Hopefully, before your pet becomes loopy, its condition will have improved.

It may be that after a few more weeks you will be able to increase the THC dose again if you aren't getting the results you desire. Some dogs, though, may be too sensitive to THC to increase that dose as much as you might need to better control their IBD.

CAVEAT: *Not all conditions are guaranteed to respond to this treatment. You may need to use some of the holistic dietary supplements I mention in the next section below or look to some diet changes, as well.*

MEDICINAL MUSHROOMS AND HEALTHY BOWEL FUNCTION

Mushrooms that are good to eat also have very powerful medicinal properties. These are mushrooms like the common white button mushrooms, crimini, and portobello mushrooms, as well as shiitake, maitake, and oyster mushrooms. They improve immune system function, support healthy digestive functions, reduce inflammation in the gut, and provide important fiber to nourish and balance the microbiome.

In the last 10 years, we have discovered that the microbiome governs more than just a healthy stool or digestive function. The microbiome speaks to all aspects of health throughout every system in the body and has a strong influence on longevity and quality of life.

DIETARY SUPPLEMENTS = DIGESTION "BOOSTERS"

One of the highest callings of dietary supplements is that they are able to address many problems of the GI tract that pharmaceuticals do not.

The digestive system is complicated, having many "moving parts." These parts of a healthy digestive system include:

- Digestive enzymes that break down ingested food; these enzymes are secreted by the salivary glands, pancreas, stomach, and small intestine.

- Intestinal bacterial populations, also known as the "microbiome"

- Liver function that produces bile acids and breaks down toxins that have been absorbed from food.

- A very vigilant and active immune system

- The "organs of digestion" include the mouth, teeth, tongue, salivary glands, stomach, gall bladder, liver, small and large intestines, cecum, colon, and rectum.

Most of our pets eat dry commercial kibble that is highly processed and manufactured from less expensive and poorer quality ingredients. Dry pet foods are so processed that they can be kept in storage for years and still, according to the manufacturer, contain vital nutrition.

Even the very expensive, made-from-human-ingredients foods

are overly processed and not as nutritionally sufficient as a wholesome whole-food diet that is freshly prepared daily or weekly.

That adage "you are what you eat" certainly applies here. Poor diets create a poorly functioning digestive system.

This is why I recommend that certain supplements be given with each meal of kibble.

Digestive Enzymes

The pancreas produces enzymes that digest our food after our teeth have ground the food down into smaller pieces in the presence of digestive enzymes in the saliva. The hydrochloric acid and enzymes in the stomach begin the process of breaking down the chewed and partially digested food into smaller pieces that can then be easily absorbed in the gut.

When digestive enzymes are added to the meal, they pre-digest the food so that when the food travels through the stomach and into the small intestine where it encounters pancreatic enzymes, the food becomes more completely digested.

Food allergies are thought to occur when certain parts of the protein molecules in the food stimulate the immune system for a variety of different reasons. The immune system reacts to the food by increasing inflammation and increasing the bowel's motility or peristalsis.

Peristalsis is the movement of food through the digestive tract caused by the contractions of the bowel. If the food moves too quickly, there isn't time for the water in the digested food to be reabsorbed. When the water in the digested food isn't reabsorbed enough, wet, liquid diarrhea results, although for some dogs the stools may simply be soft and formless.

Digestive enzymes help to break down the parts of the protein molecule that your pet is allergic to, which will reduce food allergy symptoms. There are pet diets that have their protein partially digested or "hydrolyzed," and these hydrolyzed antigen diets are considered to be less allergenic than diets that do not have their protein pre-digested.

Adding digestive enzymes to your pet's food is the equivalent of feeding a hydrolyzed protein diet if you use enough enzymes with each meal and the enzymes you are using are potent enough to digest protein.

The use of digestive enzymes can reduce soft stools and diarrhea secondary to the partial digestion of the food and can improve the absorption of the nutrients derived from a meal. Increased bowel motility, soft stools, and diarrhea result in lost nutrients.

Prebiotics, Probiotics, Synbiotics, Postbiotics, and the Microbiome

There are hundreds of strains of bacteria, yeast, protozoa, and fungi in our gut and our pets' guts. The sum total of these microorganisms is called the "microbiome." Recent research has determined that the microbiome in our gut, skin, and elsewhere is what determines our health. When the microbiome is out of balance, then we can see inflammatory bowel problems, dermatitis, allergies, immune-mediated problems, and a host of other conditions that are hard to resolve without improving the health of the microbiome.

By inoculating the bowel daily with living cultures of bacteria and other microorganisms, the health of the microbiome can be restored or maintained.

Each individual's microbiome is unique. The microbiome consists of different "classes" of microorganisms. Some people call these classes "tribes" as another descriptor for them. The health of the microbiome and the body as a whole needs to have certain tribes present in higher amounts than other tribes. This is expressed as a ratio between each of these tribes.

Other ratios of tribes are indicators of poor health and can relate to specific diseases. They have even found that when you take the microbiome from an obese person and transplant it into the bowel of a normal-weight, healthy person, that healthy, normal-weight person will then become obese! Crazy, huh?

Not all probiotics work the same, nor do they all have the same species of microorganisms. I've found a few probiotic products that seem to work for my patients, but sometimes I have to switch them up or try something new until I find the probiotic that works for that specific critter's microbiome.

It is known that all mushrooms have beneficial effects on the microbiome due to their microbiome-friendly fiber and the immune-modulating properties of their beta-glucans.[104]

Fecal transplantation is a procedure in which the healthy stool from a healthy patient is given to another patient with GI issues. Commonly, the feces is transferred by retention enema or endoscopy, but for dogs, filling capsules with healthy, fresh stool and then hiding the capsules in some tasty food is another way to get the good bugs where they belong.

They are finding amazing results with these procedures. Patients who have been on strong steroids and other energy-suppressive drugs for years to treat ulcerative colitis, for instance, are able to discontinue these drugs after successful transplants.

If you've ever wondered why dogs eat poop, perhaps this helps explain that!

(Just don't let them lick you after a tootsie roll meal!)

DIGESTIVE HERBS AND NUTRACEUTICALS

There are a few herbs that have been in use for millennia by humans for themselves and their animal's digestive health (pets and livestock). These herbs are safe and inexpensive, and they work really well.

When these herbs are combined with dietary changes and digestion boosters (digestive enzymes and probiotics)—and sometimes combined with the use of cannabis and mushrooms, as appropriate—many conditions that have been considered hopeless to treat by Western medical experts can be much better managed or even completely resolved using herbs, diet, and digestive boosters.

Ginger Root (Zingiber officinale)

One of the oldest herbs continuously in use by humans since before written history, ginger root, in addition to adding spicy flavor, and having food preservative and anti-microbial properties, has a very strong benefit to digestive function.

Ginger root has anti-nausea and anti-emetic (vomiting) properties and can stop diarrhea, as well as increase appetite. Even the culinary spice on your kitchen shelves can be used.

Ginger Root Tea Recipe

½ teaspoon of powdered dried ginger root in 6 ounces of hot water. Give this, when it cools, to your pet with nausea or vomiting. Give a few milliliters of the ginger tea with a dose syringe by mouth every hour if the vomiting continues.

If vomiting continues further, it's a good idea to take your pet to see your veterinarian.

Sometimes, dogs will chew things up that don't get digested and that stay stuck in their stomachs. Sometimes, surgery is needed to remove the object from the stomach. We call that object a "foreign body." Until it is removed, it will continue to cause your dog to vomit.

Licorice Root (*Glycyrrhiza spp.*)

We think of licorice as candy because it is 50 times sweeter than sugar. But licorice root has some very strong properties as an herb and can be very good at helping soothe the inflamed lining of the stomach and/or small and large intestines. Although very sweet, licorice does not stimulate insulin release, so it is considered to be a low-glycemic herb.

Historically, licorice root was used to help with gastric ulcers due to its protective effect on the stomach lining. A tea made from licorice root can help soothe the irritated bowel lining and provide some relief to your pet. Other than gastritis, it can also help with colitis and an irritable or inflamed bowel.

Licorice Root Tea Recipe

Tea bags of licorice root can be found commercially available. I've found it in some local supermarkets, and it can be found online.

Steeping the tea bag for about 15 minutes will infuse the hot water with the active molecules found in the licorice root, and you can take that tea, once cooled, and syringe it into your pet directly, or you can mix it with a small amount of their food and give it to them that way. I recommend giving it three times daily for the best effect.

Give 1-3 cc for pets weighing 0-25 pounds, 3-6 cc for pets weighing 25-75 pounds, and 6-10 cc for pets weighing more than 75 pounds.

Dosing an herb like licorice is approximate, and there is no problem with giving a higher dose of the licorice root, as long as you don't exceed giving it daily for more than two weeks at a time. This is because licorice root also causes sodium retention, which, over time, can lead to hypertension.

Marshmallow Root (*Althaea officinalis*)

This is not the sugary marshmallow of sweet confections. It is derived from the root of the *Althaea officinalis* plant, the marshmallow plant. It has the herbal quality of *"demulcent,"* which means that when mixed with water, it forms a mucoid gel (mucilage) that is very soothing to inflamed mucus membrane surfaces, such as we see with inflammatory conditions of the stomach and bowel.

This common herb is safe to use. Marshmallow root has very little taste, so it is well-accepted by most pets and can be mixed into your pet's food quite easily.

As a demulcent, marshmallow root is high in mucilage (slippery/slimy/soothing material) and is hydrophilic, attracting and absorbing water to form the mucilage. Therefore, for marshmallow root, slippery elm, and psyllium, plenty of water needs to be given to reduce the possibility of the mucilage creating a blockage if there is not enough liquid in it to allow it to pass through the bowel unobstructed.

Dosing marshmallow root is approximate. Usually, it comes as a powder, and you would use from ¼ to 1 teaspoon serving each time, depending on your pet's size and how severe its condition is.

Psyllium Seed (*Plantago ovata*)

The seed of the psyllium plant, *Plantago ovata*, is a rich source of both soluble and insoluble fiber. It is the active ingredient in the commercial product Metamucil™ and can help with both constipation and diarrhea.

Psyllium can also help cats who are constantly troubled with hairballs and vomiting. Psyllium seed is very similar in properties to marshmallow root and can be used interchangeably, although psyllium has more demulcent material per unit of herb than marshmallow root.

Psyllium absorbs water in the gut and will expand, thus it needs to be given with water to not cause dehydration from consuming internal fluids. If the constipation or diarrhea is due to a foreign body obstructing the bowel, psyllium may not help in that situation.

Dosing psyllium is approximate, loosely based on your pet's size. I recommend adding ¼-1 teaspoon mixed in with your pet's food and a little extra water added to that blend. It should be given two or three times daily until the desired effect is achieved: firmed-up stools or passage of the hardened, constipated stools.

Aloe Vera Juice (*Aloe barbadensis*)

Aloe vera contains a constituent that soothes inflamed skin and mucous membranes and promotes healing all at the same time. Allantoin is found both in aloe vera and also in the comfrey plant (*Symphytum officinale*). It is well known for its healing properties. Allantoin has demulcent properties but will also speed up healing.

Unfortunately, the comfrey plant also contains some compounds that are toxic to the liver, so comfrey is best used topically.

Aloe vera juice or gel, on the other hand, is absolutely safe to ingest. You can find aloe vera juice or gel sold by the gallon in some health food stores or even grocery stores.

Aloe can be used topically on rashes, wounds, and sores, but can also be ingested to benefit the inflamed mucous surfaces of the lining of the bowel, from stomach to anus. I've found it very useful for my patients with inflammatory bowel disease, oral inflammatory disease, and even peri-rectal inflammation. It is safe, well-tolerated, and fairly bland, so most animals will readily accept it when mixed with a small amount of tasty food.

I suggest giving these approximate amounts of aloe vera based on your pet's weight:

- 0-10 pounds: 1 cc 2-3 times daily

- 10-25 pounds: 2 cc 2-3 times daily

- 25-50 pounds: 3 cc 2-3 times daily

- 50-75 pounds: 4 cc 2-3 times daily

- 75-100+ pounds: 5-6 cc 2-3 times daily

Slippery Elm (*Ulmus rubra*)

Slippery elm is another herb that has demulcent properties much like psyllium, marshmallow root, and the allantoin from aloe or comfrey. The herbal material is derived from the inner bark of the slippery elm tree.

Slippery elm is becoming over-harvested, so the use of alternate demulcents is an environmentally sound idea. However, slippery elm is particularly good at soothing inflamed mucous membrane linings, so if your pet's GI inflammation is severe, I would recommend using it at first to help reduce your pet's discomfort.

Slippery elm is usually supplied as a powder, which when mixed with water, will develop its typical mucilaginous consistency as a demulcent.

Dosing of slippery elm is approximate. Add ¼-1 teaspoon mixed in with your pet's food and a little extra water added to that blend, which should be given two or three times daily until your pet's condition seems to improve.

L-glutamine

L-glutamine is an amino acid that, in addition to being a part of many protein molecules, has a beneficial effect on the lining of the bowel. I have used glutamine as a treatment for diarrhea with great success. Glutamine is the preferred food for the cells that line the small intestine and will help repair and restore the damaged lining of the gut.

It can help to overcome the problem of leaky gut, which can lead to immune system issues, and can help repair the bowel from damage done to it from cancer chemotherapy or radiation damage.

Glutamine generally can be found as a product that comes either as a powder or in 250-500 mg capsules.

Dosing glutamine by weight is ideal, and the textbooks recommend 0.25 mg/kg with food twice daily, which translates to 0.11 mg/pound with food twice daily.

N-acetyl D-glucosamine (NAG)

NAG is found in mushroom chitin-fiber, which is good for the microbiome. This is not the glucosamine we are normally used to thinking about with joint health. This form of glucosamine is a building block for connective tissue in the bowel, joint, urinary bladder, and skin. Inflammatory conditions degrade the integrity and strength of the connective tissue that holds together the matrix of the cells in a given organ.

By adding NAG as a supplement, you can help rebuild the strength of the connective tissue damaged by chronic inflammation. L-glutamine and NAG are two of my most frequent go-to supplements to help with inflammatory bowel disease entities and leaky gut syndrome.

Edible mushrooms, like the oyster mushroom, shiitake mushroom, maitake mushroom, and even the common white button mushroom, all have a high content of indigestible fiber (beta-glucan polysaccharides and chitin) that is a great food for the microbiome but which also contains a natural source of N-acetyl D-glucosamine. It's important to cook your mushrooms, as they need the heat to release the beta-glucans and chitin.

Some people don't like eating mushrooms. It might be their "umami" taste, or it might be that they are a little bit "chewy" and a bit slippery, tending to be a bit "slimy" in texture. This is the glucosamine. We use glucosamine orally because it provides a slippery nature to the joint fluid, thus reducing the friction that causes inflammation and joint pain. Similarly, when mushrooms are eaten for their chitin (think N-acetyl D-glucosamine), that slippery nature of the glucosamine coats the lining of the gut and the mucosal epithelial cells and protects them from inflammation and toxic insults. It helps to repair a leaky gut by healing the disrupted gut wall integrity.

Dosing for NAG is similar to how we dose glucosamine sulfate for joints:

<50 pounds	250-500 mg twice daily
50- 75 pounds	500-750 mg twice daily
75- 100+ pounds	1,000 mg twice daily

CONVENTIONAL PHARMACEUTICAL APPROACHES

In my 40-year career as a veterinarian, I've developed some tricks and tools for helping pets with digestive issues that I am sharing with you here.

This is in addition to blending in cannabinoids and mushrooms for digestive problems.

Conventional approaches to treat IBS/IBD, idiopathic chronic diarrhea, and colitis utilize the use of antibiotics, motility modifiers, special diets that are high in fiber, or other diets that are formulated to be limited in common antigens.

Antibiotics

Treat bacterial overgrowth that promotes inflammation

Pharmaceuticals can be used, such as metronidazole, tylosin, or cephalexin, that help reduce inflammation in the bowel and remove populations of bacteria in the bowel that might be contributing to the bowel inflammation and diarrhea.

Anti-inflammatories

Reduce pain and straining

The steroid budesonide has been shown to be effective for IBS/IBD in cats and dogs. Typically, this pharmaceutical (Entocort™) is provided in 3 mg capsules, which is more than most veterinary patients will need. Budesonide can be compounded into smaller dosages for small animals, such as cats and small dogs.

Although budesonide is a steroid, it doesn't have as many adverse effects on the liver as most steroids do. Dosing with budesonide over a prolonged period of time can affect the pituitary-adrenal axis, which can have some unwanted side effects.

Steroids like prednisone or prednisolone are much stronger than budesonide and are more commonly used to reduce the symptoms of IBS/IBD or colitis by veterinarians than budesonide. These steroids will have an adverse effect on the liver, causing your pet to drink excessively, urinate excessively, and have a huge appetite, which isn't from the "munchies." Prolonged use of prednisone or prednisolone may also cause your pet's hair to thin and fall out and may cause them to have a pot-bellied appearance.

Motility Modifiers

Slow down diarrhea or vomiting

These drugs and supplements help reduce the straining and diarrhea commonly associated with these inflammatory bowel diseases. Controlling straining reduces your pet's discomfort and pain. Motility modifiers are not commonly associated with side effects and can make your household tidier without so much loose stool to be constantly cleaned up, not to mention improving your pet's quality of life.

We don't really want to "put a cork in it" so to speak, as the function of diarrhea is to remove pathogens and inflammation from the bowel. Diarrhea can be associated with the loss of bodily fluids, leading to dehydration.

The anal glands will not get expressed with chronic diarrhea, which results in pressure and discomfort around the anus. The anal glands are normal glandular structures that secrete a smelly fluid. They are vestigial organs that evolved from the scent glands of skunks and ferrets that use them for repelling predators.

With each defecation, when the dog squeezes down to "pinch a loaf," the pressure of the anal muscles against the firm stool causes these glands to normally empty with each passage of stool. With diarrhea, that counter pressure isn't there, which results in the anal glands filling up.

The buildup of secretions in these anal glands can progress to infections and abscesses that may need to be treated by manually emptying them and with antibiotics. When your pet has full anal glands, they are uncomfortable, and they will "scoot" on their hind end, rubbing their anal area on the ground (or carpet, leaving a brown "hash mark") in an effort to release the pressure in these glands.

A "lovely," unmistakable odor will also be produced when these anal glands are expressed, either by this scooting behavior or when the vet expresses them. If your dog gets scared, it will squeeze its butt muscles in fear, and this causes these glands to empty their smelly contents. In a way, it's the smell of "fear" for a dog.

Commonly Prescribed Pharmaceuticals for Appetite and Motility Issues:

- Metoclopramide (Reglan™):
    - Promotility drug, reduces nausea and vomiting
- Loperamide (Imodium™)
    - Reduces bowel motility and decreases diarrhea
- Maropitant (Cerenia™)
    - Reduces vomiting and improves appetite
- Mirtazapine (Miratz™)
    - Improves appetite and reduces vomiting
- Capromelin (Entyce™)
    - Improves appetite
- Cyproheptadine (Periactin™)
    - Improves appetite

DIET – THE MOST IMPORTANT THING
TO CHANGE WITH DIGESTIVE PROBLEMS
(Seems obvious, but it's not always that easy.)

How I learned to make home-prepared pet diets:

I've been a veterinarian since I graduated from Colorado State University's College of Veterinary Medicine in 1982. After three years in practice, I was frustrated with my inability to help those patients with complex chronic disease issues. Think diabetes, cancer, epilepsy, inflammatory bowel disease, allergies, and so on.

In 1985, I started looking at home-prepared diets as a way to improve the health of my patients. I was doing house calls then in a mountain community near Colorado Springs, and my clients were asking me to help them by providing information about holistic alternatives and instruction in home-prepared diets. That began my lifelong journey in integrative medicine, nearly 40 years ago!

I began to educate myself about holistic and integrative approaches to pet health at that time. There wasn't much available then in terms of books, classes, or study programs, so I just started reading and talking to other like-minded veterinarians, naturopathic physicians, and veterinary nutritionists to begin my long process, which is still ongoing, of learning new and unique approaches to provide natural healing "technology" to my patients.

The first thing I learned was how to teach my clients the process of putting together a home-prepared diet that would help with their pets' diseases or, better, provide a path to "wellness." These diets needed to be complete, balanced, fairly easy for my clients to accomplish, and fit in with their pet expense budgets.

The diets I began with were much more carbohydrate-heavy than what I recommend now. As nutritional science reveals more facts about the nutritional needs of dogs and cats, so have my diet nutrient profiles adapted to the new and emerging data.

I was very surprised, and quite pleased when my clients would return months later after feeding their pets in this natural way to find that for many of them, feeding wholesome, minimally-processed food also had a beneficial effect on their chronic disease problem.

This was such amazing, positive feedback, that it really got me going with my diet recommendations, and I started sharing this information with my veterinary colleagues in presentations I was giving at veterinary medical conferences.

At that time, the natural pet diet industry was just starting to take off. Raw diets were just being introduced. As a result of my expertise with homemade and raw diets, one of the largest raw pet food diet companies at the time, Nature's Variety™, recruited me to work with them!

This section will specifically speak to the use of food to help resolve the digestive problems I've been discussing. In some cases, there may be commercial diets that can help with digestive issues. Regardless of which approach you use (commercial vs. home-prepared), when digestive issues don't resolve quickly on their own or do not respond to conventional therapeutics, the first thing I do is change the pet's diet to try to help improve things.

Our pets can develop sensitivities or allergies to ingredients in the foods we feed them. It is unknown how or why one pet will have this problem and another will not. Genetics may play a role, as well as environmental influences while they are very young puppies. Once food allergies or sensitivities are established, it's very uncommon, but not impossible, for them to resolve on their own.

My goal is to create a diet that is less reactive to the pet's digestive and immune systems. We do that by finding out which food ingredients are reactive for our four-legged friend. Once we know that, we can find a commercial diet, or more often, prepare a homemade diet, that does not contain the ingredients to which the pet is sensitive.

Pets who develop food allergies and sensitivities can eventually develop sensitivities to the foods to which they once were not reactive. With daily exposure to those non-reactive ingredients, over time, maybe a month, maybe six months, maybe a year (each dog will determine how long it takes for them), they can become reactive to that formerly non-reactive ingredient. This means you will need to eliminate that reactive food ingredient and find food to which they are not reactive. This can be a real merry-go-round of diet changing and can drive both the pet parent *and veterinarian* crazy!

FOOD SENSITIVITY AND ALLERGY TESTING

The solution to chasing that merry-go-round of ingredient sensitivities is to identify those ingredients to which your pet is **NOT** sensitive. Once you have determined that, by one of two methods that I will detail in the following paragraphs, you will want to feed one set of these non-reactive foods for a period of time, and then, before your pet establishes sensitivity to these previously non-reactive foods, change to the next set of non-reactive foods.

How do you know how long to wait before changing to the second set of non-reactive foods?

Each animal will carve out its own time interval between introducing a new set of non-reactive ingredients and the time it takes for them to become reactive. The only way to figure out how long it takes for your pet to become reactive to a set of ingredients is to measure the amount of time it takes your pet to become sensitive to the first set of non-reactive foods, and then you "sacrifice" that non-reactive ingredient to this testing process. This will tell you how long to wait before making the switch to a novel set of ingredients. (Make the switch well before the time period you have determined!)

Some vets recommend simply switching ingredients every three months to get ahead of the process whereby non-reactive ingredients become reactive.

How do you know what food ingredients are non-reactive?

The traditional approach to determining which ingredients an individual is sensitive to is the "elimination diet."

In an elimination diet, you feed a very bland, simple diet that your pet is not reactive to for three to four weeks, then start introducing food ingredients, one at a time, and look to your pet to show its reaction or sensitivity to that food ingredient.

Typical bland, non-reactive diets to feed in this initial three to four week period of time can be as simple as an all-potato diet or a similar bland, simple diet. Feeding all potatoes for a month will not cause any problems with most pets' nutritional levels, but be sure to check with your vet first to see if they think your pet's level of health can handle a month with a mono diet like all potatoes.

After adding the first ingredient to the mono diet, try a second ingredient, and so on until you've tried enough ingredients that you have a list of these ingredients. This way, you can create several different diets that are "hypoallergenic" or low sensitivity. It takes quite a bit of time and methodical work to use an elimination diet to determine non-reactive food ingredients. The method below is a test that can give you answers for 24 food ingredients within a few weeks.

Saliva Test for Food Sensitivities

The Nutriscan™ test was developed by my good friend and veterinary colleague, Dr. Jean Dodds. It uses saliva as the test fluid, and it is collected by you, in your home, using a small little rope that you place in your dog or cat's mouth to absorb saliva. You then put that saliva-soaked rope into a mailer and send it off to Nutriscan™ for analysis.

The Nutriscan™ test can analyze proteins in your dog's saliva for sensitivity to 24 different foods. This test can even tell you if your dog is sensitive to white fish versus red fish (salmon), which can be important if you are giving fish oil to help solve the allergy problem when in fact, it could be a part of the problem due to salmon or white fish sensitivity.

Once you have this list of ingredients that won't set off alarms in your pet's immune system, then you need to find food that doesn't have any of the offending ingredients in it. Pet diets, as scientifically formulated as they are, are still mass-produced commercially. They contain fixed sets of ingredients that don't change. They also are processed at high temperatures and pressures, which can change the molecular structure of the food to make it more allergenic and potentially pro-inflammatory.

There may be non-food substances in your pet's commercially processed diet or molecular changes in the food molecules that were created by the heat and pressures of processing. These secondary molecules, or non-nutritional molecules that might be used in the processing, aren't listed on the label but may also cause your pet to react.

By preparing a complete and balanced homemade pet diet, you are best able to include only those ingredients that are safe and non-reactive, which will help your pet's food issues. The wholesome nature of fresh food and its high moisture content will also provide your pet with improvements in its health and especially its digestive health.

Sometimes, the perfect solution to finding a food that is perfect for your perfect pet is to make it yourself.

HOME PREPARED MEALS (AND RAW VERSUS COOKED)

A veterinary nutritionist from whom I have learned a lot once said to me:

"The best diet in the world is a well-balanced home-prepared meal. But the worst diet in the world is an unbalanced home-prepared meal."

This means that although a wholesome, fresh, unprocessed (as much as possible) diet can promote health due to a large number of fresh nutrients and especially micronutrients present if that food is not scientifically balanced to meet the nutritional needs of your pet, it can cause a lot of nutritional problems over time.

We all need to be sure there is adequate calcium in our diets. In the wild, dogs would eat the bones of their prey and thus would get calcium, which is needed for strong bones and many other important functions in the body. Calcium is balanced in the body by phosphorus. You don't want to have too much or too little of either. There is a delicate balance between calcium and phosphorus in the body, and the dietary content of calcium and phosphorus needs to reflect this balance between these two important minerals.

If the balance between these two minerals becomes off, our bones would soften, our kidneys would fail, and the excess calcium in our blood could cause cardiac problems. Thus, it is important that homemade pet diets have adequate calcium—just enough, but not too much.

Calcium requirements vary based on the individual needs of your pet. Young animals usually need more calcium and protein, but if your dog is a large giant breed puppy, such as a Great Dane, for instance, then you need to be careful not to supplement with too much calcium, protein, or carbohydrates, thinking that a big dog needs big calcium and big nutrients. Relatively speaking, we feed giant breed puppies less calcium per body weight than a smaller dog. If we don't, then that puppy is more likely to develop problems with the formation of their bones, which could cause a lifetime of misery.

It is beyond the scope of this section to actually give recipes. In the Resource section at the end of this book, pet food preparation books and websites are listed for you.

I have found, in my 40 years of clinical practice, that diet change can be the most important "medicine" for pets with ongoing digestive problems that have not otherwise been easily solved with supplements or pharmaceuticals.

Pets with special needs can have those needs satisfied with a home-prepared diet:

- Home-prepared diets can help a pet lose weight.

- They can help control phosphorus and protein in pets with kidney disease.

- They can help if your pet has liver disease.

- Some diets can be made to be anti-inflammatory by the ingredients you are adding, such as flavonoids from brightly colored vegetables like beets, green beans, and carrots.

- Cancer patients who are on chemotherapy often lose their appetite. Home-prepared meals can get them back to eating again.

- Some pet cancer patients will respond to a ketogenic diet, which can be easily prepared fresh and wholesome in your kitchen.

- If your pet has a lot of food sensitivities, it may be impossible to find a commercially available food that meets their needs. Pets with chronic digestive issues often will improve when given fresh, wholesome home-prepared foods versus dry, processed kibble.

DOC SILVER'S HOME-PREPARED MEAL GUIDELINES

I have been recommending home-prepared pet diets for the majority of my 40+ year career as a veterinarian.

My observations over this long period of time are that pets do so much better when they get "real" food that is minimally processed, nutrient-dense, and wholesome. Whether they have a digestive complaint, full-on cancer, or just want to prevent bad things from happening from poor diets, my patients on these home-prepared diets have always done better.

I've not observed any downsides to this process other than the time, energy, attention to detail, and cost that home pet food preparation involves. For the pet parent who is fully committed to enabling their pet's optimal health, these time, energy, and financial costs are a drop in the bucket.

Creating a home-prepared meal takes time and attention to detail, but the rewards are huge. Nothing can ever replace the sheer joy your pets will have watching (maybe not so patiently) as you prepare their meal for them. There is nothing like watching your pets watch you while you are preparing their food; it is truly a wonderful bonding time for human and animal!

My approach to home preparing pet diets is more of an outline, or template, as compared to a detailed recipe with exact amounts to use per meal or week of meals. This allows flexibility in ingredients to tailor the diet to the individuality of your pet's specific needs.

I start each diet recipe with a "nutrient profile" adapted to that pet's specific and individual needs.

A *"nutrient profile" is the relative proportions of the macronutrients (protein, carbohydrates, fats, and minerals).*

Questions About Your Pet We Need to Design a Home-Prepared Diet:

- Is the pet overweight?
- What is the pet's weight and body condition score (BCS)?
- Does the pet have a specific condition that needs to be addressed with diet, such as reduced protein and phosphorus with kidney disease diets?
- What life stage is the pet in? Puppy, adult, or geriatric?
- If a puppy, is the pet a giant breed that would need to have its calcium and protein intake modified to prevent developmental bone diseases?
- Does the pet have cancer?
- Does the pet have another degenerative disease?
- How is the pet's digestive system?

I take into account these patient considerations, and from them, I design a diet recipe using percentages, or proportions, of each food category we are putting into this recipe.

CANINE NUTRIENT PROFILES

Measurements

Volume measurement in cups is not as accurate as the measured weight of these ingredients, but it is close enough for short-term use. If you measure the weight of the ingredients and then measure their volume, you can use that volume measurement to speed up the process for future food preparations.

How to Start

Initially, when you are determining the best ingredients and best nutrient profile to use for your pet, it makes more sense to put together just a few days' worth at a time of the diet. Over time, as you are more comfortable with the details of diet preparation, if your pet is thriving with the amounts you are feeding, and the nutrient profile of ingredients looks to be good, you can then begin batch preparations.

Batch Preparation Can Make Your Life Easier

A larger amount of food can be prepared at a time and then frozen into daily serving portions to simplify your time and your life. These portions can then be thawed out, warmed up, and served as meals for your pet.

Standard Diet Ratio

This diet is for a healthy adult dog with normal weight and activity.

Use this Recipe Ratio:
- Protein: 33%
- Carbohydrates: 33%
- Vegetables: 33%

How Much Healthy Fats to Add?

We add healthy fats generally as oils or powders. Flax seed meal is very rich in omega-3 and omega-6 oils, as is hemp seed meal. Fish oil provides the more potent omega-3 fatty acids. A variety of different types of fats in each meal makes for a much healthier diet.

For each meal, my suggestion is to add a teaspoon of flax seed or hemp seed meal for every 15 pounds of your pet's body weight, or 1 tablespoon for every 45 pounds of body weight in each meal.

Fish oil is added according to the amount of fish oil fatty acids present in the supplement you are using. The basic formula is 25 mg of the sum of the EPA+DHA in your supplement for each pound of body weight given in each meal twice daily. If you are only feeding once daily, then you need to give this total daily amount in that one single meal feed.

We can use nutrient profile ratios like the one above for a healthy dog, or the ones below to modify any diet to match the nutritional needs of your pooch. A pet may need a different diet ratio and specific ingredients to support their special nutritional needs if they have obesity, digestive disease, liver disease, kidney disease, heart disease, allergies, or cancer.

Lower Protein Diet Ratio

This diet is for chronic renal disease or other conditions requiring lower protein levels.

<u>Use this Recipe Ratio:</u>
- Protein: 25%
- Carbohydrate: 25-50% (use less carbohydrates if your dog is sensitive to carbohydrates)
- Vegetable: 25-50% (use more vegetables if your dog is sensitive to carbohydrates)

Higher Protein Diet Ratio

This diet is for when higher protein is needed.

This diet is beneficial to many growing dogs, except for the giant breeds, such as the Great Dane, St. Bernard, Newfoundland, Great Pyrenees, or mastiff. In other cases, there can be protein loss through the kidneys or digestive system and a higher-protein diet content can help to replace that pathological loss of protein.

<u>Use this Recipe Ratio:</u>
- Protein: 60%
- Carbohydrate: 20%
- Vegetable: 20%

D. The "Ketogenic Diet" Ratio

This diet is for cancer, epilepsy, and some types of behavior associated with epilepsy.

Ketosis is the condition where the metabolism of the individual changes from using carbohydrates for energy to using fats for energy. Carbohydrates are digested into smaller simple sugars before they are converted to energy. Fats, in the absence of sufficient carbohydrates or protein, will be metabolized for their energy into ketones, which can be measured in the urine and blood. Ketones are a good source of energy and for help control cancer and epilepsy.

Use this Recipe Ratio:

- Protein: 50%
- Carbohydrate: 0-5%
- Vegetable: 45-50%

By adding extra fat calories to this diet in the form of medium chain triglycerides (MCT), it becomes a therapeutic "ketogenic diet" (see more on this under cancer and epilepsy diets).

Published studies tell us that you need about 10-15% of the total calories of the meal to come from this special type of oil, MCT. This is true whether you are feeding a commercial kibble, canned foods, or a home-prepared meal.

Additional fat calories to make it ketogenic:

- Each teaspoon of MCT contains about 41.5 kcals.

- We want the MCT fat calories to be equal to 10-15% of total calories to create "ketosis."

- We also need to add long-chain polyunsaturated fatty acids (PUFA) like hemp seed or flax seed oils that contain both omega-3 and omega-6 fatty acids, and, of course, the fish oil omega-3 fatty acids, EPA (eicosapentaenoic acid), and DHA (docosahexaenoic acid).

Dogs are what we consider "omnivores," or more correctly, "facultative carnivores," which means that they focus on meat but can use carbohydrates nutritionally. Vegetables provide dogs with micronutrients and fiber and are not very calorie-rich, so I also use veggies to help with weight loss in dogs. They fill them up but don't contribute to weight gain.

We can feed dogs a vegetarian or vegan diet as long as we make sure to add the nutrients they normally would be getting from the meat, such as vitamin B12 and certain amino acids. (If you are interested in preparing a plant-based diet for your dog, I recommend the book *The Plant Powered Dog* for details about how to prepare this kind of diet to be complete and balanced. You can find it at www.plantpowereddog.com.)

Wolves are predators in the canine family, but most dogs are opportunistic scavengers and will eat dead and rotten animals for foods. They are able to handle scavenging for food pretty well except for maybe a little diarrhea now and then.

Cats, on the other hand, are what we call "obligate (or strict) carnivores," which means they absolutely need meat as part of their diet due to their nutritional needs as carnivores. It is not appropriate for a cat's carnivorous metabolism to not feed it meat in each meal. Vegetables can provide valuable micronutrients, antioxidants, and fiber that feeds a healthy microbiome, although they have no need for it as a macronutrient.

FELINE NUTRIENT PROFILES

A. Standard Diet Ratio

Use this Recipe Ratio:
- Protein: 75%
- Carbohydrate: 10%
- Vegetable: 15%

B. Low Protein Diet Ratio

Use this Recipe Ratio:
- Protein: 50%
- Carbohydrate: 30%
- Vegetable: 30%

C. High Protein Diet Ratio

Use this Recipe Ratio:
- Protein: 90%
- Carbohydrate: 5%
- Vegetable: 5%

D. Ketogenic Diet Ratio

Use this Recipe Ratio:
- Protein: 75%
- Carbohydrates: 0%
- Vegetables: 25%

In many ways, because cats are obligate carnivores and get the majority of their calories from protein and fats, they are already on a ketogenic-like diet. We have very little information about ketogenic diets in cats as compared to the information about using these diets in dogs and people who have similar metabolisms, which are different than the metabolism of cats.

SOURCES OF HEALTHY FATTY ACIDS

I recommend that you use flax seed meal or hemp seed meal for the oil and fat ingredients to add to your pet's diet. Flax seed meal provides about 50/50 omega-3:omega-6 fatty acids. Hemp seed meal provides 25/75 omega 3:omega-6 fatty acids. Both seed meals have the added benefit of containing both soluble and insoluble fiber.

Flax and hemp seed are superfoods, and they contain other constituents that also contribute to health and wellness, including the flax "lignans," which have been found to bind and inactivate rogue toxic estrogen molecules, as well as corticosteroids in cases of atypical Cushing's disease.

1 tablespoon of flaxseed meal or hemp seed meal
= 1 teaspoon of oil

Using the above formula then, you would add:

1 tablespoon of flax seed meal for
every 15 pounds of body weight per meal

Borage, black current seed, and evening primrose seed all yield a similar oil blend to what is found in flax and hemp seed oils, but they also contain a unique anti-inflammatory fatty acid called "gamma-linolenic acid" (GLA), which has been found in published studies to work synergistically with fish oil and flax seed oil to increase the effect on inflammation, especially with dermatitis. The remaining fatty acid in these three seed oils is mainly linoleic acid. Borage oil has the highest content of GLA of these three oils.

The other sources of fatty acids that I recommend come <u>from marine sources and algae</u>. These are the EPA and DHA commonly found in fish oil but also present in krill oil, fish roe oil, green-lipped mussel oil and found in algal EPA/DHA. Giving these active anti-inflammatory fatty acids along with the omega-3s and omega-6s in the flax seed meal gives your pet a complete range of healthy oils.

How many polyunsaturated fatty acid (PUFA) fish oils (EPA+DHA) to add?

Figuring out how many fat calories to add to a diet depends on the total calories being fed to that specific animal. This is not easy to determine without some diet calculating tools, some of which are available online. I suggest that you speak with your vet about this and see if they can refer you to a veterinary nutritionist who can help you figure out how many fat calories to add to the meal to make it a ketogenic diet.

If we aren't trying to create a ketogenic diet, then we don't need to use MCTs, but a lesser amount of them than for a ketogenic diet would still be okay. Here are easy amounts to give based on your pet's ideal weight. If your pet is overweight, we need to estimate how much its ideal weight would be and then give an appropriate amount based on that ideal weight in each and every meal.

PUFAs, like those found in hemp seed meal or flaxseed meal, are in a convenient format to provide these fatty acids to your pet. These meals also contain soluble and insoluble fiber from the seeds, which are good for digestion and the microbiome.

Both of these seed meals are sensitive to light and heat. They will degrade rapidly (think, 12 weeks) when exposed to air and room temperature. They, along with fish oils or krill meal, need to be stored in the refrigerator when not in use.

I like the meal format; it's easier to administer, less likely to cause pancreatitis, and may degrade slower than the purified oil due to the oil being contained in the seed meal as a protective coating.

If using the meal format, it has the equivalent of 30% oil by weight (this is an average based on the individual characteristics of the specific meal you source).

This means that about 1 tablespoon of seed meal contains 1 teaspoon of the oil. I recommend this over just the oil, but either is fine.

Flax or Hemp Seed Oil
Keep refrigerated!

1 teaspoon per 15 pounds of body weight per meal

Flax or Hemp Seed Meal
Keep refrigerated!

Note: Use the meal, as the whole seeds are not very digestible.

1 tablespoon per 15 pounds of body weight per meal

Fish Oil (EPA+DHA)
Keep refrigerated!

Note: Use the sum of these two fatty acids to compute the amount to add to your pet's food daily.

50 mg of EPA+DHA for each pound of body weight daily; can be divided into two meals if you feed twice daily

This is the published anti-inflammatory dosage. Almost all chronic disease has an inflammatory component, so this is important to follow. We know from published research that it may take as long as three months for the full effect of this much fish oil to be measurable. There usually are early benefits before the three months are up.

For all dogs and cats, introduce seed meals and fish oils gradually so as to not overwhelm your pet's system. Without a gradual introduction, diarrhea or pancreatitis might occur. Take it slowly over a period of two to four weeks to introduce these oils and oily foods.

HOW MUCH TO FEED?

When designing a diet, it's important to calculate how many calories it contains, so you know how many calories to feed your pet. The number of calories a pet needs is dependent on their ideal weight, age, and activity level. Even with diets that give you an exact amount to feed based on weight, you still need to recalculate how much your pet is fed depending on whether they are staying stable, gaining, or losing weight.

If your pet started at its ideal weight and is losing weight on the diet you have put together, then you will need to add another 10% more food and observe its weight after two weeks to see if it is normalizing. If it is gaining weight, then you need to do the opposite. I'm recommending 10% up or down so that it won't gain or lose too much weight. If the 10% change does not do what you need it to do after two weeks, then increase or decrease the amount of food by another 10%, making it a 20% total change from the number of calories you started with.

If your pet has a body condition score (BCS) higher than its ideal body condition score, then you need to look at reducing its calorie intake over time to achieve its ideal weight. Increasing your pet's exercise levels will also help burn off those excess calories.

You can estimate what that ideal weight is yourself, but you might want to ask your vet to help you with this determination, as it can take some experience to figure it out accurately.

If your pet has a score lower than its ideal weight, then you will need to add more food to its daily ration to increase its weight to be ideal.

DETERMINING THE BODY CONDITION SCORE (BCS)

Finding your pet's ideal weight involves assessing your pet's body condition score (BCS). The BCS score is based not on weight but on your pet's body condition: thin, normal, overweight, or obese. BCS is based on your pet's lean-to-fat ratio, which you can assess by looking at your pet and by running your fingers along its chest to assess how much spare fat is over the rib cage. The weight measurement associated with this perfect BCS is termed its "ideal weight."

An **ideal body score** is when you can look top-down on your pet's back and see that it has a defined waistline. When you look at your pet from the side, you can see its belly curving up to its groin region, not hanging down or pendulous. When you run your fingers over your dog's rib cage, you should be able to feel the ribs plainly, not covered by too much fat but also not starkly outlined.

Feline body condition scores are similar to this but adapted to the feline physique.

Although the following advice is general, one starting point for dogs that I recommend is to start with a conservative amount of 1.0-1.5 cups of homemade food for each 20-25 pounds of ideal body weight daily. This can be divided into two meals a day.

Another guideline you can use to arrive at a starting amount of food to feed your dog is to take the number of cups of dry food you are feeding daily and multiply that by 1.5 to get the number of cups of fresh food to feed. Remember that dry food is 10% moisture, whereas fresh food is about 70% moisture, which gives us about a 50-60% increase in the amount of fresh food over dry food for a similar nutrient profile.

This guidance stands for both dogs and cats. Ultimately, you will need to start somewhere, and once you start feeding, you will know from your pet's weight gain, loss, or maintenance if you can stay with the same amount or need to increase or decrease it.

Generally, your dog or cat will love this fresh, wholesome food and should eat it completely in one feeding. If you are using raw meat as your protein source and live in a warm climate, be aware that over time, this food, if uneaten, may grow food-borne pathogens like E. coli or salmonella, which could be hazardous to your pet's health and possibly even your own or your family's health if they are exposed to these pathogens.

Feeding fresh food can help with weight loss simply because fresh, wholesome food has so much more moisture in it, without adding calories. Your dog or cat should feel full after eating, and this can also help them lose weight if they need to. Diets that are higher in protein and fats also will give your pet a sense of "satiety" and reduce their food "cravings" (even for food-obsessed Labs!).

THE BODY CONDITION SCORE CHART

These Body Condition Score Charts are used with the permission of the Association for Pet Obesity Prevention (APOP), which is a great resource, especially if your pet is overweight. Their website (www.petobesityprevention.org) provides excellent tools for you to use in feeding your dog or cat to bring their weight down (or up) to their ideal weight. We are experiencing both a pet obesity and human obesity epidemic, fueled in part by the plethora of processed, high-carbohydrate, low-nutritional value foods, that are essentially empty calories but taste good. When your pet, or you, eats food that is calorie dense but contains very few other nutrients than calories, we call that "empty calories," and it promotes eating more of the high calorie food to try and get the nutrients it does not contain. These processed foods with empty calories contribute to a lot of our obesity epidemic.

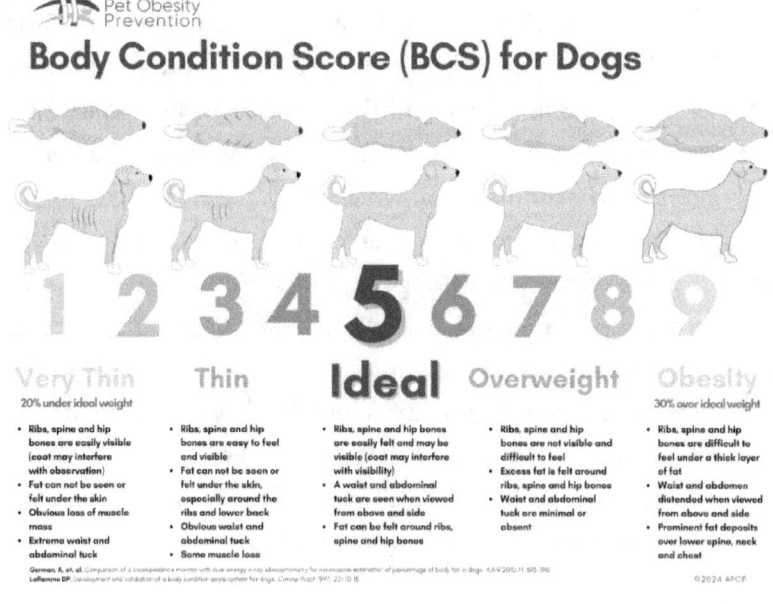

Association for
Pet Obesity
Prevention

Body Condition Score (BCS) for Dogs

1 2 3 4 5 6 7 8 9

Very Thin	Thin	**Ideal**	Overweight	Obesity
20% under ideal weight				30% over ideal weight
• Ribs, spine and hip bones are easily visible (coat may interfere with observation)	• Ribs, spine and hip bones are easy to feel and visible	• Ribs, spine and hip bones are easily felt and may be visible (coat may interfere with visibility)	• Ribs, spine and hip bones are not visible and difficult to feel	• Ribs, spine and hip bones are difficult to feel under a thick layer of fat
• Fat can not be seen or felt under the skin	• Fat can not be seen or felt under the skin, especially around the ribs and lower back	• A waist and abdominal tuck are seen when viewed from above and side	• Excess fat is felt around ribs, spine and hip bones	• Waist and abdomen distended when viewed from above and side
• Obvious loss of muscle mass	• Obvious waist and abdominal tuck	• Fat can be felt around ribs, spine and hip bones	• Waist and abdominal tuck are minimal or absent	• Prominent fat deposits over lower spine, neck and chest
• Extreme waist and abdominal tuck	• Some muscle loss			

German, A. et al. Comparison of a bioimpedance monitor with dual energy x-ray absorptiometry for non-invasive estimation of percentage of body fat in dogs. AJVR 2010;71:393-398.
Laflamme DP. Development and validation of a body condition score system for dogs. Canine Pract. 1997; 22:10-15.

©2024 APOP

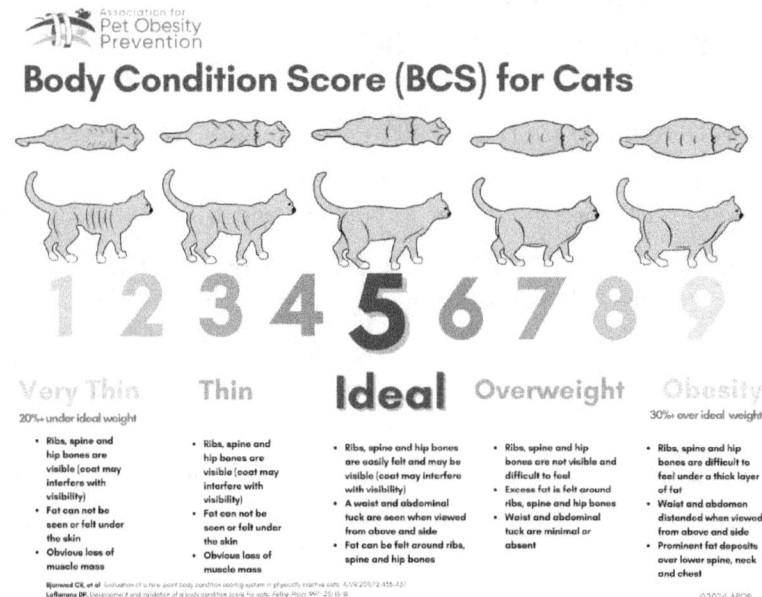

Body Condition Score (BCS) for Cats

Association for
Pet Obesity
Prevention

1 2 3 4 **5** 6 7 8 9

Very Thin   Thin   **Ideal**   Overweight   Obesity

20%+ under ideal weight   30%+ over ideal weight

- Ribs, spine and hip bones are visible (coat may interfere with visibility)
- Fat can not be seen or felt under the skin
- Obvious loss of muscle mass

- Ribs, spine and hip bones are visible (coat may interfere with visibility)
- Fat can not be seen or felt under the skin
- Obvious loss of muscle mass

- Ribs, spine and hip bones are easily felt and may be visible (coat may interfere with visibility)
- A waist and abdominal tuck are seen when viewed from above and side
- Fat can be felt around ribs, spine and hip bones

- Ribs, spine and hip bones are not visible and difficult to feel
- Excess fat is felt around ribs, spine and hip bones
- Waist and abdominal tuck are minimal or absent

- Ribs, spine and hip bones are difficult to feel under a thick layer of fat
- Waist and abdomen distended when viewed from above and side
- Prominent fat deposits over lower spine, neck and chest

Bjornvad CR, et al. *Evaluation of a nine-point body condition scoring system in physically inactive cats.* AJVR 2011;72:433-437.
LaFlamme DP. *Development and validation of a body condition score for cats.* Feline Pract 1997; 25:13-18.

©2024 APOP

Visit www.petobesityprevention.org
to learn more and download these charts.

INTRODUCING THE NEW DIET

As with anything new you are introducing to your dog that they ingest, such as supplements or a new diet, it is less likely that they will have a reaction to that supplement or new diet if you start with a much-reduced amount at the beginning.

Take out 10-25% of your dog's existing "old" diet and replace it with your new homemade food for a few days, all the while watching your dog's stools for your dog's acceptance of the food to make sure all is fine. If all is good with that smaller initial amount, then increasing that amount and reducing the amount of the old diet will allow you to fully introduce this new diet over 7-14 days.

MAKING THE DIET AS "COMPLETE" AND BALANCED AS POSSIBLE

Sources of Calcium for Healthy Bones and Metabolism

Adding calcium to the diet is important, and it is important that enough be added based on your pet's needs. When your pet is young and actively growing, or if your pet is now in that rapid growth stage, the amount of calcium it gets is very important.

If your dog is of the giant or large breed variety, then it's very important not to give them too much calcium or too much protein and carbohydrates, as these nutrients can cause bones to grow too quickly. We see developmental bone diseases arising as a result of this "over-nutrition." Your giant breed pup may wind up with unwanted developmental bone diseases, such as craniomandibular osteopathy, hypertrophic osteopathy, and osteochondritis dissecans (OCD).

As mentioned earlier, in order to provide adequate calcium to keep the bones strong, and to maintain normal nerve and muscle function, calcium needs to be added in sufficient amounts to each meal you are preparing. Sources of calcium can be as simple as dried eggshells ground up, which is an excellent source of calcium carbonate and is readily available if you also eat eggs.

Other popular sources include dried and powdered bone meal, calcium from coral reefs, dolomite, which has nearly as much magnesium as calcium, and chemicals such as dicalcium or tricalcium phosphate are all reliable sources of calcium.

Fresh, raw bones of certain types are safe to feed your dog as a source of calcium. Some dogs are better with bones than others. Some dogs have very large jaw muscles that allow them to crunch down on the bones safely and break them up into small enough pieces that can pass through the gut without causing damage.

Some types of bones, and some dogs with smaller jaw muscles, can cause serious problems, and in some cases, even death. Bones that splinter can get brittle when cooked and break into sharp, little pieces. This often happens with cooked bones, especially bones like the long bones of drumsticks, especially from turkeys and large chickens, and the rib bones of beef and pork.

Chicken neck bones, backbones that include the sacrum and pelvis, and chicken wing bones, when these bones are raw, are generally safe to feed most dogs, except for those small dogs with small jaws.

NOTE: *Due to the possibility of heavy metals such as lead, arsenic, and cadmium in mined minerals from the earth, like limestone and dolomite, be sure to check the bone meal, dolomite, and plant sources to* **see if they have been analyzed for these heavy metals,** *as these sources can often be contaminated.*

Giant breed puppies need less calcium and protein than other puppies, and those exact details are beyond the scope of this book. In the Resource section, I include contact information for veterinary nutritionists who, for a fee, will design a diet for your pet. That is one of the best ways to get a good recipe for the specific needs of your pet. There also are some websites that have calculators that will do that for a fee.

An alternative approach, if the thought of all of these calculations makes you break out in a cold sweat, is to use a commercially manufactured kibble diet, which is likely to have these calcium and protein levels accurate in the dry food, and then add healthy supplements and vegetables that are missing from the commercial dry food. This won't upset the delicate calcium-phosphorus balance or the amount of protein or carbohydrates needed to be fed.

Calcium, protein, and carbohydrates in excess can predispose a giant puppy to these "growing pains." By reducing the amount of these nutrients, we can discourage this dangerously fast growth.

IS RAW FOOD SAFE TO FEED?

There has been a lot of controversy over whether feeding complete and balanced raw food diets is nutritionally valuable and, at the same time, not dangerous due to being loaded with food-borne pathogens.

Raw meat diets may leave their manufacturing facility free of food-borne pathogens. How they are handled in transport, while on the shelf at the pet food store, or in your kitchen can introduce pathogens to the food. This is why it is important to observe hygienic food preparation practices in your kitchen. This will keep the food-borne pathogens in the food absent or as low as possible and also prevent its transmission to human members of your household.

When my daughter was crawling and just starting to walk, she watched with fascination as we prepared a homemade diet for our two dogs. She got caught up in the excitement that was generated by our dogs as they watched us prepare the meal. It followed naturally, then, that she wanted to try their food.

This is **NOT** a good idea! Dog digestive systems are generally much more resistant to food-borne pathogens than the digestive system of a one-year-old infant.

Removing the skin of chicken or turkey and rinsing off the surface of the raw meat can help remove fecal pathogens that were picked up at the slaughterhouse. Only the surface of the meat is contaminated, so rinsing it with clean water can remove most of these pathogens simply and easily.

You may be uncomfortable feeding raw food. That is not a problem.

Feeding raw food eliminates one step in the food preparation process, the cooking, which makes it easier and quicker to prepare. But there is nothing wrong with cooking your pet's meal at normal kitchen cooking temperatures that will kill food-borne pathogens. Try to avoid high heat and pressure when cooking their meals. Just as with commercial canned and dry dog foods, those high temperatures will destroy many of the delicate nutrients in the foods.

I suggest using the **meatloaf concept of food preparation** and baking up a number of meatloaves that can then be frozen and thawed out slice by slice as needed to serve a meal.

There is also a concern that raw diets may not be complete or balanced, as some are just meat and a few vegetables but are not nutritionally balanced. If you follow the ratio recipe guidelines and then add a calcium and mineral source, a fatty acid source, and a vitamin/mineral blend, you can bring the diet to become about as "complete" as a recipe can be.

There is nothing that can replace the native diet of our dogs and cats, which, to a large extent, would be raw meat, raw veggies, organs, glands, bones, and ligaments. Cats are predators, and their prey are commonly vermin and birds (although they would never turn down a tasty grasshopper, fly, moth, or even a garden snake).

But, it's impossible to create a "mouse in a can" and have it last on the shelf for two years without a substantial loss of nutrients.

You might think of me as a bit of a food nut with pets, but I've been feeding my own cats the "prey diet," which for them consists of one or two quail daily. I get the birds from a game bird producer. They have been killed and frozen. So first, I thaw them out, and then I skin the feathers off so they make less mess, and they eat the entire bird—beak, feet, guts, and all!

My last three cats lived to 19, 20, and 21 years of age, and our new Maine coon kitten is now eating two birds a day at 18 months and 18 pounds!

MEAL-BALANCING SUPPLEMENTS

Superfood Blend

I recommend mixing a blend of superfoods, whole food concentrates, and nutrient-dense powders. These are rich in vitamins, minerals, and micronutrients and **provide vitamins and trace minerals.**

One example of a **superfood blend** could contain:

Nutritional yeast	2 parts
Kelp powder	1 part
Flaxseed or hempseed meal	1 part
Sunflower lecithin	2 parts
Spirulina	½ part

This **superfood blend** will help you make your pet's homemade diet as complete and balanced as a home-prepared diet could be.

**Add 1 teaspoon of this blend
for every 15 pounds of your pet's ideal body weight.**

*When you add the superfood blend and a **variety of fatty acids** to your pet's meal in the forms recommended a little earlier, and finally, by adding enough **calcium to support healthy bones**, kidneys, and calcium metabolism, you have the makings of a complete and balanced diet.*

For **calcium supplementation,** I suggest you try the dried eggshell approach or source a powdered calcium source, such as bone meal, algae-based calcium, or even raw bones to help provide the calcium that dogs and cats need to keep their bones and kidneys healthy.

Calcium supplements that are ready-made for you to use (versus this DIY approach) are available in the marketplace, online, and in brick-and-mortar retail stores. Look for products that contain similar ingredients as I have been discussing here.

A general rule of thumb for dogs other than giant breed puppies is to give about 600 mg of calcium daily for every 10-15 pounds of ideal body weight.

Another way to look at this, with eggshell calcium, for instance, is to add ½ teaspoon of ground eggshells to each pound of food you are preparing. That is about 1 gram (1,000 mg of calcium) of calcium in those eggshells per pound of food.

Fatty Acid Blend Example:

Fish oil, krill meal, or algal oil	50 mg of oil per pound of body weight daily 1 teaspoon of krill meal per 15 pounds of body weight daily
Flaxseed or hemp seed meal	1-3 teaspoons per 15 pounds of body weight daily
Borage/black current seed/evening primrose oil (optional—best with skin problems)	1-3 teaspoons per 15 pounds of body weight daily

I have been recommending these home-prepared diets and diet-balancing supplements for the past 40 years of my career as a veterinarian. I've started puppies on it and have watched them mature into healthy adult dogs and then become geriatrics and pass away from old age. I know this diet works, that pets on it thrive, and that it is relatively easy for a pet parent to make up at home.

For ease and convenience, I recommend making the food in large batches and freezing daily serving portions that can be thawed out each night for the next day to make this process easier and less time-consuming.

There are as many approaches to pet diets as there are veterinarians, and my approach has worked for me and my patients. But if you find another approach that you resonate with more than this approach, by all means, give it a try. I do recommend discussing your desire to home-prepare meals with your veterinarian to keep them in the loop and to ask for their support and advice for the individuality of your four-legged best friend.

LIMITED ANTIGEN DIETS

These commercially available diets are an attempt at providing diets with single ingredients, thus making it less likely for many pets to have a reaction to the diet. The better limited antigen diets are made by companies that completely clean out the manufacturing equipment between each type of ingredient. It is known that ingredient residues persist in the manufacturing equipment from prior manufacturing run(s).

This residue may be sufficient in quantity to cause a pet to have an allergic reaction to that residue. The residues aren't listed on the label ingredients on the pet food bag or can but can cause a problem, nonetheless.

These can be good starter diets, and without testing for food sensitivities, can be a trial-and-error sort of thing. Some pet parents report good success with these diets when they pair them with a detailed analysis of food sensitivities, such as found with the saliva test from Nutriscan™ (www.nutriscan.org).

CHAPTER TEN SUMMARY

In Chapter Ten, we covered pet allergies and focused on Tawny's program, which can be easily adapted to your own dog or cat if they have similar issues. The use of the Nutriscan™ saliva testing has really improved my success rate with my patients while creating a diet less likely to be a risk for an immune system reaction, such as allergies. The diet information in this chapter can be applied to a pet with any need for a healthy diet.

There are many opportunities in the online marketplace and brick-and-mortar pet supply shops for a variety of already manufactured healthy diets. Once you learn what ingredients your four-legged friend is sensitive to, you can read ingredient labels to see if there is a diet already out there that is minimally processed, as in raw or lightly cooked food that doesn't contain the offending ingredients that you've determined through testing or through an elimination diet.

EPILEPSY AND OTHER NEUROLOGIC DISORDERS

TREATMENT-RESISTANT CANINE IDIOPATHIC EPILEPSY: CRYSTAL

"*Y*ou *get this terrible feeling of **helplessness** watching your fur baby in the uncontrollable throes of an epileptic 'fit.'*"

After Cheryl said that during our first appointment, I looked over at Crystal, her beautiful, pure white, American bulldog, who was one of the most regal-looking dogs I'd ever seen, and I thought to myself:

"*This is one patient that I absolutely must help.*"

(Not that I didn't absolutely want to help EVERY pet who walked through my clinic door, but Crystal was special. She had that amazingly sweet personality that I just can't resist.)

Crystal began having seizures early in her life, at two years of age. She had barely reached maturity when they began. The seizures were mild and infrequent to begin with, but over the next few years, they increased in frequency to weekly, and their severity was getting pretty bad.

The "fits" would start, Crystal would fall to the ground shaking and trembling, she wasn't responsive to Cheryl's voice or touch, and then she would start making guttural sounds and commonly lose her urine. After a minute or two, the shaking would stop, only to start back up again in a few minutes.

By the time a train of three or four of these "cluster seizures" had ended, Crystal would be exhausted and lay on the ground motionless and still, unresponsive to Cheryl's voice or touch for at least 15 minutes.

Finally, over a period of several hours, Crystal was able to get up and move around, although she never seemed to recover completely from the seizures until the next morning.

This was when Cheryl took Crystal to her veterinarian, who conducted a physical examination, including testing her neurological functions and drawing blood to send out for extensive testing in an effort to determine the cause of these violent seizures.

The neurologic testing did not reveal any abnormalities, and the blood work came back within normal limits. Her vet suggested she visit a specialist, a veterinary neurologist. Cheryl replied that she'd like to try some medication first, so she asked him to prescribe anti-epileptic pharmaceuticals to help control these seemingly uncontrollable seizures.

Crystal went home with two drugs, phenobarbital and potassium bromide, and she started right away, administering these to Crystal daily. Within a few days, Crystal seemed "out of it," and as Cheryl described:

"She was like a walking zombie, stumbling and bumping into furniture."

Cheryl, concerned, called her vet, who explained that at first, most dogs get pretty sedated from these drugs, but over several weeks, Crystal should become less affected by the two drugs. The upside, she explained to Cheryl, was that the seizures should be much better controlled on this medication.

So, Cheryl continued, reluctantly, to give these two medications. She felt that the cluster seizures were worse than the sedation from the meds. However, after about a month on the meds, Crystal had another set of cluster seizures. Not as prolonged and not as many, but she was still wiped out after they finished.

Cheryl called her vet, who suggested she continue to give these drugs a better chance to have an effect for another month or two. If the seizures continued despite the medications, her vet said that would be an indication to see the veterinary neurologist.

After several months, it was obvious that the meds were not working as hoped.

Cheryl made an appointment to see the neurologist.

At the specialty clinic, they did more blood testing and set Crystal up for an MRI to look for brain abnormalities that might explain these treatment-resistant seizures. The results of those expensive tests were all normal, with no indication of a tumor or other problem with the brain tissue. It looked normal!

Just a note: Negative findings aren't a bad thing; it meant that Crystal didn't have brain cancer or another very serious and potentially untreatable, terminal brain disease.

The neurologist added a third medication to Crystal's growing polypharmacy, gabapentin, also known as Neurontin™.

A few months went by without a seizure, and with some medication adjustments by the neurologist, Crystal was less of a "zombie," although Cheryl could still see that she had not returned to her old self.

Then another seizure occurred. Then another and another…

Frustrated with Crystal's resistance to respond to these strong drugs, Cheryl started looking for alternatives, and that's when she found my integrative clinic in Boulder, Colorado, where I practiced acupuncture, herbal and nutritional medicine, and helped clients prepare homemade diets as a part of their treatment protocol. That's in addition to treating complicated diseases with state of the art diagnostics and therapeutics. I try to blend the two together, taking the best from each to create improved outcomes. That's what I call "integrative medicine." Although some call it "holistic medicine," they are basically the same.

I have observed, over my 40 years in practice, that you can create amazing health by changing a pet's diet from the carbohydrate-rich, highly processed, commercial kibble and canned foods to a well-balanced home-prepared diet or a commercially available fresh food diet.

There are a number of choices available to pet parents for healthy, minimally processed, fresh food diets, either from raw meat and vegetables or cooked meat and vegetables. In nearly every case where I suggest to the pet parent that they improve the diet they are feeding, we have been rewarded with clinical improvement and better overall "outcomes."

As the second or third opinion on many of these difficult-to-treat epileptics, and probably the first integrative practitioner to weigh in on the patient, I never *initially* change the dosages recommended by the specialist or attending veterinarian, even if the patient is a "walking zombie."

Even with these strong pharmaceutical therapies, these animals were still seizing, and in some cases, pretty badly. My concern is that to discontinue, or even reduce the dose of the conventional pharmaceuticals, we risk creating an increase in the frequency and severity of their seizures.

My clients are eager to discontinue the "zombie meds." It takes some explaining by me for them to see the need to stay the course with the drugs until the alternative therapies have a chance to have an effect. I ask them to wait about a month or two. And when I do change the dosages of the meds, I do it very slowly, one med at a time.

I'm never sure how my epileptic patient will respond to the reduction in medication, so we "hold our breath," hoping that reducing the dose will not make things worse. Sometimes it does. In that case, we raise the dose back up to where it was for better seizure control.

We started weekly acupuncture treatments for Crystal. I suggested a change in her diet to a ketogenic diet, which studies have found can help reduce the frequency and severity of seizing. I also thought some Chinese herbs specific to Crystal's traditional Chinese veterinary medical "diagnosis" for epilepsy would be helpful, as well as some nutraceuticals supportive of the nervous system, such as the amino acid taurine, high doses of fish oil fatty acids, high doses of B vitamins, and vitamin E with mixed tocopherols.

We tested for vitamin D and found it to be insufficient, so we supplemented with vitamin D as well. Liver support was essential with the potential toxicity of the anti-convulsant drugs, so I recommended the use of the flavonoid complex silymarin, extracted from milk thistle seeds.

Cheryl came into my office weekly for Crystal's acupuncture treatment and re-assessment. I was impressed by her dedication to her four-legged family member, as it was an hour drive each way each week! Unlike standard conventional medical appointments, acupuncture treatments give the veterinarian a chance to closely observe their patient frequently, which can give insights into the most effective treatments for that patient's condition. This protocol that I used with Crystal had worked quite well with many of my other epileptic patients.

Crystal's diagnosis from her neurologist was refractory epilepsy, also known as "treatment-resistant epilepsy." It's unfortunate that modern science has not yet learned what causes this difficult-to-treat condition or what the best ways are to treat it in people or pets.

Crystal responded to the acupuncture therapy with less frequent seizing and fewer cluster seizures with less severity, but they were still occurring approximately every three or four weeks, regularly.

CBD gained its notoriety for being able to treat refractory epilepsy in children. The disease in children is called "Dravet syndrome," and it is very similar to the situation with Crystal and other dogs who have been diagnosed with this condition. CNN had a special featuring Sanjay Gupta, MD, who filmed a young child, Charlotte Figge, getting relief from CBD on camera, where you could see her having a seizure. They gave her a small amount of CBD by mouth on camera, and you could watch her stop seizing. It was very compelling, and as a result, I started to use CBD in my treatment-resistant patients and found improved success in treating this condition.

This was when I suggested we add a CBD formula I had been developing for my own company, Doc Silver Naturals. I added the minor cannabinoid, CBG, to the CBD and was hearing from pet parents who used it that they were getting excellent results for epilepsy, pain, and anxiety. With a sense of humor and a nod to my surname, I call this product "The Silver Bullet™."

There are two studies now in dogs with refractory epilepsy using cannabis extracts. The results of the first study found that CBD alone wasn't as effective to treat this difficult condition as we had hoped, even at the high dosage used in this study. This study showed some benefit to the use of CBD at higher doses for treatment-resistant epilepsy. About 67% of the dogs in this study responded to CBD. This study used a dose of about 1.5 mg of CBD for each pound of body weight twice daily.[105]

A second study in dogs with treatment-resistant epilepsy showed better effectiveness using a proprietary formulation containing a 1:1 ratio of CBD:CBDA. They used a dose of **0.5 mg of CBD/pound of body weight twice daily**. This dose of CBD also provided a dose of **0.5 mg of CBDA/pound of body weight**.[106]

I started Crystal on a dose of The Silver Bullet™, which was **0.25 mg of CBD for each pound** of her body weight twice daily.

317

Crystal weighed 65 pounds, so that came out to 16.25 mg of CBD, which translated to a little more than ¼ mL of the liquid tincture, or about seven or eight drops twice daily. Studies have shown that cannabinoids are best absorbed when given with some fatty food, so I had her put the tincture dose on a tablespoon of canned cat food, and she fed that to Crystal about 30 minutes before she fed her homemade ketogenic diet, twice daily.

At this point in time, we had been able to reduce the dose of the phenobarbital by 25%. I always try to reduce this medication first because its use is associated with the most side effects, especially with the liver and with increased appetite and weight gain.

After a month on the CBD:CBG formula, we didn't see any change in Crystal's seizure frequency or severity, so I had Cheryl double the dose to about 30 mg of CBD twice daily.

**This double dose was the equivalent of
about 0.5 mg/pound twice daily.**

I suggested Cheryl give ½ mL of The Silver Bullet™ twice daily with food and that we would see if that increased dose had any benefit over the next month.

(Since the seizure frequency was approximately monthly, I knew we had to wait at least that long to know if it was having an effect.)

When Cheryl returned a month later for a follow-up visit and an acupuncture treatment, she said that Crystal seemed to be slightly improved and the seizures she had were shorter and less severe. I felt that this result was very encouraging and suggested we wait another month and continue to observe before increasing the dosage of the CBD:CBG tincture or lowering the dose of the phenobarbital.

I am very cautious when reducing the dosage of medication that is working to reduce the seizure frequency or intensity. If I reduce the dosage too rapidly, then an excessive amount of seizing might occur, which would not be good for my patient, in this case, Crystal.

A month later, the news was still encouraging, but the seizures were still occurring monthly, even though their severity was less and the clusters were less. I suggested doubling the dose again, this time giving 60 mg of CBD twice daily. With The Silver Bullet™, each mL contains 60 mg of CBD and 30 mg of CBG. I was hopeful that with the addition of the CBG, the increased potency of the tincture would create better control of these seizures. What we were seeing in Crystal was an overall improvement in her quality of life and a reduction in seizure frequency and intensity, which told me that the addition of the CBG to this CBD formula did, in fact, improve our seizure control for Crystal.

This quadruple dose came out to about 1 mg/pound of body weight twice daily.

This dose was comparable to the doses used in the two dog studies quoted above.

It was looking like I had finally found the right combination of doses for CBD:CBG, acupuncture, nutraceutical, and Chinese herbal therapeutics for Crystal.

She didn't have a seizure for two months this time, and it was a relatively brief one.

Safety studies published for CBD in dogs showed that higher doses of CBD were safe to use for extended periods of time. Some of the dogs that received these higher doses had mild elevations in one liver enzyme, which did not indicate liver toxicity, but that the liver was working to metabolize the CBD, and that action resulted in the enzyme elevation of "serum alkaline phosphatase."

None of these safety studies lasted longer than four months.

From my practice experience with the safe use of higher doses of CBD, as many of my patients are on high doses, I was not concerned much about its safety because I hadn't seen any problems (yet). I trust my practice experience that CBD at higher doses has been safe, so far, in my patients, but trust is not enough when my patient's health is at stake. I always verify the assumptions I make about a patient from my observations of them with diagnostic blood tests. I routinely performed regular diagnostic tests to be certain the higher doses I was using were safe for my patient.

This is not where this story of Crystal ends. Managing her epileptic seizures is an ongoing process with her. We've been able to achieve much better control than with the drugs alone. We've been able to wean her off the phenobarbital and the potassium bromide completely but have continued with the gabapentin at a slightly reduced dosage.

I consider Crystal's experience to be a success story. This is why I am presenting all of these details to help you, my dear pet parent, if you have a dog suffering like Crystal. We can learn from her experience and understand that managing this treatment-resistant epilepsy is not an easy or inexpensive process. Trying to gain control over the "runaway train wreck" of refractory-to-treatment epileptic seizures is a true clinical challenge!

ABOUT TREATING NEUROLOGIC CONDITIONS

Problems with the nervous system are very challenging to treat. Often, medications for neurologic problems are themselves excessively sedating or stimulating or come bundled with other unwanted side effects. The nervous system extends throughout the entire body. It has control or influence over most bodily functions. When the nervous system is "out of whack," there are often other collateral problems that arise in other systems affected by the nervous system, such as the digestive or immune systems.

The cannabis plant contains multiple compounds that can cross the "blood-brain barrier," which is a protective function for the brain that normally excludes many compounds from entering the nervous system. CBD and THC are just two of many of these plant compounds that target the nervous system.

Historically, the cannabis plant and its extracts were used in people with seizures and other nervous system problems. This is why the first major application and the first FDA-approved drug made from CBD, Epidiolex™, is a seizure medication to treat two rare forms of pediatric epilepsy, including the Dravet syndrome that Charlotte Figge suffered from, and eventually died from at the tender age of 11 years old.

Other than epilepsy, other neurodegenerative conditions can potentially be managed with the use of cannabis extracts. There are case reports, studies, and anecdotal reports in humans with neurodegenerative conditions responding to cannabis therapeutics, such as:

- Parkinson's disease

- Alzheimer's disease

- Multiple sclerosis (MS)

- Amyotrophic lateral sclerosis (ALS or Lou Gehrig's disease)

Canine diseases that are similar in pathology to these human diseases and that, like these human diseases, have shown (anecdotally) a response to cannabinoid therapeutics:

- Degenerative myelopathy (similar to ALS and MS)

- Granulomatous meningoencephalitis (GME)

- Canine cognitive dysfunction (AD/ADHD)

UNDERSTANDING CANINE IDIOPATHIC
AND/OR TREATMENT-RESISTANT EPILEPSY

Epilepsy is a troubling condition. Watching your pet convulse uncontrollably is frightening. Epilepsy is a complex disease with many different forms and clinical manifestations. You should not try to treat this on your own. In some cases, supplements, diet, and all the other complementary therapies mentioned in this chapter just cannot address the severity of the epilepsy in an animal, and pharmaceuticals may also be needed to control the seizures.

In some forms of epilepsy, even the pharmaceuticals don't help enough. In some cases we have seen better results when we combine pharmaceuticals with complementary therapies, such as cannabis and mushrooms, Chinese herbs, acupuncture, etc.

In this section, the focus is on canine epilepsy, the most common neurodegenerative condition in the dog. Cannabis can have a beneficial impact on many forms of epilepsy when given at the appropriate dosages.

The use of cannabis for the canine neurologic conditions listed above other than epilepsy has potential but hasn't been proven yet. Cannabis may be able to help, to some degree, with each of these three neurodegenerative diseases, in addition to its well-documented benefits for canine patients with epilepsy.

Cats and horses can also get seizures, but they are much less common and more commonly caused by events such as infection, trauma, or cancer, making their treatment more complicated and beyond the scope of this book. Additionally, there are specific and unique neurodegenerative conditions in the horse and cat similar to those of the dog that may also respond positively to cannabis, but at present, there is not enough objective data to describe those in this guide.

What is Epilepsy?[107]

The term "epilepsy" describes a condition characterized by "seizure" events. It can have a number of different causes. Epilepsy is the disease itself. Seizures are the actual events characteristic of epilepsy. We see the symptoms of uncontrolled movement in this disease, caused by disorganized electrical signals in the brain, characteristic of an "epileptic episode." I liken these to a short circuit in the brain's neurologic pathways, resulting in disorganized electrical signals that cause disorganized movements of the body.

Seizures are recurrent and usually unprovoked, although there may be triggers that precipitate these events. They result from an abnormality of the brain that is often not able to be defined. That is where the medical term "idiopathic" comes from. We don't know the cause of the problem; therefore, it is termed idiopathic.

Epilepsy can be genetic (considered to be the origin of *idiopathic epilepsy*) or can be acquired through disease, trauma, or medication. There are two types of epilepsy in the dog: *"generalized"* or *"focal."*

With *generalized* seizures, usually, both sides of the brain are involved, and clinical signs are symmetric, occurring on both sides of the body due to both sides of the brain being affected. *Generalized* seizures are bilateral involuntary muscle movements or sudden losses in muscle tone.

During a *generalized* seizure, your dog may experience the following symptoms:

- Becomes less aware of its environment

- Involuntarily:
    o Salivate
    o Urinate
    o Vocalize
    o Defecate

On the other hand, *focal* seizures will have their origins in a single area of the brain. Thus, the symptoms are usually one-sided or will affect a specific part of the body.

Typical focal seizure symptoms include:

- Facial twitches

- Chewing movements

- Paddling of a leg

- Behavioral symptoms of fear and/or attention-seeking

- Dilated pupils

- Salivation

- Vomiting

- Awareness may not be impaired during *focal* seizures.

The anatomical origin of the seizures determines if they are *generalized* versus *focal* seizures. The severity of the seizures themselves dictates their duration. Most idiopathic epileptic seizures last at most 90 seconds, although it can seem like an hour if it is your dog!

Really severe cases of epilepsy may have what are called **cluster seizures**, which means that after one seizure finishes, another one begins. An epileptic patient can have multiple cluster seizures over a period of hours. The seizure can be so severe that they lose their urine or stool, and they may vocalize uncontrollably. Cluster seizures can deplete a dog's energy, and they may be totally exhausted and wiped out for a number of days following these events.

For some dogs (and people), even the use of multiple strong anticonvulsant drugs fails to stop these seizures. We call the seizures that occur even while on strong medication "**breakthrough seizures**." We call this type of epilepsy that is poorly treated by our current pharmaceuticals "**refractory epilepsy.**" Nearly 30% of human or canine seizure patients will have "**treatment-resistant epilepsy.**" The severity, frequency, and duration of the seizure episodes often dictate whether a pharmaceutical is used or not.

If the episodes occur frequently, last excessively long, or are severe enough, they will need to be medicated with anti-epileptic drugs, such as phenobarbital, potassium bromide, gabapentin, zonisamide, or levetiracetam. These types of refractory-to-treatment seizures are a real danger to your pet. The ongoing seizures pose a threat to a pet's health by depleting its energy, and the ongoing, non-resolving seizures have the potential, if left unchecked, to result in your pet's death.

It's hard to watch your own pet seizing uncontrollably. It is equally difficult to watch your pet act like a "walking zombie" due to the excessively sedative effects of these medications, which sedate but may be marginally effective against "**treatment-resistant epilepsy.**"

Cluster seizures are one sign of treatment-resistant epilepsy. "**Status epilepticus**" is a very serious form of treatment-resistant epilepsy in which the seizures never stop. It is extremely dangerous when they have this, and the only treatment we have is to use a strong barbiturate to sedate them so much that they stop seizing. Left untreated, this condition can progress to being *fatal* over a fairly short period of time.

The first study using CBD to treat refractory epilepsy was published two years ago by Colorado State University's College of Veterinary Medicine, Department of Neurology. In this study, they gave client-owned dogs with **treatment-resistant epilepsy a bit more than 1 mg of CBD/pound of body weight, fasted, twice daily** (2.5 mg/kg), and measured the frequency and duration of their seizures over a period of 12 weeks.

The CBD was in addition to their regular anti-convulsant

medications. This study found that this moderately high dose of CBD was able to reduce the severity and duration of their break-through seizures, but not as much as they had hoped. The blood levels of CBD were directly correlated to the reduction in seizure frequency.

In other words, **the CBD *did* help reduce the severity and frequency of the seizures in many of these dogs,** but the number of dogs responding to the CBD didn't meet the standards that are applied to pharmaceutical anti-convulsants in determining their effectiveness, so the study concluded that CBD didn't work for refractory seizures.[108]

This is one example of why you have to read the details in these studies to understand what they really mean. That's what I have done in this book: *I translate these complicated studies into language that anyone can understand.*

By the way, these researchers have now secured funding from the AKC Canine Health Foundation to repeat this study with a larger group of epileptic dogs and a higher dosage of CBD. This will help resolve if a higher dosage would provide the "success" they did not observe in the pilot study. The new dosage they are using is 2 mg/pound, twice daily (4.5 mg/kg).

The second study, used a product with a blend of CBD:CBA 1:1 using a 1 mg/pound dosing scheme for each cannabinoid, and they found that more than 50% of the dogs in this study achieved better control of their seizures than before they were given this product.[109]

Less severe epileptic disease may not need the use of strong anti-convulsant pharmaceuticals. If the frequency of the seizures is weekly or monthly, it might be decided, if their severity is less, to not treat with pharmaceuticals at all. Medical wisdom suggests that if the seizures are less frequent, perhaps once monthly, then the use of the strong anti-epileptic drugs may not be indicated.

Once the seizures become more frequent and more severe, such that your dog has trouble recovering from them, it then is time to start the pharmaceuticals.

For less severe cases of epilepsy, where pharmaceuticals may not be needed, these non-drug therapies may help improve your pet's quality of life:

- Cannabinoids like CBD, CBC, CBG, CBDA, CBGA, and THCA

- Neurotrophic nutraceuticals like lion's mane mushroom extract, reishi mushroom extract, fish oil, B vitamins, and l-taurine

- Regular acupuncture treatments

- Patient-specific Chinese herbal prescribing

- Other complementary therapies

CONVENTIONAL APPROACHES

The conventional therapeutic approach to epilepsy involves the use of strong drugs and needs to be under the care of a veterinarian. Your veterinarian will run a number of tests to rule out possible causes for the seizures that can be corrected with medication or diet.

Possible causes your vet will be ruling out with blood tests and possibly urine tests include:

- Poisoning

- Liver disease

- Low or high blood sugar

- Kidney disease

- Anemia

- Head injury

- Encephalitis (canine viral distemper, feline protozoal toxoplasmosis)

- Tick-borne infections (Lyme disease, anaplasmosis, etc.)

- Strokes

- Brain cancer

Although you wouldn't want your pet to have any of these other causes of seizures, some are more correctable than idiopathic treatment-resistant epilepsy. I strongly recommend that you allow your vet to run these tests to understand exactly what is going on with your four-legged friend. One rule I practice medicine by is to know what you are treating. When you have a diagnosis, it is much more likely you may have a treatment.

INTEGRATIVE/HOLISTIC APPROACHES

Cannabis & CBD have been found useful in human seizure patients for many years. Depending on the severity and type of epilepsy present, these herbs could medicate the seizures completely or could provide some increased degree of control over the seizure severity, frequency, or duration.

With the increased availability of cannabis products for human use following the legalization of cannabis and hemp, it is only natural that pet parents with critters that have a serious disease such as epilepsy would ask the question:

"If it's good for me, won't it also help my pet?"

The answer to that question is, "Maybe... Probably... Let's try it *safely* for a month and see if it can help your pet with epilepsy."

If your pet has epilepsy, as mentioned previously, I think it's important for you to see your veterinarian for this problem. They will do a physical exam and draw some blood for some tests to try and find a cause for the seizures. Sometimes, seizures can be caused by metabolic problems like low blood sugar or calcium imbalances that can be corrected nutritionally, but most of the time, seizures are what we call "idiopathic," which means we don't know the exact cause.

Most dogs with epilepsy have this form of "idiopathic" epilepsy. Some dogs with brain tumors can also have seizures. If you are following your vet's guidance in terms of anti-convulsant pharmaceuticals, it should be safe to initiate cannabinoid therapy for your pet using a low to no THC hemp product with CBD as the dominant cannabinoid. CBG, CBGA, CBDA, and THCA are four other cannabinoids that can help with seizures.

The first canine epilepsy study quoted above used just CBD

alone. As mentioned, the second study found that using a 1:1 CBD:CBDA tincture dosed at 2 mg/kg twice daily was effective in reducing the rate of seizures in this group of dogs. It's unknown if this benefit was due to the CBD, CBDA, or the combination of the two. This study was funded by the company that makes this product.

For now, most pet products contain only CBD. I am certain that in the future, we will see more products that contain CBD combined with CBDA, CBG, CBGA, or other combinations of these minor and acidic cannabinoids.

My own branded cannabinoid product line, Doc Silver Naturals contains CBD blended with the minor cannabinoid CBG in a 2:1 ratio in two different tincture strengths. In the two years these products have been available through my Well-Pet Dispensary, customer feedback has been very good regarding this formulation's ability to help with some forms of epilepsy.

I have also formulated this CBD:CBG blend in my soft chews, which also contain substantial amounts of two mushroom extracts, lion's mane, which can be helpful with brain health due to its special compounds, and cordyceps, which is good for geriatrics, and for stamina and performance, as well as protecting the kidneys and supporting the lungs.

The starting dose for an epileptic patient or a patient with one of the other neurodegenerative conditions is:

- **CBD: 0.25-0.50 mg/pound twice daily**

- *Maximum "safe" dose for CBD: 5 mg/pound twice daily*

If your dog will be on a dose this high for longer than two weeks, you should have their blood tested by your vet for liver enzymes, as we can see elevations in liver enzymes when doses are higher than 0.25 mg/pound in a few sensitive individuals. It's important to know whether there is a change in liver enzymes.

Depending on how high the elevations in liver values are, we might want to discontinue giving the CBD or add a liver-protectant herb or nutraceutical like silymarin or n-acetylcysteine (NAC) to your dog's program. Remember that some of the anti-convulsant drugs we give dogs can also increase liver enzyme values. An elevation in liver enzyme values alone is not sufficient reason to discontinue the CBD, but it is good to know so we can make an informed decision about what's best for your pet.

Ratio Products with THC

THC has the potential to spark epileptic seizures, so it is the one cannabinoid from the cannabis plant that is not recommended for seizures and may be a good reason to use a broad-spectrum hemp product with zero THC content.

The raw, acidic form of THC, known as tetrahydrocanna-binolic acid (THCA), is not intoxicating and also can be effective against seizures.

Due to the problem that we find occasionally with THC and seizures, I do not recommend ratio products with THC for sei-zures. Lower levels of THC (as in a 20:1 ratio product) might be advantageous for some of the less common neurodegenerative conditions such as degenerative myelopathy.

Remember, it's not just the *ratio*; it's also the concentration or amount of THC that is needed for safe dosing of that potentially intoxicating cannabinoid. In fact, the amount of THC that you give your dog is the limiting factor in determining the amount of cannabis your dog gets.

I think it's better to avoid a product with any significant amount of THC, but I support the use of acidic cannabinoids like THCA or CBDA (or the less commonly available CBCA and CBGA) for epileptic patients.

SUPPLEMENTS FOR EPILEPSY AND OTHER NEURODEGENERATIVE CONDITIONS

There are a number of supplements that support the structures and functions of the nervous system. No single supplement is able to treat seizures effectively. Supplements create a supportive environment for the nervous system to function in a healthier fashion.

I'm not recommending you use all of these at the same time, but rather pick and choose those that are most available to you, fit into your budget, and which your pet will tolerate being administered to them. Some pets will accept many supplements added to their food or given as treats, and some aren't so accepting. You should adapt this list of potentially supportive supplements to your own situation.

EPA/DHA fatty acids from fish oil, algal oil, and marine lipid sources.

This is the single most important supplement to give for epilepsy other than CBD.

These are dosed at 50 mg/pound of body weight daily of the sum total of EPA+DHA (50 mg/pound daily).

It takes about 12 weeks for the body to become less inflammatory as a result of being fed this amount of fish oils over time in the dog.

Reducing inflammation, as well as the direct effects of fatty acids on nervous tissue, will improve the condition of a pet with epilepsy.

L-taurine free-form amino acid makes it more difficult for the brain to have a seizure. This amino acid raises the "seizure threshold." The seizure threshold is that level that, when exceeded, results in a seizure. To better understand this concept, seizures occur when there is a "perfect storm" of conditions that, in combination, exceed this threshold, resulting in a seizure. L-taurine is an inhibitory neurotransmitter that has an influence on suppressing seizure activity by raising the seizure threshold.

B complex vitamins support healthy neurologic function and can have a calming effect on the nervous system. Higher potency B complex vitamins are often termed "stress formula." These supplements can have a beneficial effect on seizures. Vitamin B1, B3, B6, B12, and folate are important for neurodevelopment and cognitive function and have been described as helping epileptic patients reduce the severity or duration of their epileptic episodes. B vitamins are very safe, even at very high doses. A "stress formula" B complex for humans will work. B vitamins are very cost-effective supplements.

TRADITIONAL CHINESE VETERINARY MEDICINE FOR EPILEPSY

Chinese herbal formulas for epilepsy have been in use for hundreds of years in Asia to treat human epilepsy. Since the introduction of acupuncture and Chinese herbal medicine to the West in the 1970s, attention has turned to developing herbal and acupuncture protocols to treat epilepsy in veterinary patients, specifically in dogs. Human herbal formulas have been modified to address the unique needs of dogs, cats, and horses who may have seizures or neurodegenerative conditions.

Traditional Chinese Veterinary Medicine (TCVM) determines a diagnosis based on the principles of this traditional medicine of Asia. A diagnosis is achieved by looking at the color and coating of the tongue and palpating the pulses as well as taking a thorough history. Practitioners of TCVM use these diagnostic techniques to know which acupuncture points to needle and what Chinese herbal formula would be best for their patient.

For example, one formula for seizures in dogs is *Long Dan Xie Gan Tang*. This formula is used to treat seizures that are very severe, often accompanied by red eyes, red tongues, and seizures that are accompanied by extreme activity. The best way to determine which formula to use is to see a veterinarian who is skilled in TCVM diagnosis. You could try using a formula without a diagnosis, and that may work (or maybe not...).

There is another TCVM formula that is for less severe seizures, which would be more common in an older animal with deficiencies in Liver or Kidney according to the Chinese system of diagnostics. This formula is called *Tien Ma Gou Teng Yin*. This formula works better for seizures that are not as severe as the extreme seizures of the *Long Dan Xie Gan Tang* type.

A third formula is designed for epilepsy conditions in which the seizures are particularly severe and prolonged. Not necessarily treatment resistant seizures, but in the language of Traditional Chinese Medicine theses type of seizures are caused by excessive "phlegm," leading to seizures that can be prolonged, difficult to treat, and often accompanied by vocalizations. This formula is called *Ding Xian Wan*.

If you would like to find a veterinarian skilled in the use of Chinese herbs and acupuncture for epilepsy, there are several membership lists of veterinarians you can check to see if there is a vet near you who can do this TCVM diagnosis to more accurately prescribe the right formula for your pet's epilepsy. Check our Resource section in the back for a website with directories of holistic veterinarians.

VITAMIN D AND VITAMIN E[110,111]

High dosages of vitamin D have been found to be supportive of the patient with epilepsy. Most people don't know that vitamin D in dogs and cats is not created in their skin under the influence of UV light from the sun like with humans, but is only provided in their food. Many diets are deficient in adequate amounts of vitamin D, and it has been found that vitamin D levels in epileptics are usually quite low. Supplementing with adequate vitamin D has been found to have a beneficial effect in a few published studies in humans.

In a study in humans with epilepsy, 400 IU of d-alpha-tocopherol (the natural form of one isoform of vitamin E) daily for three months reduced seizure frequency by 60%. I suggest using the full spectrum vitamin E, which is called "mixed tocopherols."

MEDICINAL MUSHROOMS

Poria or Tuckahoe (*Poria pararadicis*) is a fungus that grows around the roots of trees. The fungal mycelium grows near the tree root and forms a hard, woody "sclerotium," which looks kind of like a potato. The center part of the sclerotium is the part of this fungus that has calming and anti-epileptic properties. The other parts of the fungus are for digestive, urinary, and other types of applications. It is used extensively in a number of Traditional Chinese Herbal formulas.

Lion's mane (*Hericium erinaceous*) is a medicinal mushroom that is a part of traditional Chinese herbal medicine. It has beneficial properties to improve the healthy functioning of the brain. A published study found that lion's mane can provide healthy support to the nervous tissue in the brain of epileptics.[112]

This mushroom, and every other mushroom as well, contains a pre-vitamin D source, ergosterol, which is converted to vitamin D_2 under the influence of UV light. This was found to help protect nerve cells in the brain following prolonged seizures in *status epilepticus*.[113]

Reishi (*Ganoderma lingzhi*) is considered the "mushroom of immortality." It contains antioxidants and other nutrients such as terpenes and triterpenes, like ganoderic acid, that have proven to support the nervous tissue in the brain following the damage that can occur from excessively strong and prolonged seizures.

Ergothioneine, from the oyster mushroom (*Pleurotus ostreatus*), is a unique fungal antioxidant that is also found in substantial amounts in other edible mushrooms, such as the shiitake, lion's mane, and maitake mushrooms. A study with the oyster-mushroom-derived ergothioneine found that it served a protective function to reduce and reverse the damage caused by excessive seizuring.[114]

ACUPUNCTURE FOR EPILEPSY

Acupuncture for epilepsy works on the same principles as Traditional Chinese Veterinary Medicine herbal therapies. Acupuncture needles are inserted into spots over the skull that can directly help to reduce abnormal electrical activity. Acupuncture needles are also placed on the arms, legs, and back. Adding microampere electrical stimulation of certain acupuncture points can create a powerful treatment that is able to reduce seizure events, frequency, and severity of the epileptic episodes.

Acupuncture is practiced by veterinarians who have taken a course with a minimum of 150-200 hours of classes and practical laboratories. They achieve certification in veterinary acupuncture after completing the course work and a written and practical examination that tests the veterinarians' skills on dogs, cats, horses, and cattle.

The links to find members of these various veterinary acupuncture training programs can be found in the Resource section at the end of this book.

KETOGENIC DIET

Diet has been found to have a very strong influence on patients with epilepsy. The diet that has the most research supporting its value to the epileptic patient is the ketogenic diet that was discussed in the sections under cancer and bowel diseases.

The discussion of this diet deserves repeating because its benefits can be huge for your pet with epilepsy.

The ketogenic diet is based on providing ingredients in your pet's diet that force the metabolism of fats versus carbohydrates. With carbohydrate metabolism, we get lactic acid as a by-product. Lactic acid has been found to feed cancer cells, but it also will feed nerve and brain cells, which gives them enough energy to have a seizure. High carbohydrate diets also tend to be pro-inflammatory, and it is inflammation that is driving the seizures.

On the other hand, the ketogenic diet forces the patient to develop a fat-based metabolism by feeding it less than 5% carbohydrates, moderate protein amounts (25%), and high fat levels (70%). It has been found in multiple studies in dogs that adding medium chain triglycerides (MCT) as a major source of fat (10% of total calories and 67% of calories from fat in the ketogenic diet) will increase the formation of the ketone bodies that are characteristic of this diet.[115,116,117]

Ketone bodies nourish the nerve cells and brain cells in such a way as to prevent them from having the disorganized electrical signals that are fundamental to the major symptom of epilepsy, the seizure. Ketone bodies will not nourish cancer cells either, which is why this diet can be good for cancer patients.

Currently, Purina™ is the only company with a ketogenic diet formula that has been measured to reliably produce ketone bodies after several weeks of consuming it, in the absence of consuming other sources of carbohydrates. Ketogenic diets and the studies that validate them are so new that the marketplace hasn't caught up with them by offering many "keto" products for pets. If you find a product that claims to be ketogenic, ask the company to supply you with the study(s) that support its ability to create ketosis in your pet.

A workaround to not have to use the Purina™ diet is to find another diet formula with similar amounts of energy and protein and then to add additional MCT to the diet's fat content to transform it into a ketogenic diet. You can buy urine strips online or at your pharmacy (KetoStix™) that will measure the development of ketone bodies in your dog's urine from the diet you are feeding.

NOTE: *There are some contraindications for the use of the ketogenic diet, including ketoacidotic diabetes and low body weight. The high-fat content could affect digestive function or precipitate pancreatitis if your dog is sensitive to fats. Prolonged use of a ketogenic diet may cause deficiencies in trace minerals, so it's good to check the blood for these deficiencies and supplement with additional dietary minerals like selenium, copper, and zinc if needed.*

CHAPTER ELEVEN SUMMARY

Epilepsy, like cancer, can be a life-threatening ailment that can take a huge toll on the pet and their family. Some forms of epilepsy are very difficult to treat, even with strong anti-convulsant medication. Often epileptics also suffer from behavior problems like ADHD or cognitive issues.

Anti-convulsant medications often leave the pet groggy or slowed down, due to their strong sedative effects. Even with the sedation, some pets will still have breakthrough seizures.

With the emerging therapies of cannabis and medicinal mushrooms, combined with new research into supplements like fish oil and medium chain triglycerides, and with the historically successful herbal and acupuncture treatments from the use of Traditional Chinese Veterinary Medicine, more dogs and cats are finding relief and remission from their seizures and convulsions.

Of great interest in the treatment of epilepsy is the influence of diet on the risk of seizures. Research in the past 15 years has found that the ketogenic diet can have a beneficial influence on reducing the frequency and severity of epileptic seizures, as well as having a benefit to both cognition and behavior.

CHAPTER TWELVE

OLLIE'S HEALTHY PET WELLNESS PROGRAM

My own lovable, but nervous Labrador, "Ollie," provides us with a good example of a wellness program that any healthy dog can follow.

But first, let me speak to the value of wellness and what it is and what it isn't.

The earlier you get your pet started with a wellness program, the sooner they can achieve substantial benefits, and the longer those benefits will be on board to create vibrant and optimal health. "Optimal health" *is* "wellness."

There is a relatively new concept being expressed that you can "**train**" your immune system to work more quickly and efficiently.[118] This concept is based on the use of a good diet, exercise, herbs, and mushrooms, all regularly and for sufficiently long enough to train the immune system. Once primed with immuno-modulating substances like beta-glucans, the immunocytes (immune cells) better retain the "memory" of pathogens it has encountered in the past, which allows these immune cells to respond better and more quickly to challenges. Those pets who did not receive the benefit of taking healthy supplements will take more time to respond to immune system challenges and may not respond with adequate strength to "do the job."

It is said that an "ounce of prevention" is worth a "pound of cure."
I have found this to be very true when it comes to the
value of wellness programs for pets.

Treating a disease early usually has much better outcomes than waiting until the eleventh hour. "**Wellness**" is defined as the condition in which the body's systems are functioning at their most efficient and optimal levels, which helps prevent your pet from becoming ill. And if your pet does become ill, it will recover quickly.

"Wellness," or "health," is much more than just *the absence of disease*. It is the desired state of optimal existence and well-being, in addition to being free of disease.

Wellness won't necessarily prevent illness, but it will reduce the chance that illness will occur by optimizing the body's metabolism and its immune and cognitive functions. The tools we use to create wellness can also help mitigate and reduce the incidence and severity of disease when it unavoidably happens.

To establish wellness, we need to provide support to these systems in the body, all of which together contribute to health and wellness. What follows is the Wellness Program that I have been recommending for years, with the addition of some new supplements and nutrients.

12-POINT WELLNESS PROGRAM
FOR YOUR DOG OR CAT

1. Support the microbiome with healthy probiotics and wholesome, minimally processed foods

2. Support the digestive system's optimal functioning with digestive enzymes, prebiotics, probiotics, and balanced, wholesome minimally processed foods

3. Antioxidant support, which helps reduce tissue damage from free radicals in our environment and which occur from normal metabolic processes

4. Detoxification support for the liver to help keep toxicity down

5. Cognitive function and neurologic support with healthy oils, B vitamins, and mushrooms with ergothioneine

6. Endocannabinoid system support with extracts of the cannabis plant and palmitoylethanolamide (PEA) from food sources or as extracts

7. Anti-inflammatory diet to keep inflammation down

8. Anti-inflammatory supplements to keep inflammation under control

9. Healthy oils are the key to a healthy life.

10. Moderate exercise

11. Clean water and fresh air

12. Emotionally stable home environment

This seems like a lot of stuff to do, but don't worry, it's not as complicated as it seems!

HOW TO ACHIEVE WELLNESS FOR YOUR PET: A SIMPLE SUMMARY

<u>Feed food that is not pro-inflammatory</u>. This means low carbo-hydrates, higher protein, and healthy fats. Preferably, feed food that is as unprocessed as possible. Dry kibble dog food is excessive-ly processed and is not as healthy a diet as home-prepared, com-mercial raw diets, or commercially prepared cooked diets.

Recent research has documented the value of intermittent fast-ing, even when that means just one meal daily. It can help regulate insulin levels, promote a healthy weight, and includes behavioral and cognitive benefits. Medium-chain triglycerides (MCT) can be added to your pet's morning meal to enhance its metabolism. I suggest you start at 40 mg of MCT for each pound of your pet's body weight. See how your dog reacts to the MCT oil. Some may have digestive sensitivity to excessive fats and oils, others may be overweight. If your pet is overweight, you can use the MCT oil as part of a weight loss program, or a ketogenic diet. But if you just give the MCT oil without regard for your pet's caloric needs, it might also cause them to gain weight! You may be able to work up to as much as 125 mg of MCT for each pound of your pet's body weight, if your dog is tolerating the extra MCT without digestive upset. The extra fat from the MCT oil, like protein, can create a sense of fullness and satiety in your dog, and help to reduce its ap-petite if it is too ravenous, contributing to its weight.[119,120]

<u>Give supplements daily</u>, such as fish oils, antioxidants, and probiotics; these three categories of supplements will provide support for cognitive function, neurological function, digestive sys-tem health, and antioxidant support.

<u>Maintain a healthy home environment</u> and provide clean air and water; provide moderate exercise daily for you and your pet. ☺

Quarterly, do a detoxification with herbs like milk thistle, dandelion, and curcumin; I've found that intermittent fasting by feeding a single daily meal, and during detox, to reduce the amount of food being fed to 30% of what is usually fed, are all very helpful aids to detoxification.

As compared to completely fasting or starving, I suggest feeding fewer calories and more fiber as a form of a modified fast to assist the digestive system in its work.

Use CBD to help support a slow or low endocannabinoid system (eCS). **Not all dogs and cats need CBD daily.**

CBD can work in the body when the body's naturally-occurring endocannabinoids are low. When they are low, there may be some manifestation of clinical disease. Trauma can also cause the endocannabinoids to get reduced so that is also a place where CBD can help, as can THC.

If you give CBD and your pet doesn't need it, it's a waste of your money. CBD is great if there is a need, such as epilepsy, anxiety, mild-moderate pain and arthritis, issues with appetite, or cancer.

If your pet has specific weaknesses in its system, such as a poorly functioning digestive system, then adding some digestive supplements like digestive enzymes, digestive aids like ginger root, or psyllium seed can help a lot. Address your pet's specific weakness with the appropriate herb(s) or nutraceutical(s) for that problem.

I don't have a specific, generic wellness program here for you to follow. I think that each animal is an individual that needs to have its own wellness program tailored to its specific needs.

Check out "**Ollie's Wellness Program**" below, as it could serve as a good model for your own pet's wellness program. Keep in mind, you may need to make some specific changes, especially customized for your four-legged family member.

OLLIE'S WELLNESS PROGRAM

Take a look at my narrative here regarding Ollie and his individualized wellness program designed to address the problems he came "bundled with" and, at the same time, strengthen his immune system, improve his attitude, and deal with the orthopedic surgery he had when found as an injured stray puppy.

Trigger, my chocolate rescue lab before Ollie, passed away from a pulmonary carcinoma at age 12. After he passed away, I had taken enough time to "recycle my emotions" to be ready for my next four-legged companion. I started looking at Labrador rescue groups in my area in Colorado. (I'm a confessed "Labaholic," although there are no 12-step programs for people with my breed addiction.) I'm a veterinarian and I've always tried to find a "Labby" rescue dog that my unique veterinary training and skills can help.

One day, I saw the cutest picture of a little lab puppy in an email offered by Safe Harbor Lab Rescue in Golden, Colorado. (Safe Harbor Lab Rescue is a really great rescue group, by the way.) I showed the picture to my wife and daughter, and they agreed that this was a super, way-cute little pup!

So, we arranged to see this cute pooch at the home where they were fostering him. I kept telling myself that I would show restraint. I would check him out and then go home and think about it. In the past, I would just make that decision impulsively, based on my compassion for the dog, without considering the long-term consequences of adopting that rescue pup. In the past, I would commit to a pup on the spur of the moment. I wanted this time to be different—no spur-of-the-moment decisions for me anymore!

Well, you can guess what happened next. Ollie came home with us that same day! (I have so little control when it comes to rescues!)

His story is a sad one, as was Trigger's before him. Ollie had been found as a stray puppy of three to four months of age with a dislocated hip and fractured thigh bone (femur). He had been a stray so long that the broken bone had healed back together! (Although not exactly straight.)

A good Samaritan had gone by the shelter where he was and saw him. The shelter was a "kill" shelter, which meant they put to sleep most of the dogs there, and they didn't have a vet on duty to provide pain management. Ollie's dislocated hip and broken bone had to have been painful to him. He was scheduled to be put to sleep the very next day, as well.

The good Samaritans at Safe Harbor Lab Rescue Group in Golden, Colorado, sent a pilot down to pick him up, along with several other labs, also all slated to be put to sleep. They flew them all back to Colorado. Safe Harbor Lab Rescue took him to their veterinarian, who performed orthopedic surgery to correct the dislocated hip.

The surgeon left the broken bone alone because it had healed fairly straight, and to rebreak it and reset it would not be humane to this poor little puppy, who had wandered alone with a broken bone and dislocated hip for probably a month!

Ollie was just recovering from the surgery when I adopted him. So, I gave him some Chinese herbs I knew would help with wound healing, and I put him on some CBD to help with the pain he was experiencing. CBD is also known to help stimulate bone growth, so I thought it would be perfect to help him with the healing from the surgery, as well as with the pain.

It didn't take long for Ollie to become part of our family, but his trauma was not forgotten by him. He was super happy to be in our family, but he had fears and timidity, especially to loud voices and men. Although he bonded immediately with me, he would "slink" away, for instance, if he heard me raise my voice at one of my cats if they were on the kitchen counter trying to eat some of our food.

I continued the CBD with Ollie in the hopes that its anxiolytic effect would help his emotions settle down so he would be less fearful. I also felt that just spending time with our loving family and feeling our love and kindness would help. I enrolled Ollie and my 10-year-old daughter in a local training program for dogs at the Boulder Humane Society.

Dogs feel more safe, comfortable, and loved when they have the clear boundaries that training provides. They want to please us, and training provides that education to them and actually teaches them to understand us when we are asking them to do things. Training is high on the list of wellness program practices.

I am a strong proponent of feeding dogs and cats the most unprocessed food possible, and I have had concerns about the highly processed nature of commercial dry food (kibble). I do believe that "you are what you eat" and that the most important thing you can do for yourself or for your pet is to eat food that is as wholesome and unprocessed as possible.

For Ollie (my light-yellow lab), and for Trigger before him (my chocolate lab), and for Bean (my black lab) before him, I have fed all of my dogs a homemade diet. I know this isn't for everyone. The process takes time, attention to detail, and an understanding of hygienic food handling since we are using raw meat and want to be careful about food-borne pathogens. I will say, though, that after feeding all of my dogs this way, with raw food for years, I've never seen a problem with this diet making them sick. This is the same diet I've taught to my clients, and none of their dogs ever had an adverse reaction either.

What Ollie actually eats on a daily basis for his 65 pounds of ideal body weight:

- ½ pound of ground turkey served raw

- 1 cup of chopped-up raw broccoli or green beans, usually from a package of frozen veggies from our supermarket

- Vitamin D liquid drops in the right amount for him, based on Vitamin D testing

- 1 tablespoon of fish oil with lecithin to provide an anti-inflammatory dose

- 3 tablespoons of flax seed meal that has been in the refrigerator to keep the delicate oils in it fresh

- Calcium in the right amounts for him from a powdered product that contains a high concentration of calcium derived from seaweed, egg shells, and/or bone meal

- 1 teaspoon of powdered medicinal mushroom extract rich in beta-glucans and antioxidants

- 1 tablespoon of a product that contains a lot of powdered veggies and seaweed to provide micronutrients and food-bound antioxidants

- 1 teaspoon of a mushroom/seaweed/probiotic meal topper

- Enough vitamin-mineral blend to make the diet more complete and balanced

These are the amounts I use for Ollie. The amounts you use for your own dog may be different based on its weight and needs.

I use boiling hot water to bring the frozen veggies up to a warm temperature, and then I blend the veggies and hot water into the rest of the supplements and ingredients. I serve this to him once daily. If the frozen veggies are too large, after they are warmed up in the hot water, I use scissors to cut them into smaller mouth-sized pieces while they are in the hot water. I defrost them in a 32-ounce measuring cup and cover them so there is an inch of hot water above the level of the frozen veggie.

You should see how excited he gets as I put the diet together, knowing that at the end of this process will be a tasty meat and veggie stew! The extra water in the food from warming up the veggies also helps to make sure he is getting enough water to maintain a healthy state of hydration.

Needless to say, this diet has caused him to thrive, and as a Labrador retriever, he is a true foodie. With food in his belly and the promise of regular meals (unlike his starvation diet while he was a stray) Ollie's sweet personality began to blossom.

Other wellness supplements that I add to his diet include digestive enzymes and probiotics to help create a healthy digestive system and gastrointestinal tract.

WELLNESS PROGRAM ADDITIONS SPECIFICALLY FOR CATS

Cats are a different story entirely from dogs when it comes to home-prepared diets. This is because, unlike dogs, they are obligate carnivores and need a lot of fresh meat. Cats have no nutritional need for carbohydrates, as their metabolism is not adapted to using carbohydrates. I have observed, though, that some cats have a "sweet tooth" for carbs, like potato chips and such.

I think raw meat diets for cats are very appropriate, given their basic nature as predators. Still, many cats can develop an "addiction" to the processed dry foods they are fed. This can make them very picky about trying any other food that doesn't look like dry kibble. This "bonding" with dry, high-carbohydrate kibble diets begins at the time they are first introduced to them as weanling kittens.

If you start by feeding your kitten a variety of different foods that are fresh and wholesome as part of a homemade diet, or a commercial frozen raw or cooked meat diet, they are less likely to become junk food junkies for their dry kibble. With this increased flexibility in what they consider edible food, kittens and cats won't develop the "pickiness" about what they eat compared to when they started out feeding just kibble, and being fed that almost exclusively.

These cats who are "easy-eaters," who aren't as picky, are also easier to give supplements to or to get to eat supplements hidden in some tasty fresh or canned food.

Still, other than the differences in what dogs eat versus what cats eat due to their differences in metabolism, cat supplements and cat lifestyle choices are very similar to dog supplements and lifestyle choices.

Your cat's wellness program is quite similar to a dog's wellness program, like the one I've developed for Ollie. The main differences are that most cats will not be accepting of very many supplements added to their food, and even fewer cats will accept pills being administered directly to their mouth.

So you have to be efficient with the administration of your cat's wellness supplements, fine-tuning what you are giving to be not too many cause you don't want to overwhelm the kitty with too many administrations and additions to their food. Some cats will accept more supplements than others.

Whole food supplements can be very effective for cats. For instance, fish oil is usually accepted by many cats. Adding **flax seed meal** to your cat's food will help with hairballs, as well as adding healthy omega-3 and omega-6 oils to your cat's program. B vitamins are very important to cats, and they have an absolute requirement for a few B vitamins, so I recommend using a **nutritional yeast** powder, which is usually tasty to cats, and which has good levels of many B vitamins, glucose tolerance factor, chromium, zinc, and other essential nutrients.

Cordyceps militaris mushroom extract is something I also recommend, **specifically for cats**, due to its ability to help protect the kidneys. Cats are very prone to having problems with their kidneys, and reluctant to eat new tasting things. If your cat will accept the cordyceps powder, and most do, it will benefit them, especially if you provide it over a long period of time, if not for the life of your cat.

Have fresh water always available. Due to our feline friends' increased risk of developing kidney disease, it's really important to always have multiple sources of fresh water around the house. When one of my older cats was suffering from increased kidney values on his blood test, and his thirst had increased while his body was trying to compensate for decreased kidney clearance of his toxins, I left glasses of fresh water all around the house. Chance wasn't getting around as well as he used to, so having those glasses of fresh water so he could access water everywhere really helped him, in my opinion.

Keep litter boxes clean. The ammonia from the urine build up in litter boxes can be caustic to upper respiratory membranes, and cause problems. Some cats are reluctant to use litter boxes when they are dirty, and will either urinate or defecate in the house, or not urinate, thus leading to bladder retention and increased risk of infections and lower urinary problems like crystals and bladder stones. Keep several boxes in the house and keep them clean.

Avoid feeding dry food. Dry food needs to have at least 50% carbohydrates in it so that it can be formed into those nuggets on heat and pressure extrusion. Cats are obligate carnivores and have no nutritional need for carbohydrates. When carbohydrates are fed constantly, the risk of obesity and type 2 diabetes increases greatly. Occasional dry food as a treat or a junk food meal is okay from time to time, but a higher protein and lower carbohydrate diet with moderate to high fats and oils is the best nutrient profile for most cats.

CAT-FRIENDLY SUPPLEMENTS for WELLNESS

1. EPA+DHA from fish oil, algal oil, or krill meal
   - Give 50 mg/pound of EPA+DHA daily
2. l-taurine (if taurine has been included in the food already may not need this)
   - 50-150 mg daily
3. B-complex (as found in nutritional yeast)
   - ¼-½ teaspoon per meal
4. Cordyceps mushroom 1:1 extract
   - ¼ teaspoon per meal
5. Probiotics
   - *Saccharomyces boulardii* (providing at least 2 billion colony forming units per day)
   - Multi-strain probiotic (providing at least 2 billion colony forming units per day)
   - Each of the above is good on its own, but with gut health issues, giving both is even better.
6. Flax seed meal
   - ¼ teaspoon per meal for the omega-3 and omega-6 fatty acids and for the soluble and insoluble fiber
7. Green foods (give ⅛ to ¼ teaspoon per meal of any or each of these):
   - Cracked cell chlorella
   - Spirulina
   - Powdered herbs like nettle leaf and alfalfa

DOC ROB'S WELLNESS PROGRAM FOR YOUR FOUR-LEGGED FAMILY MEMBER

C hecking off the boxes for each of the different wellness supplement categories can help to ensure you are building an effective wellness program for your pet.

☐ **Healthy food**, minimally processed with a nutrient profile matched to your pet's metabolism and life stage and fed with portion control to create an optimal body condition and weight in your pet

☐ **Probiotics** (healthy bowel bacteria) and digestion boosters like digestive enzymes and soluble and insoluble fiber sources

☐ **Healthy oils** to include both marine lipids, such as EPA/DHA, and the omega-3 and omega-6 fatty acids found in flax seed oil and hemp seed oil (ALA), which provide a broad spectrum of a variety of fatty acids

☐ **Antioxidants** from brightly colored fruits, vegetables, and herbs. Small amounts of fruits are okay to add to your pets' diet (especially berries, apples, and pears). Cats, with their lack of a metabolic need for sweets or carbohydrates, will still have a sweet tooth, as mentioned above. My Maine coon kitty loves cantaloupe, which is something I had often heard when in practice from my clients about their cats.

☐ Moderate daily **exercise**, **fresh air**, and **clean water**

☐ **Early obedience training** so your dog will mind you. Cats can be "sort of" trained, but not quite in the same way as dogs. Training techniques for cats are beyond the scope of this book, but if you feel you need something like that for your cat(s), there are behavioral specialists, many of whom are veterinarians, who can help you.

☐ The appropriate **herbal and nutraceutical supplements** based on your pet's needs. I've listed below some of the more commonly suggested and widely available supplements for wellness.

There are many great herbal, mushroom and nutraceutical supplements in addition to the ones I list below.

- **Turmeric** (find a highly bioavailable format of this culinary spice)

- **Silymarin** (best if standardized to 80% from milk thistle seed)

- **Medical Mushrooms** for wellness. I recommend a blend of several mushrooms, like a wellness "shotgun" approach. I recommend 5 Defenders™ for pets from Real Mushrooms pet product line. Mushrooms, in addition to containing beta-glucans and other immune-modulating compounds, also contain non-digestible fiber and chitin, which support the microbiome and the health of the gut lining. I consider mushrooms to be a keystone supplement for wellness but also for most medical problems that affect our four-legged family members.

☐ **Cannabinoid** use daily if your pet responds to its use (I recommend my Doc Silver Naturals tinctures: Sterling Silver™ and The Silver Bullet™, or my Doc Silver Naturals soft chews: SilverDog™ Savory chews and SilverCat™ Savory chews that contain both a broad spectrum CBD blended with CBG in a 2:1 ratio; these tasty dosage-form treats also contain two potent mushrooms, cordyceps and lion's mane.)

☐ **Nutritive green foods** like spirulina or chlorella, and nutritional herbs, such as nettles and alfalfa. Nutritional yeast and seaweeds, such as kelp or bladderwrack, round out my recommendations for wellness supplements.

NOTE TO THE READER

It is really important for you to find an integrative veterinarian who can guide you in your pet's wellness by virtue of a physical examination, thorough history taking, and the use of an alternative approach to pet health, like Traditional Chinese Veterinary Medicine, to understand your pet from a different perspective. Regular examinations and blood work are important to be able to catch problems early before they become more difficult to treat.

Although self-help books are great, and it's great to empower yourself so you can better care for your pet, veterinarians who are skilled in integrative medicine have the experience and skills to help you create a healthy, vibrant, long, and happy life for you and your pet.

RESOURCE GUIDE

In this Resource section, I have listed several directories for veterinarians who practice acupuncture and Chinese herbal therapies. Take a look to see if any are near you and what it's all about, schedule an appointment, and let them help you and your pet reach a new level of wellness that you may never have thought possible.

I have also listed both veterinarian and lay pet health consultants who can help you with your diet questions for your pets. This list is by no means complete.

You will also find a list of books I have found useful in my journey of learning about medicinal mushrooms, cannabis and integrative medicine. Some of these books are written for humans versus pets, but much of the information they contain holds true for our four-leggeds.

FIND A HOLISTIC VET

Integrative and Holistic Veterinarian listing:
www.AHVMA.org

Veterinary Herbalists
www.VBMA.org
www.AHVMA.org

Veterinary Acupuncturists
www.AAVA.org
www.IVAS.org

LIST OF PET NUTRITION CONSULTANTS
WHO CAN HELP WITH FORMULATING DIETS

List of veterinary nutritional specialists who may be able to help you with formulating a specific diet for your pet's health)
www.vetspecialists.com/specialties/nutrition

Veterinary Nutritional Consultants, founded by Dr. Rebecca Remillard, DVM has 5 veterinary nutritionists on staff
www.petdiets.com/about

Dr. Laura Gaylord, DVM nutritional service
www.wholepetprovisions.com

Raw Feeding Veterinary Society (UK based)
This is a group of veterinarians, veterinary nurses and other paraprofessionals with a common interest in raw feeding and species appropriate nutrition for dogs and cats.
www.rfvs.org

Diet consultations with Lindsey Hadfield, a pet nutrition consultant, with a certificate in Companion Animal Nutrition from the University of Illinois. Her website also has listings of other Nutrition Professionals you may want to browse through to find the right person for your pet.
www.clovisandcompany.com/professionals

Directory of Canine and Feline nutritional consultants both do-mestic and international, includes both veterinarians as well as paraprofessional pet health consultants.
www.freshfoodconsultants.org

Directory of Board Certified Veterinary Nutritionists both Domestic and International
www.balance.it/dacvim

Automated diet recipes, you factor in your pet information and requirements for the diet and the diet formulator provides you with a diet for home preparation. Very cool!
www.balance.it/recipes

The Feed Real Institute
Provides courses and education for pet parents and health consult-ants who want to learn more about creating healthy diets for pets.
www.feedreal.com

BOOKS

Pet Diets and Recipes

Fresh Food & Ancient Wisdom: Preparing Healthy and Balanced Meals for your Dogs. Ihor John Basko DVM, CVA. (2013) Makana Kai Publishing.

The Forever Dog: Surprising New Science to Help Your Canine Companion Liver Younger, Healthier and Longer. Rodney Habib and Dr Karen Shaw Becker (2021) Harper Wave: Harper Collins, NYC, NY.

The Forever Dog Life: 120+ Recipes, Longevity Tips, and New Science for Better Bowls & Healthier Homes. Dr. Karen Shaw Becker & Rodney Habib. (2024) Harper Collins Publishers, NYC, NY.

The Plant Powered Dog: Unleash the healing powers of a whole-food plant-based diet to help your canine companion enjoy a healthier, longer life. Diana Laverdure-Dunetz (2023) Dogwise Publishing Wenatchee, WA.

The Modern Dog Parent Handbook: The Holistic Approach to Raw Feeding, Mental Enrichment and Keeping your Dog Healthy and Happy. Bryce and Kenzie Francois (2023) Page Street Publishing, Salem, MA.

Home-Prepared Dog & Cat Diets. Patricia Schenck (2010) Wiley-Blackwell Publishing, Ames, IA.

Mushrooms

Christopher Hobbs's Medicinal Mushrooms - The Essential Guide: Boost immunity, Improve memory, Fight Cancer, Stop Infection, and Expand your Consciousness. Christopher Hobbs (2020) Storey Publishing, North Adams, MA.

The Rebel's Apothecary: A Practical Guide to the Healing Magic of Cannabis, CBD, and Mushrooms. Jenny Sansouci (2020) Tarcherperigee, Random House, LLC.

The Mushroom Cultivator: A Practical Guide to Growing Mushrooms at Home. Paul Stamets and J.S. Chilton (1983); Agarikon Press, Olympia, WA.

Entangled Life: How Fungi Make Our Worlds, Change Our Minds and & Shape our Futures. Merlin Sheldrake (2020) Random House, NY.

The Fungal Pharmacy: The Complete Guide to Medicinal Mushrooms & Lichens of North America. Robert Rogers (2011) North Atlantic Books, Berkeley, CA.

Mushrooms Demystified: A Comprehensive Guide to the Fleshy Fungi. David Arora (1986) Ten Speed Press; Berkeley.

All That the Rain Promises, and More… : A Hip Pocket Guide to Western Mushrooms. David Arora (1991) Ten Speed Press, Berkeley; BioSystems Books, Santa Cruz.

How to Forage for Mushrooms without Dying: An Absolute Beginners Guide to Identifying 29 Wild, Edible Mushrooms. Frank Hyman (2021) Storey Publishing, North Adams, MA.

Medicinal Mushrooms: A Clinical Guide. Martin Powell (2010), Mycology Press, East Sussex, UK.

Mushrooms: An Illustrated Field Guide. Niko Summers (2022) Appleseed Press Book Publishers, LLC., Nashville, TN.

Organic Mushroom Farming and Mycoremediation: Simple to Advanced and Experimental Techniques for Indoor and Outdoor Cultivation. Tradd Cotter (2014) Chelsea Green Publishing, White River, VT.

Cannabis and CBD

Handbook of Cannabis for Clinicians: Principles and Practice. Dustin Sulak, DO (2021) W.W. Norton & Company, NYC, NY.

CBD: What Does the Science Say? LA Parker, EM Rock and Raphael Mechoulam (2022) MIT Press, Cambridge, MA.

Cannabis Therapy in Veterinary Medicine: A Complete Guide. Cital, Kramer, Hughston and Gaynor, ed. (2021) Springer Nature, Switzerland.

INDEX

A

abdomen, 188, 190, 199, 205, 244–45

abscesses, 47–50, 96, 252, 280

absorption, 173, 226, 239, 269

acetaminophen, 169

acetylcholine, 156

acid group, 36, 174

active components, 101

active compounds, 34–35, 43, 81, 86, 108

active constituents, 18, 23, 81

active ingredients, 44, 48, 53, 59, 65, 70, 73, 78–79, 92, 96, 100, 102–3, 197, 254, 273

activity, 26, 165–66, 181–82, 201, 236–38, 255, 291

acupuncture, 12, 115, 162–64, 176, 183–86, 319, 322, 333–34, 336, 357

adaptogens, 55, 58, 66, 143, 240, 242

addiction, 77, 169–70, 349

adenocarcinomas, 209

adenosine, 41, 229

Adequan injections, 186

ADHD, 321, 338

agar, 29

agaratines, 48

Agaricus, 24, 45–50, 73, 77, 86–89, 230

    agaritine, 23

    arvensis, 46

    bisporus, 21, 23, 29, 39, 46–47, 85

    campestris, 46

aggressiveness, 148

aging, 38, 139, 162, 185

alcohol, 79

alfalfa, 352–55

algae, 35, 297

alkaline phosphatase, 319

allantoin, 274–75

allergic, 37, 85, 113, 116–17, 119, 124–31, 131, 133, 135, 253, 268

    dermatitis, 94, 107, 121, 126, 132–33

    rhinitis, 56

    skin disease, 118

allergies, 7–8, 12, 54–56, 82–84, 94, 107, 113–19, 122–32, 133–38, 269, 281–82, 285

    food, 128, 255

    inhalant, 128

    seasonal, 15, 107

    shots, 114, 127

    symptoms, 10, 116–20, 124–27, 135, 137

    testing, 283

aloe vera, 274–75

Althaea officinalis, 273

Alzheimer's disease, 62, 65, 82, 321

Amanita muscaria, 75
amino acids, 48, 156–60, 276, 294, 332
amputation, 192, 194, 200
Amyotrophic, 321
analgesic, 55, 84, 175, 263
anandamide, 153, 169
anaplasmosis, 328
anemia, 99, 169, 217–18, 328
    sickle cell, 38
angiogenesis, 215
animal DNA, 17
anti-aging, 55, 59, 75, 84–86, 91–93
anti-allergenic, 91
anti-allergic, 37, 132
anti-anxiety, 84, 145, 155
    pharmaceuticals, 145
anti-arthritic, 71
antibiotics, 123, 140, 258, 278–80
antibodies, 129–30, 213
    monoclonal, 125
anti-cancer, 36, 49, 55, 64–65, 69, 83–87, 96, 98, 100, 220
    herbs, 205
    molecules, 204, 229
anti-cholesterol, 50, 55
anti-convulsant, 329, 338
anti-depressant, 69, 84
anti-emetic, 271
anti-epileptic drugs, 325–26
anti-fatigue, 55, 58
anti-fungal, 61, 263
antigens, 127, 257, 278
    environmental, 128
anti-hepatotoxic, 81
antihistamines, 79, 100, 105, 114, 124
anti-hyperlipidemic, 38, 53
anti-inflammatory, 62, 95, 119, 175, 177–78, 278

diet, 121, 186, 342
    supplements, 342
anti-leukemia, 61
anti-Lyme's disease, 61
anti-microbial, 47–49, 64, 69, 86–88
anti-nausea, 271
anti-neoplastic, 81
anti-obesity, 71
antioxidants, 37–38, 50, 55, 70, 83, 95, 175, 232–34, 246, 335, 343, 348, 353
    amino acid, 38, 234
    compounds, 232
    drinks, 234
    extracts, 234
    food-bound, 348
    fungal, 336
    plant-bound, 233
anti-parasite, 20, 55
antiseptic soap, 123
anti-tuberculosis, 53
anti-tumor, 38, 53, 81
anti-viral, 47–55, 58–61, 69–71, 83–87
anus, 128, 256, 261, 275, 279
    anal gland, 128, 280
anxiety, 5–7, 10–15, 67, 76–77, 100, 141, 144–49, 153–56, 160–61, 258, 261, 317, 344
    disorders, 42, 76–78
    separation, 148, 157
aphrodisiac, 58
apoptosis, 37–38, 241
Apoquel, 113–15, 126–27
apples, 246, 263, 353
arabinogalactans, 239
arthritis, 7–8, 70, 80, 97, 162–63, 165–68, 171–73, 175–76, 179–80, 186, 344
    bony, 163, 165, 176
    cat, 186

juvenile, 166
pain, 174
rheumatoid, 163, 166, 176, 178
symptoms, 167
ascomycete, 58
ascorbic acid (vitamin C), 246
ash, 24
Ashwagandha, 236, 240–41
Asia, 80, 90–91, 119, 197, 333
asthma, 41, 57–62, 80, 92
bronchial, 56
Astragalus root, 236, 240–41
atherosclerosis, 91
athletes, 41, 59, 162, 165, 181
equine, 57
world-class, 181
atopic dermatitis, 55, 90–94, 126, 133
feline, 133
atopy, 124, 132
Auricularia auricula, 21, 91
autoimmune, 118
azurescens, 77

B

bacteria, 13, 18, 136, 246, 259, 269, 278
bowel, 353
healthy, 135
probiotic, 258
barbiturate, 325
bark, 18, 38, 51–52, 239
inner, 275
tree's, 51
Basidiomycota, 47, 69, 73, 77, 80, 86, 91, 95
beans, 160, 347
green, 287, 348
beech, 69, 86
beef, 128, 160, 305

behavior, 140–41, 144–46, 148–54, 157–60, 168, 170, 293, 339
aggressive, 160
anxious, 149, 155, 158
destructive, 123, 148
fear-based, 153
good, 150
negative, 157
scooting, 280
stress-related, 148
territorial, 152
behavioral disorders, 77
behavioral problems, 139–40, 148–49, 153, 156, 185, 338
Benadryl, 125
benign tumors, 209
beta-caryophyllene, 263
beta-glucans, 23–24, 29–31, 35–37, 39–41, 48, 52–53, 57–59, 70–75, 78–82, 94–96, 100, 102–6, 118, 219, 229, 236–37
compounds, 40
molecules, 36, 94–95, 229
peptide-enhanced, 36
polysaccharides, 277
structures, 37
unique, 68
beta-sitosterol, 81, 96
betulin, 53
betulinic acid, 38, 51–53
Bhutan, 57
bile, 40, 267
bioactive components, 23
bioavailability, 103, 135, 226, 239, 354
biochemical, 17, 213
biomass, 31–33
mycelial, 30
bipolar disorder, 42
birch tree fungus, 51–54

birds, 307
bite, 56
black currant, 135
black forest, 85
black gum, 69
bladder
    bladderwrack, 355
    retention, 351
    stones, 351
bleeding, 96, 113, 169, 188, 190,
    196, 205, 242–43, 259
blood, 48–50, 88, 154, 173,
    237–39, 241–43, 245, 248–
    50, 253, 286, 293, 313–14,
    329–30
    abdominal, 243
    clotting, 196, 242
    fats, 64
    glucose, 23
    loss, 188, 190, 199
    stagnation types, 244
    sugar, 23, 47–50, 64, 69, 94,
        327–29
    tests, 127, 129–30, 163, 167–
        69, 211, 237, 259, 313,
        320, 327, 351, 355
    thinners, 93
    vessels, 93
blood-brain barrier, 36, 38, 42,
    321
bloodstream, 154
blueberries, 234
Body Condition Score (BCS),
    289, 300–301
body language, 148
body weight, 104–6, 118, 131,
    133, 154, 172, 198, 241, 287,
    291, 296, 298, 309, 317, 325,
    343
bone meal, 305, 308, 348
    powdered, 304
bones

broken, 142, 346
    chicken, 178, 305
    cooked, 305
    formation, 40
    marrow, 61, 105, 218
    rib, 305
    spurs, 163–66
bony deposits, 163
bony swelling, 168
borage, 296
    black, 309
    oil, 120
bowel, 62, 135–36, 256–62,
    268–70, 273–76, 278–79
    diseases, 337
    hyperpermeability, 261
    inflammation, 261–62, 272,
        278
    lining, 272
    lower, 259
    motility, 261, 280
    problems, 136, 258
brain, 36, 42, 51, 60–67, 82, 92,
    174, 240, 258, 261, 321, 323–
    24, 332, 335
    abnormalities, 314
    cells, 314, 337
    health, 330
    tumors, 210, 329
break, 19, 23, 117, 162, 242, 244,
    255, 267–68, 304–5
breast, 49, 53, 89
broad-spectrum CBD tincture,
    226–28
broad-spectrum hemp products,
    173, 224, 331
bronchitis, 57, 61
budesonide, 278–79

C

caerulescens, 77

caffeine, 145, 158, 234–35

calcium, 286–87, 289, 304–9, 348

  algae-based, 308

  deposits, 165

  eggshell, 309

  excess, 286

  imbalances, 329

  metabolism, 308

  supplements, 308–9

calcium carbonate, 304

California poppy, 159

calming, 36–37, 66, 71, 82–84, 94, 100, 105, 140, 145, 149, 155–58, 161, 170, 175, 335

calories, 22, 179–81, 195, 249–50, 296, 299–302, 337, 344

Canada, 31, 52, 69, 174, 191, 214, 221, 254

cancer, 6–9, 12–16, 36–38, 51–56, 58–60, 71, 80–94, 96–100, 189–92, 195–200, 202–6, 209–24, 228–32, 235–43, 245–51, 289–93

  bladder, 245, 250

  bone, 200, 213

  brain, 314, 328

  breast, 47, 71

  carcinoma-type, 209

  cells, 36–37, 38, 41, 195, 205, 209, 210, 211, 212, 213, 219–22, 222, 223, 229, 232, 233, 234, 235, 236, 237, 238–40, 241, 245–48, 337

  chemotherapy, 233, 276

  connective tissue, 71

  cytotoxicity, 233

  diagnosis, 191, 202–3, 215, 219

  diet, 203, 234, 247, 251

  gastric, 63

  growth, 6, 158, 198, 204–5, 218, 220–23, 229, 234, 237, 238–42

  lung, 142, 188

  malignant, 209

  markers, 259

  patient, 62, 216, 224, 231, 246–47, 249, 287, 337

  prevention, 64

  side effects, 220, 223

  splenic, 16, 98, 191

  supplements, 203, 232

  support, 45, 51, 62, 66–67, 71

  terminal, 251

  therapies, 13, 50, 187, 189, 191–92, 199, 211, 214, 220, 223, 232–34, 238, 245

  treatment, 20, 192–93, 195, 211, 213–14, 220, 229

  tumors, 51, 242

canker, 51–52

cannabigerol, 155

cannabinoids, 123, 131–32, 145, 154–55, 169, 172–73, 175, 221, 256, 261, 318, 321, 326–31

  acidic, 155, 174, 330, 331

  individual, 175

  intoxicating, 331

  minor, 155, 173, 261, 317

  receptors, 261

  with mushrooms, 148, 256, 259, 278

cannabis, 2–3, 6–13, 16, 109–11, 131, 175–78, 191, 220–23, 232–33, 260–61, 262–63, 322, 329, 359–61

  adult-use, 204

  compounds, 5

extracts, 37, 131, 175, 222–23, 317, 321
fiber, 3
for arthritis, 173
full-spectrum, 191
legislation, 191
medical, 187, 214
plant, 220, 321, 331, 342
products, 2, 329
therapeutics, 321
canned tuna fish, 160
Capromelin, 280
capsules, 101, 243–44, 270, 276, 278
carbohydrates, 22, 23, 29, 160–61, 180, 195, 247–48, 249–50, 287, 289–95, 295, 304, 305, 337, 343, 349, 351, 353
high carbohydrate diets, 180, 337, 349
carcinogens, 48, 210
carcinomas, 209
cardiac arrest, 45, 141
cardiomyopathy, 141
cardioprotective, 64, 97
cardiotonic, 58–61
cardiovascular, 53, 60–61
care, end-of-life, 188
carnivores
facultative, 294
obligate, 296, 349, 351
carotenoids, 73
carprofen, 155, 169
cartilage, 166, 177–78, 209
cat fights, 139
catalase, 73
caterpillar mushroom, 56
catnip, 146, 159

cats, 12–15, 39–40, 116–18, 122, 125–27, 132–34, 139–41, 151–52, 207, 211–12, 237, 259–60, 294–96, 301–2, 307–9, 334–36, 342–44, 349–54
adult, 139
female, 152
mouth, 285
urine, 141, 152
CBA, 326
CBC, 174, 327
CBCA, 331
CBD, 11–12, 117, 123, 131–32, 140–41, 145–46, 153–56, 172–76, 178–79, 204–5, 220–24, 227–28, 234, 261–65, 317–21, 325–32, 344, 346–47, 359–61
blood levels, 154, 326
broad-spectrum, 131, 195, 222, 264
full-spectrum, 153
idiopathic epilepsy, 10
spectrum, 355
unprocessed, 172
CBD and THC, 6, 174, 204, 209, 214, 220, 221–23, 228, 265, 321
CBD/CBDA, 131
CBDA, 117, 122–23, 131–32, 155, 172–74, 223, 317, 327–30, 331
salve, 123
tincture, 330
CBG, 63, 117–18, 123, 140, 145–46, 149, 155, 164, 173–74, 256, 261, 317, 319, 327–30, 330, 355
formula, 318
tincture, 140, 253, 318
CBGA, 155, 174, 327–30, 331

CCD (Canine cognitive disorder), 63–66
cell death, 241
    programmed, 37
cell lines
    canine cancer, 71
    epithelial, 209
cell migration, 37
cells, 37–38, 41, 119, 123, 133, 159, 209–11, 212–13, 235–37, 239, 246, 276
    allergy, 119
    cancerous, 210
    dendritic, 36
    healthy, 212, 240, 247–48
    mast, 36, 37, 119–20, 122–24, 135
    mucosal epithelial, 277
    neoplastic, 95
    new, 38
    non-cancerous, 209, 239
    pre-cancerous, 236
    pro-inflammatory, 259
    walls, 35, 94, 237
    white blood, 36
cellular membrane, 159
Central America, 20, 76
chaga, 36–38, 45, 51–52, 62, 67, 100, 102, 118–19, 176, 197, 230
    extract, 32
chamomile, 156
cheese, 160
chemotherapy, 16, 50, 61, 83, 89, 99, 105, 188–90, 195, 197, 199, 211–18, 231–33, 287
    agents, 209, 211–13, 233, 250
        individual, 213
        oral, 215
        Taxol, 18
    aggressive, 190
    chemotherapeutic agents, 212

drugs, 204
    metronomic, 215
    protocols, 218
    side effects, 212, 231
chest, 162, 196, 244, 300
chicken, 50, 253, 255, 305
    liver, 255
Chihuahua, 103
China, 2, 21, 64, 69, 78, 86, 216, 242
Chinese herbal medicine, 98, 106, 191, 196, 200, 204, 241–42, 245, 316, 319, 322, 327, 333–35
    cancer, 205
    hemangiosarcoma, 196
chiropractic, 12, 183
chitin, 23, 79, 92, 118, 136, 276–77, 354
chlorpheniramine, 125
cholecalciferol, 238
cholesterol, 39–41, 47–49, 73, 86–87, 91, 238
    levels, 40–41, 53, 75, 82–85, 93, 100
    molecules, 40, 237–38
    synthesis, 81
choline chloride, 156, 159
chondroitin, 165
chondroitin sulfate, 177–78
chromosomes, 28
chronic inflammatory granulomatous condition, 133
circulation, 19, 60, 74, 86, 94, 97, 222
citrinopileatus, 72
CLA (conjugated linolenic acid), 48
Claritin, 125
claws, 141
clinic, 207, 312, 314–15, 322
clinical trial, 71, 116, 203, 217

Clinker polypore, 52
clomipramine, 149
cognitive dysfunction, 39, 63–66, 90–94, 321
colds, 47–50
colitis, 89, 136, 257–59, 263, 270–72, 278–79
collagen, 177
colon, 49, 267
Colorado, 142–43, 162, 181, 281, 314, 325, 345–46
Columbia, 221
commercial diets, 180, 234, 249–50, 260, 282
    kibble, 267, 293, 315
components
    isolated, 89
    multiple, 102
compounds, 2–3, 18, 36, 40–42, 100, 123, 125, 153, 175, 220, 232, 246, 274, 321
    anti-cancer, 48
    bioactive, 118
    cytotoxic, 232
    extracellular, 33
    fiber-bound medicinal, 106
    hallucinogenic, 42
    hydrazine, 23, 48
    immune-modulating, 95, 354
    individual, 43
    low-toxicity, 23
    multiple, 16, 35, 321
    pro-inflammatory, 125
    psychoactive, 1, 42
    toxic, 23
congestive heart failure, 196, 244
Congress, 107
conjugated linolenic acid (CLA), 48
conjunctivitis, 83
constipation, 74, 93, 274

constituents, bioactive anti-cancer, 229
consumption, 38, 51, 197
contact dermatitis, 126, 129
contamination, 39, 105
convulsions, 339
coral, 27, 62, 304
cordycepin, 41, 59, 229
cordyceps, 41, 45–46, 56–57, 63, 176–77, 230, 240, 330, 355
    extract, 32, 146
    militaris, 41
    powder, 351
Cordyceps militaris, 57
coriolus versicolor, 95
corticosteroids, 124–26, 134, 296
cosmetics, 91, 119
cough, 47, 50, 57–61, 91–96
COX1, 71
COX2, 71, 155, 169
cracked cell chlorella, 352
craniomandibular osteopathy, 304
crimini, 46, 266
Crohn's disease, 259
cubensis, 77
cultivation, 21, 29, 68
cultures, 2, 21, 67, 76, 197, 269
Curcuma zedoaria, 244
curcumin, 198, 233, 236, 238–39, 344
Cushing's disease, 120, 296
cyanescens, 77
cyanobacteria, 38
cyanthane derivatives, 65
cyclooctasulphur, 81
cyclosporin, 115, 124
cyproheptadine, 280
cytokines, 87, 125–26
cytopoint, 113–15, 126

cytotoxicity, 71, 219, 233, 241, 246

D

d-alpha-tocopherol, 335
dandelion, 137, 344
death, 71, 147, 194, 202, 305, 325
decaffeinate, 235
defecation, 193–94, 265, 279, 323, 351
dehydration, 279
dementia, 15, 63–67
demulcent, 273–75
dental problems, 257
Denver, 156, 214
depression, 42, 67, 76–77, 82
dermatitis, 113, 122, 126, 132–34, 269, 297
detoxification, 137, 344
devil's claw, 178
dexamethasone, 113–15
D-fraction, 70–71
DHA, 119, 134–35, 195, 294, 297
diabetes, 47–53, 58, 69–71, 84–86, 97, 207–8, 248, 281, 351
  ketoacidotic, 338
  mellitus, 248
  support, 55
  treatment, 208
diagnosis, 9, 167, 199, 217, 219, 316, 328, 333–34
diagnostics, 9, 188, 211, 258, 314, 333–34
dialkyl tryptamines, 42
diarrhea, 121, 198, 252–60, 262–63, 269, 274, 276, 278–80, 294, 299
diet, 128–29, 160–61, 179–80, 247–52, 254–55, 259–62, 268–69, 278, 281–99, 301–4,

305–11, 315–16, 334–43, 347–49, 357–58
  canned, 248
  changes, 260, 262, 266, 287
  elimination, 128, 284, 311
  fiber, 24, 239
  healthy, 205, 247, 291, 311
  high protein, 160, 180
  hydrolyzed protein, 269
  hypoallergenic, 128–29
  ketongenic, 10, 160, 180, 195, 200–201, 204, 245, 247–50, 287, 293–97, 316, 318, 337–39, 343
  low-carbohydrate, 250
  mono, 284
  native, 307
  non-inflammatory, 121
  non-reactive, 284
  preparation, 248, 289–90
  starvation, 349
  vegan, 294
Dietary Supplement Health and Education Act (DSHEA), 107
digestion, 19, 28–29, 70, 156, 253–55, 258, 260–61, 267–68, 269, 271, 288, 297, 344, 353
  disorders, 7–8, 252, 256–60, 278, 281–82
  enzymes, 28, 253–58, 260, 267–69, 269, 271, 342, 344, 349, 353
  herbs, 271
digestive
  system, 17, 20, 122, 229, 254–57, 260–61, 267, 289, 292, 306, 342–44, 349
  tract, 257, 261, 268
dilated pupils, 324
Ding Xian Wan, 334

diphenhydramine, 125
discomfort, 84, 169, 176, 186, 275, 279
diseases, 12, 18, 35, 40, 107–8, 165–67, 231, 235–36, 256, 259, 322–23, 329, 341
  autoimmune, 83, 163, 166
  bone, 289, 304
  brain, 314
  canine, 321
  cardiovascular, 38
  chronic, 8, 282, 299
  clinical, 344
  degenerative, 289
  digestive, 291
  gastro-esophageal reflux, 263
  human, 321
  immune-mediated, 224, 236
  infectious, 45, 90
  lower urinary tract, 55
  neurological, 38, 322
  pulmonary, 96
  renal, 292
  terminal, 13, 72, 198, 214, 231
  viral, 15, 85
dispensaries, 10, 174, 191, 204, 223–25, 228, 264–65
distemper, 72, 328
distillate, 224, 226–27
  hemp oil, 262
diterpenes, 36, 63, 175
diuretic, 69, 74
Doc Silver Naturals, 145, 317, 330, 355
dolomite, 304–5
Dong Chong Xia Cao, 57
dosage, 97–99, 102–3, 131, 134–36, 153–54, 172–73, 195–96, 197–98, 220–21, 224, 227–28, 240, 262, 264–66, 277–78, 315–19, 330

cannabis, 191
  high, 132, 145, 153–54, 170, 174, 198, 215, 238, 264, 273, 317, 319–20
  lethal, 206
  marshmallow root, 273
  maximum tolerated dose (MTD), 212, 215
  microdosing, 1, 76
  PEA, 133
  psyllium, 274
  slippery elm, 275
Dravet syndrome, 317, 321
dried mushrooms, 90, 101, 102, 108
drugs
  anti-allergy, 126
  anti-convulsant, 316, 331
  anti-inflammatory, 123
  cholesterol-lowering, 40
  energy-suppressive, 270
  immunomodulatory, 127
  narcotic, 169
  pharmaceutical, 145, 149
DSHEA (Dietary Supplement Health and Education Act), 107
dust, 118, 122

E

E. coli, 301
ears, 128, 140, 148–50
edible mushrooms, 20, 21, 67, 72, 85, 108, 277, 336, 360
education, 187, 347, 358
effects
  additive, 120
  antihistamine, 55
  anxiolytic, 155, 347
  intoxicating, 174
  pro-oxidant, 249
  sickening, 212

efficacy, 40

eggs, 116, 123, 132, 160, 304
  shells, 304, 309, 348

Egypt, 2, 20

eicosapentaenoic acid (EPA),
  119, 134–35, 177, 248, 291–
  94, 297–99, 332, 352–53

elbows, 171
  dysplasia, 166

electrical stimulation, 336

electromagnetic waveforms, 157,
  185

elm, 69, 246

emotions, 144, 153, 206–7, 256,
  347

encephalitis, 328

endocannabinoids, 261, 342–44

endophytes, 17–18

endoscopy, 242, 270

energy, 57–58, 83, 89–91, 195,
  201, 202–3, 245, 247–48,
  256, 288, 293, 324–25, 337–
  38
  cellular, 205
  energetics, 88–92, 97, 245
  mental, 256
  nervous, 256
  support, 59

Entocort, 278

Entyce, 280

environment, 122, 148, 162, 259,
  323, 342–43

enzymes, 40, 117, 151, 169, 255,
  262, 267–69
  cholesterol-lowering, 40
  elevation, 319
  pancreatic, 255–56, 268

Epidiolex, 321

Epigallocatechin gallate (EGCG),
  234–35

epilepsy, 7–9, 12, 36, 46, 82–84,
  249, 281, 293, 316–17, 321–
  24, 325, 327–30, 332–38,
  338, 339, 344
  idiopathic, 10, 323, 329
  patients, 160, 249, 312, 315–
    16, 324, 330–33, 335–37
  refractory, 249, 316–17, 325
  seizures, 170, 250, 313–14,
    316, 320, 324–25, 327,
    331, 339
  treatment-resistant, 316–17,
    320, 325, 328

ergocalciferol, 39, 68, 72, 238

Ergostane, 65

ergosterol, 39–40, 48, 53, 59, 65,
  68–73, 78, 81, 92, 96, 103,
  238, 335

ergothioneine (ERGO), 24, 38–
  39, 48, 59, 73, 92, 175, 336,
  342

erinacines, 65

eritadenine, 41, 87

eryngii, 72

esophagus, 65, 257

ethnobotany, 1, 4, 47

Europe, 64, 69, 246

euthanasia, 126, 194, 201, 206–8

examination, 112, 253, 313, 355

exercise, moderate, 342–43

exocrine pancreatic insufficiency
  (EPI), 255–56

extracts, 43, 57, 79, 95, 98, 102–
  3, 196–97, 254, 262–63, 342,
  352
  broad-spectrum, 173, 261–62
  individual, 197

F

facial twitches, 324
fasting, 173, 344
  intermittent, 343–44
fatigue, 54, 80
fats, 22–24, 36, 68, 74, 113, 116, 162, 180–81, 195, 247, 249–50, 289–93, 296, 301, 337–38
  excess, 50
  healthy, 48, 180, 291, 343
  metabolism, 195, 248, 337
fatty acids, 120, 134–35, 248, 291–94, 296–99, 308, 316, 332, 352–53
  anti-inflammatory, 120, 297
  polyunsaturated, 294, 297
fatty molecule, 116, 133
FDA (Food and Drug Administration), 107, 133, 216, 239, 265
feathers, 307
fecal transplantation, 270
feline eosinophilic granuloma, 133
Feline Immunodeficiency Virus (FIV), 88
feline protozoal toxoplasmosis, 328
femoral head ostectomy, 171
femur, 142, 144, 184, 346
fermentation, 18, 136
fertility, 58
fevers, 69–71, 96
fiber, 2, 22–23, 68, 101, 118, 136, 254, 266, 270, 278, 294, 344
  healthy, 25
  indigestible, 23, 94, 253, 277, 354
fibromyalgia, 56
fireworks, 157

First Amendment, 108
fish, 40, 160, 195, 248, 285
fish oil, 115, 119–20, 134–35, 164–65, 179, 233–34, 291, 297–99, 327, 332, 338, 343, 348, 350–52
  high doses, 177, 249, 316
  omega-3, 294
flagella, 17
flavonoids, 68, 118, 120, 135, 159, 175, 220, 229, 287, 316
flax, 119–20, 291–94, 296–97, 298, 348, 350, 352–53
flesh of the gods, 21
fluid, 166–68, 194, 225, 262, 274, 279
  intravenous, 245–47
Fluoxetine, 145
Fomes fomentarius, 20
food, 18–23, 101–2, 115–18, 121–22, 127–33, 135–40, 160–61, 173, 179–81, 233–34, 253–55, 265–69, 270–77, 282–86, 288–90, 299–303, 306–10, 343–44, 346–47, 349–52
  allergies, 127–30, 268, 282–83
  antioxidant-rich, 234
  cancer, 245
  canned, 260, 293, 315, 318, 350
  cooked, 311
  digesting, 255, 261, 268
  fatty, 131, 145, 198, 318
  fermented, 18
  fresh, 285, 301, 358
  home-prepared, 267, 288
  hygienic handling, 306, 347
  intolerance, 130, 254
  metabolizing, 245
  minimally-processed, 282

moist, 140, 181
non-reactive, 283–84
oily, 299
processed, 161, 302, 342
reactive, 283
sensitivities, 55, 130, 253,
    283–85, 288, 311
supplements, 350
unprocessed, 315, 347
Food and Drug Administration.
    See FDA.
foraging, 197
forests, 19, 21, 203
fruit bodies, 26–28, 30–33, 51,
    56, 90
    grain-free, 57
fruits, 2, 26, 135, 175, 234, 262,
    353
fungal, 15
    endophyte, 18
    enzymes, 255
    extract, 31
    forms, 19, 28
    mycelia, 3
    mycelium, 18–19, 38, 51–52,
        56, 335
fungi, 1, 2, 3, 6, 13, 17–20, 27,
    34–35, 38–40, 51, 56, 76, 90,
    94, 136, 269, 335
    braided, 68
    caterpillar, 57
    jelly, 90
    kombucha, 19
    medicinal, 1, 6
    parasitic, 56
    snow, 90, 119

G

G. oregonensis, 80
GABA, 65
gabapentin, 149, 170, 314, 320,
    325

gait exam, 167
gall bladder, 267
Galliprant, 169
gamma-linolenic acid (GLA),
    120, 135, 297
ganoderic acids, 81, 335
Ganoderma, 79–80
    lingzhi, 79, 335
    lucidum, 79, 149
Ganodosterone, 81
gas chromatography, 262
gastritis, 51–56, 63–66, 90–93,
    272
gastroenterology, 256, 263, 349
gastro-esophageal reflux disease
    (GERD), 263
gastrointestinal problems, 53,
    64–67, 93, 258, 262–64, 267
genetics, 133, 166, 209, 213, 258,
    282
geochemistry, 17
geriatrics, 63, 206, 289, 310, 330
German shepherd, 255
giant mastiff, 103
ginger root, 255, 258, 271, 344
    powdered dried, 271
ginseng, 242
glands, 209, 280, 307
    adrenal, 59, 240
    anal, 252–53, 279–80
    endocrine, 240
    salivary, 267
    scent, 140–41, 279
glaucoma, 141–42
glucan chain, 36
glucosamine, 107, 164–65, 177–
    78, 186, 276–77
glucose, 229, 350
glutamine, 276
glutathione, 38, 73
GME, 321
golden oyster, 72–73

gonorrhea, 69
grain, 29–30, 31, 34–36, 39, 52, 57, 137, 237
  carbohydrates, 30
  grain-free diet, 30
  myceliated, 29–31, 105
  mycelium, 29–33
  spawn, 29–30
granulomatous meningoencephalitis, 321
Great Dane, 286, 292
Great Pyrenees, 292
green tea, 51, 145, 158, 233–35
  extracts, 233
Grifolan, 68–70
groggy, 149
groin, 300
ground turkey, 348
gut, 136, 170, 253, 256, 266–69, 274, 276–77, 304
  inflamed, 260
  leaky, 136, 260, 276–77
  lining, 354
Gymnopilus junonius, 77

H

hair, 122
  hairballs, 274, 350
  haircoat, 10, 113, 118
  loss, 50, 138
hallucinations, 1
head injury, 328
health
  benefits, 15–16, 72, 108
  digestive, 136, 271, 286
  intestinal, 50
  joint, 176, 276
  mental, 42, 75–76
  optimal, 288, 340
heart, 16, 66, 70, 83, 92, 97, 112, 190

hemangiosarcoma, 16, 98–99, 188–91, 195–200, 204–5, 216–17, 242–44, 251
  cancer cells, 243
  naturally-occurring, 217
  treatment, 188, 217–18, 251
hematocrit, 99, 217–18
hemorrhoids, 69
hemostatic, 96
hemp, 153, 173–74, 222, 224, 264, 291–94, 296–97, 309, 329, 353
  broad-spectrum, 174
  cultivar, 228
  full-spectrum, 173–74, 222
  products, 263
  seed meal, 298
  seed oil, 298
Hemp Farming Act, 172
hen of the woods, 67
hepatitis, 58, 80, 89, 96, 245
hepatoprotective, 37, 50, 58–61, 64, 69–71, 84–92, 97
herbs, 134, 137, 158–61, 177–79, 186–88, 196, 198, 232–33, 241–45, 258–60, 262, 271–75, 339–40, 344, 353–54
  liver-protectant, 331
  low-glycemic, 272
  soothing, 260
Hericium erinaceus, 63, 149, 335
herpes virus, 87–88
hip, 142–44, 147, 166, 171, 184
  dislocated, 142, 184, 346
  dysplasia, 171
histamine, 37, 119–20, 124, 135
  chemical, 119
  release, 37, 81, 119–20, 122, 135
histopathology, 212
Hobbs, Christopher, 2

holistic, 7, 12, 137, 152, 188, 219, 266, 281, 315, 356

homemade diet, 8, 12, 180–81, 234, 281–83, 286–89, 293, 301, 306, 308–10, 314, 347, 349–50

homeopathy, 13, 115

homeostasis, 236

hormones, 120, 152, 240
    reproductive, 152

horses, 15, 40, 57, 122, 132, 166, 176, 211–12, 226, 322, 333, 336

hospice, 202

Houston, 142

HPA-Adrenal Axis, 240

HSA cancer cells, 196

Hui Shu Hua, 68

Huisheng Xie, 196, 241

human
    civilization, 20
    patients, 62, 212

human immunodeficiency virus (HIV), 87–89

hydration, 90–93, 119, 194, 349

hydrochloric acid, 268

hydrochloride, 177

hydrogen peroxide, 246

hydrophilic, 273

hyperlipidemia, 48–50, 74, 88

hypersensitivity, 114, 122, 128, 138, 236, 259

hypertension, 56, 80–83, 273

hypertrophic osteopathy, 304

hyphal tubes, 28–29

hypoallergenic, 39, 128–29, 284

hypoglycemic, 81

I

IBD (Inflammatory Bowel Disease), 12, 53–56, 63, 97, 136, 228, 257–59, 263, 266, 275, 277–79, 281

IBD (inflammatory bowel disease), feline, 258

IBS (irritable bowel syndrome), 256–59, 278

ibuprofen, 155

idiopathic, 259, 278, 323, 328–29

IgE, 130
    antibodies, 129–30

IgG, 130

IgM antibodies, 130

IL-12, 87

IL-31, 126

IL-31 cytokine, 126

imaging, 167

immune
    activation, 37
    cells, 122, 125–26, 135, 229, 246, 340
        allergy-activated, 125
        pro-inflammatory, 258
    defense, 96
    dysfunction, 86, 96–97, 116
    enhancement, 36, 50, 235
    function, 58, 74, 115, 202, 235
    modulation, 74, 81–82, 89, 93, 118, 126, 235–36, 260
    response, 72, 133
    support, 2, 45, 55, 60, 65, 75, 82, 175
    suppressive therapies, 124
    system, 118–19, 121–22, 124, 127, 136–38, 163, 166, 210, 213, 219, 235–37, 245, 268, 282, 340
        healthy, 235
        over-active, 236

immunocompromised, 72

immunocytes, 340

Imodium, 280
implants, 222
I'mYunity, 36, 98, 197, 203, 204, 216–17
India, 2
Indian ginseng, 240
indigestion, 47
indole alkaloid, 42
infections, 13, 47, 83, 88–91, 100, 105, 132, 253, 280, 322, 328, 351
   acute, 105
   bacterial, 96, 140
   fungal, 12–13, 17
   viral, 88–89, 97
infiltration, 258
inflammation, 117, 122, 134–35, 136, 155, 157, 169, 172, 175–79, 180, 241, 260, 261–64, 277–79, 342
   chronic, 276
   decreasing, 121, 125
   excessive, 121
   increasing, 268
   joint, 180
   peri-rectal, 275
   reducing, 36, 120–22, 178, 332
Inflammatory Bowel Disease. See IBD.
inflammatory dermatitis, 113
inflammatory diseases, 258–59
   oral, 275
inflammatory infiltrates, 259
ingestion, 108, 259, 274, 303
   repeated, 85
ingredient labels, 311
ingredients
   allergenic, 129
   fat, 296
   hypoallergenic, 129
   non-reactive, 129, 283–84

residues, 310
sensitivities, 283
inhibition, 37
inhibitory neurotransmitter, 332
injections, 126–27, 246
   injection therapy, 128
   mistletoe, 246
Inonotus obliquus, 52
Inositol, 54
Inositol hexaphosphate, 236, 239
Inositol-1,2,3,4,5,6-hexaphosphate, 239
inotodiol, 37, 51–54
insects, 17–18, 28, 56
insoluble fiber, 120, 273, 296–97, 352–53
insulin, 23
intervention, 67, 231
intestines, 169, 196, 267, 272
   small, 267–68, 276
intoxicating, 174, 264, 331
ionizing radiation, 90, 210
IP-6, 239–40
irritable bowel syndrome. See IBS.
ISY-15, 48
Italian Alps, 20
itching, 116–23, 126, 131–35

J

Japan, 47, 64, 69, 80, 86, 123, 136
Japanese alder, 86
Japanese evergreen oak tree, 85
jaw muscles, 305
joints, 163–67, 179, 277
   bad, 176
   cartilage, 163, 166, 177–78
   elbow, 166
   fluid, 165–66, 177–79, 277
   pain, 178, 277
      chronic, 176

pained, 185
pet's, 165
replacement surgery, 171
supplements, 176–78

K

kelp, 355
ketoacidosis, 248
ketones, 195, 247–50, 293, 337–38
ketosis, 248–49, 293, 338
KetoStix, 338
kibble, 137, 234, 249–50, 260, 267–68, 301, 305, 343, 347, 349–50, 350, 351
kidney beans, 62
kidney disease, 57–61, 62, 287, 289–91, 327, 351
Kidney Jing, 92
Kidney Qi, 60
kidneys, 15, 54, 57–62, 66, 92–93, 99, 169, 230, 286, 292, 308–9, 330, 334, 351
king oyster, 72–73
knees, 142, 163

L

labels, 31, 105, 310
laboratory animals, 62, 71, 84, 89, 93, 240
Labrador retriever, 141–43, 162, 179, 184–87, 200–201, 251, 340, 345–47, 349
lactic acid, 248, 337
lactones, 54
lanosteroid triterpenoids, 53
lanosterols, 51–53
larch arabinogalactan, 236
Larix occidentalis, 239
lateral sclerosis, 321
lavender, 153, 175

leaf, 28, 56
leaky gut syndrome, 261, 277
lectins, 48
legalization, 172, 220, 329
legs, 57, 144, 163, 168, 184, 324, 336
broken, 142
damaged, 147
diseased, 200
lemon balm, 146
lentinan, 86–89
leukemia, 64
levetiracetam, 325
L-glutamine, 276
Liberty cap, 77
licking, 114, 120, 122–23, 128
licorice, 137, 258, 272–73
life cycle, fungal, 27–28, 34
lifespan, 179, 259
ligaments, 74, 167, 307
lignans, 120, 296
limb, painful, 179
limonene, 229, 263
limp, 163, 168, 181–82
linalool, 153
terpene, 175
linoleic acid, 119, 297
gamma, 135
lion's mane, 45–46, 51, 62–63, 136, 140, 145, 149, 155, 254, 256, 327, 330, 335–36
liquid culture, 36, 63, 87, 197, 203
liquid tinctures, 146, 318
liver, 13–15, 39, 49, 53–54, 59–62, 70, 74, 82–83, 89, 169–70, 218, 230, 235–38, 278–79, 318–19
detoxification, 61
disease, 287, 291, 327
enzymes, 319, 330
function, 84, 267

support, 46, 53, 316
toxicity, 319
local, 101, 264, 272
longevity, 8, 12, 38, 57–59, 75, 78, 80–84, 91–96, 179, 267
loopy, 196, 266
lower bowel problems, 257
lower doses, 131, 134, 145, 153–54, 172, 198, 215, 223–24, 262
lower urinary problems, 351
lower urinary tract disease (LUTD), 55
l-taurine, 327, 332, 352
l-theanine, 234
Lung Yin, 60, 92
lungs, 49, 53, 57–60, 66, 70, 82–83, 88–93, 97, 99, 211, 218, 230, 235
deficiency, 92
disorders, 61
function, 41, 59
support, 15, 59
tonic, 59
Lyme disease, 328
lymph nodes, 189
regional, 211, 218
lymphoma, 71, 230, 251, 259
cells, 71
feline, 258
intestinal, 259
malignant, 71
patients, 245
small cell, 258, 259
LZ-8, 81

M

macronutrients, 289, 294
magnetic resonance imaging (MRI), 314
Maine coon kitty, 353

maitake, 24, 31–32, 39, 45, 51, 62, 67–68, 72, 89, 176, 197, 230, 266
extracts, 32, 71
fruiting body, 68
malformations, 166
malignant tumors, 209, 235
malnutrition, 255
mammals, 38, 123, 132, 156, 238
mangos, 153, 263
manure, 28, 56
maple, 69, 86
marijuana, 75, 220
marrow, 60, 66
mass, 28, 188, 201, 211
massages, 147, 184–86
mast cell tumors, 55, 242, 244–45, 251
Matricaria recutita, 159
maturity, 312
sexual, 141, 152
MCT (medium chain triglycerides), 195, 226, 234, 249–50, 293, 297, 337–38, 343
additional, 338
extra, 343
oil, 250, 343
meal, 298
flaxseed, 296–97
hempseed, 308
krill, 298, 309, 352
meat, 160, 294, 306–7, 349
cooked, 315
fresh, 349
muscle, 255
mussel, 177
mechanical help, 194
medication, 9, 16, 21, 98–99, 113–15, 169, 176, 185, 206, 208, 313–15, 318–22, 323–27

anti-cholesterol, 72
anti-convulsant, 338
antifungal, 13
anti-infection, 20
euthanasia, 208
immune-suppressive, 115
new allergy, 114
steroid, 131
medicines, 2, 18, 20–21, 112,
  115, 145, 187, 215, 287
  functional, 105
  modern, 113
  sports, 182
  traditional, 333
  veterinary herbal, 137
medium chain triglycerides. *See*
  MCT.
melanin, 54
melanoma, 89, 242, 244, 251
  malignant, 213, 244
meloxicam, 155, 169
membrane receptors, 37, 41, 132,
  153, 156
  proteins, 159
memory, 62–64, 69, 93–94, 144,
  156, 159, 199, 340, 359
mental calmness, 253
mental clarity, 92
mental health, 76
mental stability, 76
metabolic disorders, 47, 88
metabolic energy production, 59
metabolic processes, 342
metabolism, 40, 47–49, 66, 73–
  74, 87, 245, 247–48, 293,
  296, 304, 319, 343, 349–50
  carbohydrate, 337
metals, heavy, 305
Metamucil, 274
metastasis, 58, 99, 190, 222, 235
methylsulfonylmethane (MSM),
  164, 177–78

metoclopramide, 280
metronidazole, 278
mevinolin, 40–41, 72–75
Mexico, 76
mice, 93, 307
microampere, 336
microbiome, 118, 136, 254, 266–
  67, 269–70, 276–77, 297,
  342, 354
  support, 64–65, 69, 82–84,
    97, 118, 135
microdosing, 1, 76
micro-ecology, 19
micro-exposures, 138
micronutrients, 286, 294, 308,
  348
microorganisms, 118, 135, 269–
  70
microtrauma, 186
milk, 160
milk thistle, 137, 233, 344, 354
  seeds, 316
milk, production, 47
millet, 29–30
milo, 29–30
minerals, 22, 68, 286, 289, 305,
  308, 338
Mirtazapine, 280
mistletoe, 246
mobility, 64, 172, 194
modulators, 235–36
molecules, 1, 18, 35, 41–44, 63,
  117, 125, 132, 174, 175, 229,
  237–38, 241, 257
  active, 17, 41, 51–52, 237,
    272
  bioactive, 39, 68
  cell signal, 159
  fat-soluble, 79
  hallucinogenic, 42
  hydrocarbon, 36
  immune-active, 118

inflammatory, 166–67
neuroprotective, 132
non-nutritional, 285
rogue toxic estrogen, 296
volatile, 257, 262
monoclonal antibody treatments, 125–26, 213
montmorillonite clay, 253
mortality, 38
motility, 261, 278–80
movement, 19, 167, 184, 201, 222, 268, 323, 324
mucilage, 273
Mucolytic, 61
mucous membranes, 274
Multiple sclerosis (MS), 65, 321
muscles, spasms, 256
mushroom blends, 45
mushroom chews, 146
mushroom extracts, 11, 16, 31, 101–6, 216–17, 236, 254, 330, 348
  cordyceps militaris, 351
  lion's mane, 140, 155
  PSP, 216
mushroom fiber, 136, 261
mushroom of immortality, 80, 335
mushroom powder, 39, 103
  dried unprocessed, 106
  extracted, 106
Mushroom Quality Product Analysis Study, 30
mushrooms
  adaptogenic, 240
  calming, 145
  cooked, 108
  cordyceps, 28, 56–57, 352
  magic, 42, 75–77
  maitake, 67, 71, 277, 336
  psilocybin, 42, 76
  rehydrated, 101

reishi, 37
shiitake, 31, 41, 85, 277
snow, 90
species, 6, 40, 42–46, 68, 100, 102, 105–6
spores, 28
tree of life, 80
mutations, 209–10, 235
mycelial
  culture, 36
  networks, 19
myceliated
  brown rice, 32
  grain products, 30
mycelium, 19, 23, 28–36, 51–56, 63, 87, 99, 137, 196–97, 219
mycobacteria, 38
mycologist, 2
mycorrhizae, 17–18
myelopathy, 321, 331
myrcene, 153

N

n-acetyl d-glucosamine (NAG), 276–77
n-acetylcysteine (NAC), 331
narcotics, 170
nausea, 223, 238, 258, 261, 271, 280
negative reinforcement, 150, 161
Nepal, 57–58
Nephritis, 80
nerves, 64, 174, 304, 335–37
  tonic, 65
nervous system, 10, 19, 56, 63–67, 99, 153, 156, 159, 218, 316, 320–21, 332–33
nervousness, 157
nettle, 352
neuralgia, 69
neurasthenia, 64, 80
NeuroCare, 249–50

neurodegeneration, 39, 82–84, 321–22, 330–33

neurodevelopment, 333

neurogenesis, 77, 258

neurology, 65, 313–14, 316, 325
   adverse effects, 205
   disorders, 38, 312

Neurontin, 314

neuropathic pain, 170

neurotransmitters, 149, 153, 156

neurotropic effect, 327

neutering, 140–41

New Jersey, 246

Newfoundland, 292

NF-kappa-beta, 241

nitrogen, 17

non-steroidal anti-inflammatory drugs (NSAIDs), 155, 169–70, 186

North America, 64, 360

northern hemisphere, 73

nose, 12, 114, 138
   nasal passages, 242

Nosema ceranae, 50

nucleoside adenosine, 41

nucleosides, 41, 44, 59, 118, 229

nursing mothers, 47

nutraceuticals, 134, 158, 176, 186, 198, 232–33, 251, 271, 316, 319, 331, 344

nutrients, 18–19, 27, 136, 177, 241, 257, 269, 286–87, 294, 302–4, 305–7, 335, 341, 350
   profiles, 180, 248, 289–90, 301, 351–53

Nutriscan, 121, 127, 254, 285, 311

nutrition, 22–23, 38, 85, 180, 248, 257, 267, 281–82, 284–86, 291, 294, 314, 349, 351, 355

nuts, 160

O

oak, 69, 86–90, 246

oak mushroom, 85

oats, 29–30, 40, 160

obesity, 97, 142, 179–81, 270, 289–91, 297, 300, 343, 351

obsessive compulsive disorder (OCD), 76–77, 304

Oclacitinib maleate, 126

odor, 114, 141, 151, 280

oils, 120, 135, 159, 173, 226, 234, 250, 256, 291–93, 296–99, 343, 351
   algal, 195, 309, 332, 352
   borage, 135, 297
   carrier, 226–27
   delicate, 348
   fatty acid, 120
   fish roe, 297
   green-lipped mussel, 134, 177, 297
   healthy, 138, 297, 342, 353
   high DHA, 134
   krill, 297
   medium chain triglyceride, 226
   olive, 226
   palm, 226
   primrose, 135
   purified, 298
   safflower, 226
   seed, 120, 135, 294, 296–97, 353
   seed/evening primrose, 309

oleic acid, 81

omega-3, 120, 180, 291–94, 296–97, 350, 352–53

omega-6, 120, 180, 291–94, 296–97, 350, 352–53

omnivores, 294

oncology, 16, 193, 211–14, 216, 218–19, 232–33, 246

Ophiocordyceps sinensis, 41, 57
opioids, 169–70
oral, 173, 220, 246
Oregon, 19, 80
organisms, 3, 7, 100
organs, 62, 189–90, 199, 211,
    218, 276, 279, 307
orthopedics, 167–68
    surgery, 345–46
osteoarthritis, 163, 165, 170–72,
    176
osteochondritis dissecans, 304
osteosarcoma, 200, 213, 242
oxygen, 194, 205, 245–46
oyster mushrooms, 24, 40, 45,
    72–73, 230, 266, 277, 336
ozone therapy, 13, 205

P

Pacific yew tree, 18
pain, 142–43, 145, 153, 157,
    162, 163–72, 174, 176–77,
    180–82, 185, 200–201, 261–
    63, 278–79, 346
    chronic, 5, 169, 176
    management, 170, 194, 346
    mild-moderate, 344
    severe, 224, 228
palmitoylethanolamide (PEA),
    116, 120, 123, 132–34, 342
pancreas, 50, 255–57, 267–68
    pancreatitis, 55, 299, 338
Paneolus cyanescens, 77
parasites, 2, 20, 90, 253
Parkinson's disease (PD), 38, 62,
    65, 82, 321
paroxetine, 145
parvovirus, 72
passion flower, 146, 159
pathogens, 18, 36, 257, 279, 301,
    306, 340, 347
    fecal, 306

fungal, 19, 88
    microbial, 229
pathology, 134, 167, 321
Pawspice, 193–94
Paxil, 145, 149
pelvic osteotomy, 171
peppermint, 256
peptides, 36
    polysaccharide, 98
Periactin, 280
peristalsis, 268
petri dishes, 29, 213, 223
Phellinus, 32
phenobarbital, 313, 318, 320,
    325
phenols, 92, 118, 175, 229
pheromones, 141
    feline, 141, 152
phlegm, 49, 60, 83, 242, 334
phosphatidylcholine, 156, 159
phospholipids, 87, 156
phosphorus, 17–18, 286–87,
    289
photosynthesis, 18
Phyllanthus emblica, 234
physical exam, 167, 329
physical rehabilitation, 182
pileus, 26
Ping Gu, 73
pituitary gland, 240
pituitary-adrenal axis, 279
Plantago ovata, 273
plants, 2–3, 17–19, 26–27, 51,
    62, 94, 102, 122, 159, 175,
    220, 239, 244, 273, 305
    comfrey, 274
    compounds, 321
    DNA, 17
    extract, 220
    mind-altering, 1
    psyllium, 273
    semi-parasitic, 246

Pleurotus ostreatus, 40, 72, 336
poison, 327
pollen, 118, 122
polymers, 35–36, 237
polypore, 20, 67, 69, 80, 95
    birch, 20
Polyporus obliquus, 52
Polysaccharide Krestin (PSK),
    96, 196–97
polysaccharides, 22–23, 53, 59,
    65, 70, 87, 93, 239
    non-digestible, 239
polysaccharopeptide (PSP), 96–
    99, 197, 217–19
    Coriolus, 81, 203–4, 216
    extract, 98–99, 204, 216–17,
    219
polyunsaturated fatty acids
    (PUFA), 294, 297
Poria, 52, 335
Poria obliqua, 52
pork, 146, 160, 305
portobello, 46
postbiotics, 136–37, 269
post-traumatic stress disorder
    (PTSD), 76–78, 143–44,
    146–49
potassium bromide, 313, 320,
    325
potato, 128, 284
powders, 29, 39, 101–4, 273,
    275–76, 291, 352
    kelp, 308
    nutritional yeast, 308, 350
prebiotics, 136, 239, 258, 260,
    269, 342
predators, 171, 279, 294, 307,
    349
prednisolone, 113–15, 279
prednisone, 115, 124, 279
prescription, 170, 241, 252
preservatives, 128

pressure extrusion, 351
pressure sores, 194
prey, 286, 307
primordia, 30–33
probiotics, 135–36, 138, 253,
    258, 260–62, 269–71, 342–
    43, 349, 352–53
    cultures, 136
    fungal-based, 136
    lactic acid bacteria, 136
properties
    antibacterial, 20
    anti-microbial, 271
    anti-neoplastic, 55
    aphrodisiac, 57
    cytotoxic, 235
    fever-reducing, 20
    immune-modulating, 68, 270
    oxidizing, 246
prostate, 230
protein, 22–24, 68–70, 180, 195,
    219, 247–50, 258, 269, 285,
    286–87, 289–96, 301–4, 305,
    338, 343
    inflammatory, 259
    molecules, 36, 268, 276
proteoglycans, 48
Prozac, 145, 149
pruritus, 117, 120, 122, 131,
    133–34
pseudoginseng, 196, 242
Psilocin, 42, 78
psilocybin, 21, 29, 42, 75–78
psoriasis, 53, 118
psychotropic, 21, 25
psyllium, 262, 273–75, 344
pulmonary carcinoma, 345
pulmonary inflammation, 61
Purina, 249, 337–38

Q

QoL. *See* Quality of life.
quality of life, 5, 8, 10–13, 100, 125, 133–34, 192–95, 198, 206, 209, 267, 279, 319, 327
quercetin, 120, 135

R

rabies, 72
radiation, 58–61, 83, 93, 105, 188, 213, 215–16, 231–33, 240, 276
radix notoginseng, 242
rainbow bridge, 142, 194
raspberries, 234
ratio, 173–74, 180, 204, 220, 224, 228, 264–65, 270, 307, 330, 331, 355
   cannabinoids, 173
   high-THC, 224
   low-THC, 224
   nutrient profile, 291
   products, 173–74, 191, 196, 220–25, 226–28, 263–65, 331
   tinctures, 174
rats, 40, 97, 233
raw, 161, 172–74, 181, 250, 286, 305, 311, 331, 348
   bones, 304, 308
   diets, 282, 307, 343
   frozen, 350
   meat, 301, 306–7, 315, 347, 349
   veggies, 307, 348
reactions
   adverse, 121, 126, 206, 215, 220, 228, 247, 347
   allergy-positive, 121
   antihistamine, 119
   low-oxygen, 245

rectum, 245, 252–53, 267
   rectal exam, 253
   rectal insufflation, 245
red clover, 137
rehabilitation, 182–84
reishi, 31–32, 36–37, 45–46, 78–82, 94, 100, 102, 118–19, 145, 149, 176–77, 197, 230, 240, 335
   anti-histaminic effect, 55
   bitter, 102
   extract, 32, 79, 327
   red, 79–80
   triterpenes, 37
Relax Mushroom Chews, 145
relief, symptomatic, 258
remission, 133, 196, 204, 220–22, 231, 249, 339
renoprotective, 58–61, 64, 84–88
repetitive motion, 165
reproduction, 34
rescue, 61, 141, 150, 184, 345
respiratory
   problems, 2, 62
   upper respiratory illnesses, 75, 351
retention enema, 270
rheumatic fever, 132
rheumatism, 96, 163
rhinitis, 83
rhizome, 238, 244
rib cage, 300
rice, 29, 253, 254
   flour, 30
   growth medium, 57
   substrate, 57
   white, 253, 255
rickets, 40
Romans, 20
roots, 18–19, 238, 244, 273, 335
   marshmallow, 273–75

Russia, 52
rye, 29

S

Saccharomyces boulardii, 352
Safe Harbor Lab Rescue, 142, 345–46
saliva, 268, 285, 323–24
    test, 128, 130, 285, 311
salmon, 146, 285
salmonella, 301
salmoneostramineus, 72
sarcomas, 209
Scandinavia, 52
schizophrenia, 42
sclerotium, 335
scratching, 113–14, 116, 120–23, 138, 140, 150–51
sea cucumbers, 177–78
Seattle, 156
secretion, 253
sedate, 63, 153, 156, 170, 313, 320, 325, 338
seed meal, 119–20, 291, 296–99, 309, 350, 352
seeding, 29, 190
seeds, 26–27, 160, 297–98
seizure, threshold, 332
seizures, 36, 160, 175, 194, 312–15, 317–19, 321–34, 336–39
    breakthrough, 324
    focal, 324
    frequency, 318–19, 326
        reduced, 335
    generalized, 323
    medication, 321
    non-resolving, 325
    ongoing, 325
    refractory, 326
    resistant, 334
    severe, 329, 334
self-medicate, 2

semilanceata, 77
serotonin, 42, 153, 156–58
    receptors, 42, 100
sesquiterpenes, 36, 95
sesterpenes, 36, 175
shamanic medicine, 76–77
sheep lanolin, 238
sheep's head, 67
Shiia tree, 85–86
Shittake, 21, 24, 32, 36, 39, 45–46, 72, 85–87, 176, 197, 266, 336
Shockwave Therapy, 186
Siberia, 52
side effects
    adverse, 124, 198, 205, 222, 227, 264
    cardiovascular, 222
    steroid, 125
Silver Bullet, 145, 174, 317–19, 355
Silver, Robert, 3, 253
SilverDog Chews, 146–47
Silymarin, 233, 316, 331, 354
single-celled organism, 17
sinusitis, 47–50
skin, 10, 38, 93, 113–14, 115–22, 126, 131–32, 136, 138, 166, 237–38, 269, 276, 306–9, 334
    allergies, 122, 131–35
    dry, 93
    greasy, 113
    infections, 2
    inflammation, 70, 274
    intradermal, 127
    lesions, 131–32
    moisture, 119
    naked, 122
    red, 116
    shiny, 80
    sores, 123, 131, 135

skull, 210, 336
sleep, 156, 188, 192, 200, 206–7, 346
sleep aid, 84
slippery elm, 273–75
sneeze, 107, 138
sodium ascorbate, 246
sodium retention, 273
soft chews, 102, 146, 156, 173, 330, 355
soil, 18, 56
sores, 113, 133, 274
    ulcerated, 122
South America, 20, 76
soy sauce, 136
Sparganium stoloniferum, 244
specialist, 149, 252, 313–15
species
    fungal, 22, 34
    intestinal probiotic, 239
spectrum product, 221
spinal cord, 82
spirulina, 308, 352–55
spleen, 16, 49, 54, 66, 70, 74, 88, 97–98, 188–90, 196, 199–200, 201, 203, 216, 243
    blood-filled, 188
    diseased, 99, 199
    splenectomy, 190–91, 216
spores, 25–29, 34, 56–58
    germinate, 28–29
sporocarp, 27–28
St. Bernard, 292
stagnation, 242, 244–45
stamina, 15, 59, 86–89, 330
Star Trek, 185
starch, 22–24, 29–31
starve, 248
Stasis Breaker, 196, 205, 242–44
statins, 72
stem cell, 61
Sterling Silver, 174, 355

steroids, 113–14, 123, 126, 134, 205, 278–79
sterol, 39, 53
stipe, 26
stomach, 49, 53–54, 64–66, 74, 88–92, 99, 169, 255, 261, 267–68, 272–75
Stomach Yin, 92
stools, 28, 193, 253–55, 262, 264–65, 268, 270, 274, 279–80, 303, 324
    healthy, 267, 270
    soft, 256, 258, 269
    straining, 252, 264–65, 278–79
stratosphere, 17
strays, 72–75, 142–43, 184, 345–46, 349
strength, 203, 276, 340
stress, 15, 18, 37, 38, 55, 59–62, 72, 148, 161, 165, 199, 240, 258–60, 333
    management, 65
    relief, 105
    support, 59, 69
stroke, 82–84, 328
structure
    chemical, 41
    fungal, 26
    glandular, 279
    joint, 177
    spore-bearing, 62, 91
    thin-walled tubular, 28
substances, 1–2, 3–6, 118
    abuse, 42
    hallucinogenic, 42
    immunomodulating, 340
    innocuous, 138
substrates, 27–29, 33, 56
success, 121, 171–72, 180, 192, 197–98, 203–5, 226, 233, 246, 276, 311, 317, 320, 326

sugars, 18, 22, 29, 272–73
  simple, 195, 229, 234, 247–48, 293
superfood, 105, 108, 296, 308
supplements, 11–12, 107–12, 119–21, 134, 142–44, 176–77, 198, 201–3, 231–34, 287, 291, 303, 332–33, 338, 343, 350
  anti-anxiety, 155
  antioxidant, 211
  calming, 158, 256
  dietary, 9, 106–7, 266–67
  diet-balancing, 310
  digestive, 262, 344
  healthy, 305, 340
  human, 176
  turmeric, 239
surgery, 141, 143, 171, 179, 184–85, 188–89, 192, 195, 199, 211–12, 250, 272, 346
survival, 40, 99, 190, 199, 218
sweet, 13, 49, 54, 60, 66, 70, 74, 83, 86–92, 97, 142, 272–73, 353
symptoms, 119, 123–31, 138, 167–68, 212, 279, 323–24, 337
synergy, 35, 43, 173, 220–22
syringe, 225–26, 272
systems
  cardiovascular, 82
  circulatory, 209
  lymphatic, 209
  respiratory, 122

T

taste, 23, 36, 49, 54–56, 60, 66, 70–74, 83, 88–92, 97, 101, 302, 351
  bitter, 37, 54, 79, 83, 97, 102, 229, 244
  bland, 226
  fishy, 63
  toasty, 59
  umami, 277
taurine, 316
Taxus brevifolia, 18
tea, 18, 156, 234–35, 272
  ginger, 271
  peppermint, 256
teeth, 267–68
telehealth, 214, 246
tendons, 74, 167
terpenes, 36–37, 79, 95, 100, 159, 175, 220, 229, 236, 262–63, 335
  analyses, 262
  important, 37–38
  molecules, 229, 263
  sedating, 153
  volatile, 175
terpinolene, 263
testosterone, 140
tests, 121, 129–30, 213, 249, 254, 284–85, 314, 320, 327–29, 336
tetrahydrocannabinolic acid, 331
THC, 153, 154, 173–74, 191, 195–96, 204–5, 209, 214, 220–28, 261, 263–66, 331
  adverse effects, 224
  distillate, 225–27
  dose, 227, 266
  hemp product, 329
  ratio product, 174, 204, 224
THCA, 155, 174, 327–31
theanine, 145, 158, 235
therapies, 124–26, 134, 147, 176, 182–88, 192, 198, 204, 215, 232, 246
  adjunctive, 94
  cannabinoid, 329
  drug, 11, 315

emerging, 260, 338
herbal, 185
hyposensitization, 127
immune-based, 125
immune-supportive, 115
monoclonal antibody, 126
non-drug, 327
physical, 12, 182, 186
surgical, 9
Thunderphobia, 157
Thundershirts, 147, 157
Tibet, 57–58
tincture, 145–46, 226–28, 319, 330
tinder conk, 20
tissues, 38, 154, 166, 209, 238
connective, 209, 276
culture, 213
damage, 342
mesenchymal, 209
nasal, 13
oxygenation, 41
TNF (Tumor necrosis factor), 87
tocopherols, 316, 335
toes, 128
webbed, 162
tofu, 128, 160
tolerance, 169–70, 222, 224, 227–28, 264
tongue, 220, 267, 333
toxic, 22–23, 41, 134, 215, 277, 316
toxicity, 21–23, 169, 212, 342
toxins, 257, 267, 351
trademark, 183
Traditional Chinese Veterinary Medicine (TCVM), 44, 49, 54, 60, 66, 70, 74, 83, 88–92, 97, 333–36, 339
training, 147, 150, 161–63, 181–82, 347

Tramadol, 170
trametenolic acid, 53
trametes versicolor, 16, 95
transformation, 90
transmission, 306
trauma, 91, 114, 144, 149, 165, 176, 322–23, 344, 346
traumatic injury, 82
tree ear, 91
tree root, 335
trees, 38, 51, 246, 335
birch, 20, 38, 51–52
broadleaf, 86
western larch, 239
tremella, 45–46, 91–93, 118–19, 230
Tremella mesenterica, 91
triamcinolone, 113–15
tricalcium phosphate, 304
triglycerides, 48–49, 87, 250, 343
triple helixes, 229
triterpenes, 36–37, 44, 51, 68–70, 82, 95, 100, 103, 118–19, 175, 335
lanostanic, 37
triterpenoid content, 79
triterpenoids, 38, 55, 79–81, 96
pentacyclic, 38
truffle, 56
tryptophan, 42, 145, 156–60
tuberculosis, 88–89, 96
tumor, 141, 188, 190, 199, 201, 210–13, 218, 220–22, 231, 235, 241–42, 244, 314
blood stagnation, 244
blood-filled, 188
cells, 190, 212
excised, 212
experimentally-induced, 71
growth, 69, 190
mass, 245
metastatic, 190, 196, 200, 222

painful, 200
splenic, 189
turkey tail, 16, 30–33, 36–38,
    45, 94–98, 197, 203–4, 219,
    229–30
    extract, 16, 98–99, 197, 203–
    4, 219
    hemangiosarcoma study, 189,
    216
    mycelium, 36, 98, 204, 216,
    219
    triterpenes, 102
turmeric, 137, 164, 178, 198,
    233, 236, 238–39, 241, 244,
    258, 354
Tylenol, 169

U

ulcers, 53, 64, 93, 122, 169, 259
    gastric, 80, 272
United States, 191
Upper Respiratory Infections
    (URI), 83, 91, 96
urinary, 88, 139, 141, 148, 151,
    276, 327
Urinary Tract Infections (UTI),
    96
urination, 148, 151–52, 193–94,
    207–8, 279, 323, 351
urine, 141, 148, 151–52, 193,
    211, 249, 293, 313, 324, 338,
    351
UV light, 238, 334–35
UVB light, 39, 238

V

vaccines, 72, 82, 105, 213
valerian root, 159
varnished conk, 79

vegetables, 19, 135, 175, 180,
    234, 262, 291–95, 305–7,
    315, 348–49, 353
veterinarians, 3–8, 13–16, 112,
    182–83, 187–88, 191–92,
    196–97, 237, 241–42, 278–
    79, 310, 315–16, 327–29,
    334, 336, 345–46, 355–58
    medicine, 5, 7, 182–83, 187,
    211, 216, 281, 325, 361
    neurology, 313–14
    nurses, 183, 357
    specialists, 242
Veterinary Botanical Medical
    Association, 137
Viet Cong, 242
Vietnam, 242
vitamins, 22, 39–40, 48, 68, 156,
    233, 236–38, 247, 308, 316,
    327, 333–35, 348, 350
    spectrum, 335
    vitamin B, 156, 316, 350
    vitamin B1, 333
    vitamin B12, 294, 333
    vitamin B3, 333
    vitamin B6, 333
    vitamin C, 246
    vitamin D, 237, 316, 334, 348
    vitamin D2, 39–40, 68, 72,
    81, 238, 335
    vitamin D3, 39–40, 237–38
    vitamin E, 233, 316
vizsla, 252, 256
volva, 26
vomiting, 121, 198, 223, 258–60,
    261, 271–74, 279–80, 324

W

water, 18, 22, 226, 244, 253, 256,
    268, 273–74, 275, 306, 342–
    43, 349, 351–54
    fresh, 351

weakness, 47, 80, 176, 188, 201,
  344
Wei Qi Booster, 196, 205, 236,
  241–42
weight, 103, 179–81, 184, 265,
  272, 276, 287, 290, 298–302,
  343, 348, 353
  excessive, 166
  healthy, 343
  losing, 176, 179–80, 186, 260,
    294, 299, 301, 343
wellness, 7–9, 15, 94, 103–5,
  281, 296, 340–41, 352, 354–
  56
  program, 340–41, 344, 350
Well-Pet Dispensary, 145, 330
Western equine encephalitis, 87–
  88
Western medicine, 1, 3, 271
white blood cells, 218
white button mushrooms, 23,
  45–48, 85, 266, 277
white jelly mushroom, 90
white tree jellyfish, 90
white willow bark, 178
white wood ear, 90
wildcrafters, 67–68
witch's butter, 91
Withania somnifera, 240

wolf, 294
wound, 20, 140, 194, 274

X

XFZYT (Xue Fu Zhu Yu Tan),
  196, 244–45
Xiao Chai Hu Tang, 245
Xie Gan Tang, 333
X-rays, 163, 167

Y

yang, 60
yeast, 13–15, 35, 90, 136, 236–
  37, 269
yucca root, 178
Yun Zhi, 95
Yunnan Pai Yao, 196, 205

Z

zen, 145, 158, 234
Zheng Qi, 54
Zhu, 196, 244
zinc, 338
  chromium, 350
Zyrtec, 125

REFERENCES

Section One

[1] Brown, D. C., & Reetz, J. (2012). Single agent polysaccharopeptide delays metastases and improves survival in naturally occurring hemangiosarcoma. *Evidence-based Complementary and Alternative Medicine, 2012*, Article ID 384301. https://doi.org/10.1155/2012/384301

Chapter One

[2] Hawksworth, D. L., & Lucking, R. (2017). Fungal diversity revisited: 2.2 to 3.8 million species. *ASM Journals, 5*(4). https://doi.org/10.1128/microbiolspec.FUNK-0052-2016

[3] Wainright, P. O., Hinkle, G., Sogin, M. L., & Stickel, S. K. (1993). Monophyletic origins of the Metazoa: An evolutionary link with fungi. *Science, 260*(April 16), 340–342.

[4] Chang, S-T., & Miles, P. G. (2004). *Mushrooms: Cultivation, Nutritional Value, Medicinal Effect, and Environmental Impact* (Chapter 2, pp. 55-60). CRC Press. ISBN: 0-8493-1043-1.

[5] Rogers, R. (2011). *The Fungal Pharmacy: The Complete Guide to Medicinal Mushrooms and Lichen of North America*. North Atlantic Books.

[6] Chang, S-T., & Miles, P. G. (2004). *Mushrooms: Cultivation, Nutritional Value, Medicinal Effect, and Environmental Impact* (Preface). CRC Press. ISBN: 0-8493-1043-1.

[7] Chang, S.-T., & Miles, P. G. (2004). *Mushrooms: Cultivation, Nutritional Value, Medicinal Effect, and Environmental Impact* (Overview, pp. 1-6). CRC Press. ISBN: 0-8493-1043-1.

[8] Cheung, P. C. K. (2013). Mini-review on edible mushrooms as a source of dietary fiber: Preparation and health benefits. *Food Science & Human Wellness, 2*, 162-166.

[9] US Department of Agriculture. (2023). USDA Nutrient Database. Retrieved from https://fdc.nal.usda.gov/fdc-app.html#/ (Accessed August, 2023).

Chapter Two

[10] Chang, S.-T., & Miles, P. G. (2004). *Mushrooms: Cultivation, Nutritional Value, Medicinal Effect, and Environmental Impact* (Overview, pp. 1-6). CRC Press. ISBN: 0-8493-1043-1.

Chapter Three

[11] Vetvicka, V., & Vetvivkova, J. (2010). 1,3-glucan: Silver bullet or hot air? *Open Glycoscience, 3*, 1-6.

[12] Chen, M-L., Hsieh, C-C., Chiang, B-L, & Lin, Bi-F. (2015). Triterpenoids and polysaccharide fractions of Ganoderma tsugae exert different effects on anti-allergic activities. *Evidence-Based Complementary and Alternative Medicine*, Article ID: 7534886.

[13] Nguyen, T. M. N., Le, H. S., Le, V. B., Kim, Y. H., & Hwang, I. (2020). Anti-allergic effect of inotodiol, a lanostane triterpenoid from chaga mushroom, via selective inhibition of mast cell function. *International Immunopharmacology, 81*, 106244. https://doi.org/10.1016/j.intimp.2020.106244

[14] Beelman, R. B., Kalaras, M. D., & Richie, J. P. (2019). Micronutrients and bioactive compounds in mushrooms: A recipe for healthy aging? *Nutrition Today, 54*(1), 16–22.

[15] Beelman, R. B., Kalaras, M. D., Phillips, A. T., & Richie, J. P., Jr. (2020). Is ergothioneine a "longevity vitamin" limited in the American diet? *Journal of Nutritional Science, 9,* e52, 1-5. https://doi.org/10.1017/jns.2020.44

[16] Halliwell, B., Cheah, I. K., & Tang, R. (2018). Ergothioneine — a diet-derived antioxidant with therapeutic potential. *FEBS Letters, 592*(20), 3357–3366. https://doi.org/10.1002/1873-3468.13123

[17] Hatano, T., Saiki, S., Okuzumi, A., Mohney, R. P., & Hattori, N. (2016). Identification of novel biomarkers for Parkinson's disease by metabolomic technologies. *Journal of Neurology, Neurosurgery, and Psychiatry, 87*(4), 295–301.

[18] Tang, R. M. Y., Cheah, I. K., Yew, T. S. K., & Halliwell, B. (2018). Distribution and accumulation of dietary ergothioneine and its metabolites in mouse tissues. *Scientific Reports, 8,* 1–15.

[19] Cheah, I. K., Feng, L., Tang, R. M. Y., Lim, K. H. C., & Halliwell, B. (2016). Ergothioneine levels in an elderly population decrease with age and incidence of cognitive decline; a risk factor for neurodegeneration? *Biochemical and Biophysical Research Communications, 478*(1), 162–167.

[20] Hazewinkel, H. A., How, K. L., Bosch, R., Goedegebuure, S. A., & Voorhout, G. (1987). Inadequate photosynthesis of vitamin D in dogs. Nutrition, malnutrition, and dietetics in the dog and cat: Proceedings of the international symposium held at Hanover, September 3 to 4, 1987. British Veterinary Association in collaboration with the Waltham Centre for Pet Nutrition.

[21] How, K. L., Hazewinkel, H. A., & Mol, J. A. (1994). Dietary vitamin D dependence of cat and dog due to inadequate cutaneous synthesis of vitamin D. *General and Comparative Endocrinology, 96,* 12-18.

[22] Smith, C., Bucca, G., Penson, S., Chope, G., Hypponen, E., Berry, J., Vieth, R., & Lanham-New, S. (2012). Comparison of vitamin D_2 and vitamin D_3 status: A systematic review and meta-analysis. *The American Journal of Clinical Nutrition, 95*(6), 1357-1364.

[23] Biancuzzo, R. M., Clarke, N., Reitz, R. E., Travison, T. G., & Holick, M. F. (2013). Serum concentrations of 1,25-dihydroxyvitamin D_2 and 1,25-dihydroxyvitamin D_3 in response to vitamin D_2 and vitamin D_3 supplementation. *Journal of Clinical Endocrinology & Metabolism, 98*(3), 973-979.

[24] Kala, K., Kryczyk-Poprawa, A., Rzewinska, A., & Muszynska, B. (2020). Fruiting bodies of selected edible mushrooms as a potential source of lovastatin. *European Food Research and Technology, 246*(4), 713-722. https://doi.org/10.1007/s00217-020-03435-w

[25] Du, J., Kan, W., Bao, H., Jia, Y., Yang, J., & Hongxiao, J. (2021). Interactions between adenosine receptors and cordycepin (3'-deoxyadenosine) from *Cordyceps militaris*: Possible pharmacological mechanisms for protection of the brain and the amelioration of COVID-19 pneumonia. *Journal of Biotechnology and Biomedical Science, 4*(2), 26-62.

[26] Moldavan, M. G., Grodzinskaya, A. A., Solomko, E. F., Lomberh, M. L., Wasser, S. P., & Storozhuk, V. M. (2000). Neurotropic effect of extracts from the hallucinogenic mushroom *Psilocybe cubensis* (Earle) Sing. (Agaricomycetideae): In vitro studies. *International Journal of Medicinal Mushrooms, 2*, 329-338.

[27] Hobbs, C. (2020). *Medicinal Mushrooms: The Essential Guide*. Storey Publishing.

[28] Zied, D. C., & Pardo-Gimenez, A. (2017). Mushrooms and human civilization. In D.C. Zied & A. Pardo-Gimenez (Eds.), *Edible and Medicinal Mushrooms: Technology and Applications*, 1-3. Wiley Blackwell.

[29] Lowe, H., Toyang, N., Steele, B., Valentine, H., Grant, J., Ali, A., Ngwa, W., & Gordon, L. (2021). The therapeutic potential of psilocybin. *Molecules, 26*(10), 2948.

[30] MacCallum, C. A., Lo, L. A., Pistawka, C. A., & Deol, J. K. (2022, December 1). Therapeutic use of psilocybin: Practical considerations for dosing and administration. *Frontiers in Psychiatry*, *13*, 1040217. https://doi.org/10.3389/fpsyt.2022.1040217

Chapter Four

[31] Rogers, R. (2011). *The Fungal Pharmacy: The Complete Guide to Medicinal Mushrooms and Lichen of North America*. North Atlantic Books.

[32] Giannenas, I., Tontis, D., & Tsalie, E. (2010). Influence of dietary mushroom *Agaricus bisporus* on intestinal morphology and microflora composition in broiler chickens. *Research in Veterinary Science*, *89*(1), 78-84.

[33] Glavinic, U., Rajkovic, M., Vunduk, J., Vejnovic, B., Stevanovic, J., Milenkovic, I., & Stanimirovic, Z. (2021). Effects of agaricus bisporus mushroom extract on honey bees infected with *Nosema ceranae*. *Insects*, *12*(10), 915. https://doi.org/10.3390/insects12100915

[34] Zhang, M., Huang, J., Xie, X., & Holman, C. D. J. (2009). Dietary intake of mushrooms and green tea combine to reduce the risk of breast cancer in Chinese women. *International Journal of Cancer*, *124*, 1404-1408.

[35] Chang, S-T., & Miles, P. G. (2004). *Mushrooms: Cultivation, Nutritional Value, Medicinal Effect, and Environmental Impact* (Chapter 2, pp. 55-60). CRC Press. ISBN: 0-8493-1043-1.

[36] Konno, S. (2004). Potential growth inhibitory effect of Maitake D-Fraction on canine cancer cells. *Veterinary Therapeutics*, *5*(4), 263-270.

[37] Griessmayr, P. C., Gauthier, M., Barber, L. G., & Cotter, S. M. (2007). Mushroom-derived Maitake PETfraction as single agent for the treatment of lymphoma in dogs. *Journal of Veterinary Internal Medicine*, *21*, 1409-1412.

[38] Kodama, N., Komuta, K., Nanba, H., & Saito, N. (2005). Maitake D-Fraction enhances anti-tumor effects and reduces immunosuppression by mitomycin-C in tumor-bearing mice. *Nutrition, 21*(5), 624-629.

[39] Haladová, E., Mojžišová, J., Smrčo, P., Ondrejková, A., Vojtek, B., Prokeš, M., & Petrovová, E. (2011). Immunomodulatory effect of glucan on specific and nonspecific immunity after vaccination in puppies. *Acta Veterinaria Hungarica, 59*(1), 77-86.

[40] Alberts, A. W., Chen, J., Kuron, G., Hunt, V., Huff, J., Hoffman, C., Rothrock, J., Lopez, M., Joshua, H., Harris, E., Patchett, A., Monaghan, R., Currie, S., Stapley, E., Albers-Schonberg, G., Hensens, O., Hirshfield, J., Hoogsteen, K., Liesch, J., & Springer, J. (1980). Mevinolin: A highly potent competitive inhibitor of hydroxymethylglutaryl-coenzyme A reductase and a cholesterol-lowering agent. *Proceedings of the National Academy of Sciences, 77*(7), 3957-3961.

[41] Hobbs, C. (2020). *Medicinal Mushrooms: The Essential Guide.* Storey Publishing.

[42] Mendonça, C. N., Silva, P. M., Avelleira, J. C., Nishimori, F. S., & Cassia, F. deF. (2015). Shiitake dermatitis. *Anais Brasileiros de Dermatologia, 90*(2), 276-278. https://doi.org/10.1590/abd1806-4841.20153396

[43] Xu, W., Shen, X., Yang, F., Han, Y., Li, R., Xue, D., & Jiang, C. (2012). Protective effect of polysaccharides isolated from *Tremella fuciformis* against radiation-induced damage in mice. *Journal of Radiation Research, 53*(3), 353–360.

[44] Xie, L., Yang, K., Liang, Y., Zhu, Z., Yuan, Z., & Du, Z. (2022). *Tremella fuciformis* polysaccharides alleviate induced atopic dermatitis in mice by regulating immune response and gut microbiota. *Frontiers in Pharmacology, 13*, 944801.

[45] Barros, A. B., Ferrao, J., & Fernandes, T. A. (2016). Safety assessment of *Coriolus versicolor* biomass as a food supplement. *Food & Nutrition Research*, 60, 29953.

[46] Brown, D. C., & Reetz, J. (2012). Single agent polysaccharopeptide delays metastases and improves survival in naturally occurring hemangiosarcoma. *Evidence-based Complementary and Alternative Medicine*, 2012, Article ID 384301. https://doi.org/10.1155/2012/384301

[47] Gedney, A., Saleh, P., Mahoney, J. A., Krick, E., Martins, R., Scavello, H., Lenz, J. A., & Atherton, M. J. (2022). Evaluation of the anti-tumor activity of *Coriolus versicolor* polysaccharopeptide (I'mYunity™) alone or in combination with doxorubicin for canine splenic hemangiosarcoma. *Veterinary and Comparative Oncology*. https://doi.org/10.1111/vco.12823

Chapter Six

[48] Clayton, P., Hill, M., Bogoda, N., Subah, S., & Venkatesh, R. (2021). Palmitoylethanolamide: A natural compound for health management. *International Journal of Molecular Sciences*, 22(10), 5305. https://doi.org/10.3390/ijms22105305

[49] Noli, C., Della Valle, M. F., Miolo, A., Medori, C., Schievano, C., & Skinalia Clinical Research Group. (2015). Efficacy of ultra-micronized palmitoylethanolamide in canine atopic dermatitis: An open-label multi-centre study. *Veterinary Dermatology*, 26(6), 432-e101. https://doi.org/10.1111/vde.12250

[50] Mogi, C., Yoshida, M., Kawano, K., Fukuyama, T., & Arai, T. (2022, April). Effects of cannabidiol without delta-9-tetrahydrocannabinol on canine atopic dermatitis: A retrospective assessment of 8 cases. *Canadian Veterinary Journal*, 63(4), 423-426

[51]Lowinger, M., Wakslag, J. J., Bowden, D., Peters-Kennedy, J., & Rosenberg, A. (2022). The effect of a mixed cannabidiol and cannabidiolic acid. *Veterinary Dermatology*, 33, 329-e77.

[52] Jastrzab, A., Jarocka-Karpowicz, I., & Skrzydlewska, E. (2022). The origin and biomedical relevance of cannabigerol. *International Journal of Molecular Sciences, 23*(14), 7929. https://doi.org/10.3390/ijms23147929

[53] Yin, C., Noratto, G. D., Fan, X., Chen, Z., Yao, F., Shi, D., & Gao, H. (2020).The impact of mushroom polysaccharides on gut microbiota and its beneficial effects to host: a review. *Carbohydrate Polymers, 250,* 116942.

[54] Cho, H. W., Choi, S., Seo, K., Kim, K. H., Jeon, J. H., Kim, C. H., Lim, S., Jeong, S., & Chun, J. L. (2022). Gut microbiota profiling in aged dogs after feeding pet food contained *Hericium erinaceus. Journal of Animal Science and Technology, 64*(5), 937–949. https://doi.org/10.5187/jast.2022.e66

[55] Vetvicka, V., & Vetvivkova, J. (2010). 1,3-glucan: Silver bullet or hot air? *Open Glycoscience, 3,* 1-6.

[56] Nguyen, T. M. N., Le, H. S., Le, V. B., Kim, Y. H., & Hwang, I. (2020). Anti-allergic effect of inotodiol, a lanostane triterpenoid from chaga mushroom, via selective inhibition of mast cell function. *International Immunopharmacology, 81,* 106244. https://doi.org/10.1016/j.intimp.2020.106244

[57] Mueller, R. S., Fieseler, K. V., Fettman, M. J., Zabel, S., Rosychuk, R. A., Ogilvie, G. K., & Greenwalt, T. L. (2004). Effect of omega-3 fatty acids on canine atopic dermatitis. *Journal of Small Animal Practice, 45,* 293-297.

[58] Mueller, R. S., Fieseler, K. V., Fettman, M. J., Zabel, S., Rosychuk, R. A., Ogilvie, G. K., & Greenwalt, T. L. (2004). Effect of omega-3 fatty acids on canine atopic dermatitis. *Journal of Small Animal Practice, 45,* 293-297.

[59] Beynen, A. C. (2020). Beynen, A.C., 2020. Quercetin for dogs. 30-37.

[60] Mogi, C., Yoshida, M., Kawano, K., Fukuyama, T., & Arai, T. (2022, April). Effects of cannabidiol without delta-9-tetrahydrocannabinol on canine atopic dermatitis: A retrospective assessment of 8 cases. *Canadian Veterinary Journal, 63*(4), 423-426.

[61] Lowinger, M., Wakslag, J. J., Bowden, D., Peters-Kennedy, J., & Rosenberg, A. (2022). The effect of a mixed cannabidiol and cannabidiolic acid. *Veterinary Dermatology, 33*, 329-e77.

[62] Mogi, C., Yoshida, M., Kawano, K., Fukuyama, T., & Arai, T. (2022, April). Effects of cannabidiol without delta-9-tetrahydrocannabinol on canine atopic dermatitis: A retrospective assessment of 8 cases. *Canadian Veterinary Journal, 63*(4), 423-426.

[63] Lowinger, M., Wakslag, J. J., Bowden, D., Peters-Kennedy, J., & Rosenberg, A. (2022). The effect of a mixed cannabidiol and cannabidiolic acid. *Veterinary Dermatology, 33*, 329-e77.

[64] Clayton, P., Hill, M., Bogoda, N., Subah, S., & Venkatesh, R. (2021). Palmitoylethanolamide: A natural compound for health management. *International Journal of Molecular Sciences, 22*(10), 5305. https://doi.org/10.3390/ijms22105305

[65] Scarampella, F., Abramo, F., & Noli, C. (2001). Clinical and histological evaluation of an analogue of palmitoylethanolamide, PLR 120 (comicronized Palmidrol INN) in cats with eosinophilic granuloma and eosinophilic plaque: A pilot study. *Veterinary Dermatology, 12*, 29-39.

[66] Noli, C., Della Valle, M. F., Miolo, A., Medori, C., Schievano, C., & Skinalia Clinical Research Group. (2015). Efficacy of ultra-micronized palmitoylethanolamide in canine atopic dermatitis: An open-label multi-centre study. *Veterinary Dermatology, 26*(6), 432-e101. https://doi.org/10.1111/vde.12250

[67] Scarampella, F., Abramo, F., & Noli, C. (2001). Clinical and histological evaluation of an analogue of palmitoylethanolamide, PLR 120 (comicronized Palmidrol INN) in cats with eosinophilic granuloma and eosinophilic plaque: A pilot study. *Veterinary Dermatology, 12,* 29-39.

[68] Noli, C., Della Valle, M. F., Miolo, A., Medori, C., Schievano, C., & Skinalia Clinical Research Group. (2015). Efficacy of ultra-micronized palmitoylethanolamide in canine atopic dermatitis: An open-label multi-centre study. *Veterinary Dermatology, 26*(6), 432-e101. https://doi.org/10.1111/vde.12250

[69] Scarampella, F., Abramo, F., & Noli, C. (2001). Clinical and histological evaluation of an analogue of palmitoylethanolamide, PLR 120 (comicronized Palmidrol INN) in cats with eosinophilic granuloma and eosinophilic plaque: A pilot study. *Veterinary Dermatology, 12,* 29-39.

[70] Noli, C., Della Valle, M. F., Miolo, A., Medori, C., Schievano, C., & Skinalia Clinical Research Group. (2015). Efficacy of ultra-micronized palmitoylethanolamide in canine atopic dermatitis: An open-label multi-centre study. *Veterinary Dermatology, 26*(6), 432-e101. https://doi.org/10.1111/vde.12250

[71] Noli, C., Della Valle, M. F., Miolo, A., Medori, C., Schievano, C., & Skinalia Clinical Research Group (2019). Effect of dietary supplementation with ultramicronized palmitoylethanolamide in maintaining remission in cats with non-flea hypersensitivity dermatitis: a double-blind, multicenter, randomized, placebo-controlled study. *Veterinary Dermatology, 30*(5), 387–e117. https://doi.org/10.1111/vde.12764

[72] Mueller, R. S., Fieseler, K. V., Fettman, M. J., Zabel, S., Rosychuk, R. A., Ogilvie, G. K., & Greenwalt, T. L. (2004). Effect of omega-3 fatty acids on canine atopic dermatitis. *Journal of Small Animal Practice, 45,* 293-297.

[73] Taugbøl, B. B., Vroom, M. W., Nordberg, L., & Leistra, W. H. G. (2004). A randomized, double-blinded, placebo-controlled, multicenter study on the efficacy of a diet with high levels of eicosapentaenoic acid and gamma linolenic acid in the control of canine atopic dermatitis. *Veterinary Dermatology, 15*(Suppl. 1), 1-19.

[74] Beynen, A.C. (2020). Beynen, A. C., 2020. Quercetin for dogs. 30-37.

[75] Yin, C., Noratto, G. D., Fan, X., Chen, Z., Yao, F., Shi, D., & Gao, H. (2020). The impact of mushroom polysaccharides on gut microbiota and its beneficial effects to host: a review. *Carbohydrate Polymers, 250,* 116942.

[76] Cho, H. W., Choi, S., Seo, K., Kim, K. H., Jeon, J. H., Kim, C. H., Lim, S., Jeong, S., & Chun, J. L. (2022). Gut microbiota profiling in aged dogs after feeding pet food contained *Hericium erinaceus. Journal of Animal Science and Technology, 64*(5), 937–949. https://doi.org/10.5187/jast.2022.e66

Chapter Seven

[77] Jastrząb, A., Jarocka-Karpowicz, I., & Skrzydlewska, E. (2022). The origin and biomedical relevance of cannabigerol. *International Journal of Molecular Sciences, 23*(14), 7929. https://doi.org/10.3390/ijms23147929

[78] Takeda, S., Misawa, K., Yamamoto, I., & Watanabe, K. (2008). Cannabidiolic acid as a selective cyclooxygenase-2 inhibitory component in cannabis. *Drug Metabolism and Disposition: The Biological Fate of Chemicals, 36*(9), 1917–1921. https://doi.org/10.1124/dmd.108.020909

[79] Nagano, M., Shimizu, K., Kondo, R., Hayashi, C., Sato, D., Kitagawa, K., & Ohnuk, K. (2010). Reduction of depression and anxiety by 4 weeks *Hericium erinaceus* intake. *Biomedical Research (Tokyo, Japan), 31*(4), 231–237. https://doi.org/10.2220/biomedres.31.231

[80]Silver, R. J., & Paiss, Z. R. A. (2023). The positive behavioral impact of a CBD-containing nutraceutical formulation on privately-owned dogs. *Okoa Pets*. Retrieved from https://www.dropbox.com/scl/fi/ka81lyhzf4fbmdfqza1x6/OkoaPet_D rSilverSidewalkDog_BehaviorStudy_04.pdf?rlkey=pjnjs4igqspe5dcg8js 4x4hfs&dl=0 (Accessed March 16, 2024).

Chapter Eight

[81] Takeda, S., Misawa, K., Yamamoto, I., & Watanabe, K. (2008). Cannabidiolic acid as a selective cyclooxygenase-2 inhibitory component in cannabis. *Drug Metabolism and Disposition: The Biological Fate of Chemicals*, 36(9), 1917–1921. https://doi.org/10.1124/dmd.108.020909

[82] S.2667 - 115th Congress (2017-2018): Hemp Farming Act of 2018. (2018). Congress.gov. Retrieved from https://www.congress.gov/bill/115th-congress/senate-bill/2667/text (accessed 8-1-23).

[83] Gamble, L. J., Boesch, J. M., Frye, C. W., Schwark, W. S., Mann, S., Wolfe, L., Brown, H., Berthelsen, E. S., & Wakshlag, J. J. (2018). Pharmacokinetics, safety, and clinical efficacy of cannabidiol treatment in osteoarthritic dogs. *Frontiers in Veterinary Science*, 5, 165. https://doi.org/10.3389/fvets.2018.00165

[84] Wang, K., Wang, Z., Cui, R., & Chu, H. (2019). Polysaccharopeptide from Trametes versicolor blocks inflammatory osteoarthritis pain-morphine tolerance effects via activating cannabinoid type 2 receptor. *International Journal of Biological Macromolecules*, 126, 805-810.

[85] Kealy, R. D., Lawler, D. F., Ballam, J. M., Mantz, S. L., Biery, D. N., Greeley, E. H., Lust, G., Segre, M., Smith, G. K., & Stowe, H. D. (2002). Effects of diet restriction on life span and age-related changes in dogs. *Journal of the American Veterinary Medical Association*, 220(9), 1315-1320.

Chapter Nine

[86] Wendelburg, K. M., Price, L. L., Burgess, K. E., Lyons, J. A., Lew, F. H., & Berg, J. (2015). Survival time of dogs with splenic hemangiosarcoma treated by splenectomy with or without adjuvant chemotherapy: 208 cases (2001-2012). *Journal of the American Veterinary Medical Association, 247*(4), 393-403.

[87] Gedney, A., Saleh, P., Mahoney, J. A., Krick, E., Martins, R., Scavello, H., Lenz, J. A., & Atherton, M. J. (2022). Evaluation of the anti-tumor activity of *Coriolus versicolor* polysaccharopeptide (I'mYunity™) alone or in combination with doxorubicin for canine splenic hemangiosarcoma. *Veterinary and Comparative Oncology.* https://doi.org/10.1111/vco.12823

[88] Wendelburg, K. M., Price, L. L., Burgess, K. E., Lyons, J. A., Lew, F. H., & Berg, J. (2015). Survival time of dogs with splenic hemangiosarcoma treated by splenectomy with or without adjuvant chemotherapy: 208 cases (2001-2012). *Journal of the American Veterinary Medical Association, 247*(4), 393-403.

[89] Gedney, A., Saleh, P., Mahoney, J. A., Krick, E., Martins, R., Scavello, H., Lenz, J. A., & Atherton, M. J. (2022). Evaluation of the anti-tumor activity of *Coriolus versicolor* polysaccharopeptide (I'mYunity™) alone or in combination with doxorubicin for canine splenic hemangiosarcoma. *Veterinary and Comparative Oncology.* https://doi.org/10.1111/vco.12823

[90] Villalobos, A. E., & Kaplan, L. (2018). *Canine and Feline Geriatric Oncology: Honoring the Human-Animal Bond.* John Wiley & Sons.

[91] Gedney, A., Saleh, P., Mahoney, J. A., Krick, E., Martins, R., Scavello, H., Lenz, J. A., & Atherton, M. J. (2022). Evaluation of the anti-tumor activity of *Coriolus versicolor* polysaccharopeptide (I'mYunity™) alone or in combination with doxorubicin for canine splenic hemangiosarcoma. *Veterinary and Comparative Oncology.* https://doi.org/10.1111/vco.12823

[92] Villalobos, A. E., & Kaplan, L. (2018). *Canine and Feline Geriatric Oncology: Honoring the Human-Animal Bond*. John Wiley & Sons.

[93] Gedney, A., Saleh, P., Mahoney, J. A., Krick, E., Martins, R., Scavello, H., Lenz, J. A., & Atherton, M. J. (2022). Evaluation of the anti-tumor activity of *Coriolus versicolor* polysaccharopeptide (I'mYunity™) alone or in combination with doxorubicin for canine splenic hemangiosarcoma. *Veterinary and Comparative Oncology*. https://doi.org/10.1111/vco.12823

[94] Gedney, A., Saleh, P., Mahoney, J. A., Krick, E., Martins, R., Scavello, H., Lenz, J. A., & Atherton, M. J. (2022). Evaluation of the anti-tumor activity of *Coriolus versicolor* polysaccharopeptide (I'mYunity™) alone or in combination with doxorubicin for canine splenic hemangiosarcoma. *Veterinary and Comparative Oncology*. https://doi.org/10.1111/vco.12823

[95] Henry, J. G., Shoemaker, G., Prieto, J. M., Hannon, M. B., & Wakslag, J. J. (2020). The effect of cannabidiol on canine neoplastic cell proliferation and mitogen-activated protein kinase activation during autophagy and apoptosis. *Veterinary Comparative Oncology*. https://doi.org/10.1111/vco.12669

[96] Buonomo, A. R., Scotto, R., Nappa, S., Arcopinto, M., Salzano, A., Marra, A. M., D'Assante, R., Zappulo, E., Borgia, G., & Gentile, I. (2019). The role of curcumin in liver diseases. *Archives of Medical Science, 15*(6), 1608-1620.

[97] Tao, L., Qu, X., Zhang, Y., Song, Y., & Zhang, S. X. (2019). Prophylactic therapy of silymarin (Milk thistle) on tuberculosis drug-induced liver injury: A meta-analysis of randomized controlled trials. *Canadian Journal of Gastroenterology, 2019*, 3192351.

[98] Colas, S., Paon, L., Denis, F., Prat, M., Louisot, P., Hoinard, C., Le Floch, O., Ogilvie, G., & Bougnoux, P. (2004). Enhanced radiosensitivity of rat autochthonous mammary tumors by dietary docosahexaenoic acid. *International Journal of Cancer, 109*, 449-454.

[99] Vannucci, L., Krizan, J., Sima, P., Stakheev, D., Caja, F., Rajsiglova, L., Horak, V., & Saieh, M. (2013). Immunostimulatory properties and antitumor activities of glucan. *International Journal of Oncology, 43,* 357-364.

[100] Pope, K.V. (2020). The role of vitamin D in veterinary oncology: A literature review. *Journal of the American Holistic Veterinary Medical Association, 60,* 18-29.

[101] Kumar, P. Sharma, R., Garg, N. (2022). Withania somnifera – a magic plant targeting multiple pathways in cancer related inflammation. *Phytomedicine 101,* 154137.

[102] Ogilvie, G. K., Fettman, M. J., Mallinckrodt, C. H., Walton, J. A., Hansen, R. A., Davenport, D. J., Gross, K. L., Richardson, K. L., Rogers, Q., & Hand, M. S. (2000). Effect of fish oil, arginine, and doxorubicin chemotherapy on remission and survival time for dogs with lymphoma: A double-blind, placebo-controlled study. *Cancer, 88*(8), 1916-1928.

[103] Vail, D. M., Ogilvie, G. K., Wheeler, S. L., Fettman, M. J., Johnston, S. D., & Hegstad, R. L. (1990). Alterations in carbohydrate metabolism in canine lymphoma. *Journal of Veterinary Internal Medicine, 4,* 8-11.

Chapter Ten

[104] Yin, C., Noratto, G. D., Fan, X., Chen, Z., Yao, F., Shi, D., & Gao, H. The impact of mushroom polysaccharides on gut microbiota and its beneficial effects to host: a review. (2020) *Carbohydrate Polymers, 250,* 116942.

Chapter Eleven

[105] McGrath, S., Bartner, L. R., Rao, S., Packer, R. A., & Gustafson, D. L. (2019). Randomized blinded controlled clinical trial to assess the effect of oral cannabidiol administration in addition to conventional antiepileptic treatment on seizure frequency in dogs with intractable idiopathic epilepsy. *Journal of the American Veterinary Medical Association, 254*(11), 1301-1308.

[106] Garcia, G. A., Kube, S., Carrera-Justiz, S., Tittle, D., & Wakshlag, J. J. (2022). Safety and efficacy of cannabidiol-cannabidiolic acid rich hemp extract in the treatment of refractory epileptic seizures in dogs. *Frontiers in Veterinary Science, 9,* 939966.

[107] Mariani, C., Muñana, K., Patterson, N., & Smith, M. (Eds.).Understanding canine epilepsy. AKC Canine Health Foundation | Understanding Canine Epilepsy. https://www.akcchf.org/canine-health/top-health-concerns/epilepsy/understanding-canine-epilepsy.html (Accessed August 2023).

[108] McGrath, S., Bartner, L. R., Rao, S., Packer, R. A., & Gustafson, D. L. (2019). Randomized blinded controlled clinical trial to assess the effect of oral cannabidiol administration in addition to conventional antiepileptic treatment on seizure frequency in dogs with intractable idiopathic epilepsy. *Journal of the American Veterinary Medical Association, 254*(11), 1301-1308.

[109] Garcia, G. A., Kube, S., Carrera-Justiz, S., Tittle, D., & Wakshlag, J. J. (2022). Safety and efficacy of cannabidiol-cannabidiolic acid rich hemp extract in the treatment of refractory epileptic seizures in dogs. *Frontiers in Veterinary Science, 9,* 939966.

[110] Wakshlag, J. J., Rassnick, K. M., Malone, E. K., Struble, A. M., Vachhani, P., Trump, D. L., & Tian, L. (2011). Cross-sectional study to investigate the association between vitamin D status and cutaneous mast cell tumors in Labrador retrievers. *British Journal of Nutrition, 106,* S60-S63.

[111] Kim, J-E., & Cho, K-O. (2019). Functional nutrients for epilepsy. *Nutrients, 11*(6), 1309. https://doi.org/10.3390/nu11061309

[112] Jang, H-J., Kim, J-E., Jeong, K. H., Lim, S. C., Kim, S. Y., & Cho, K-O. (2019). The neuroprotective effect of *Hericium erinaceus* extracts in mouse hippocampus after pilocarpine-induced status epilepticus. *International Journal of Molecular Sciences, 20,* 859.

[113] Kim, J-E., & Cho, K-O. (2019). Functional nutrients for epilepsy. *Nutrients, 11*(6), 1309. https://doi.org/10.3390/nu11061309

[114] Ishimoto, T., & Kato, Y. (2022). Ergothioneine in the brain. *FEBS Letters, 596,* 1290-1298.

[115] Law, T. H., Davies, E. S., Pan, Y., Zanghi, B., Want, E., & Volk, H. A. (2015). A randomized trial of a medium-chain TAG diet as treatment for dogs with idiopathic epilepsy. *British Journal of Nutrition, 114,* 1438-1447.

[116] Packer, R. M., Law, T. H., Davies, E., Zanghi, B., Pan, Y., & Volk, H. A. (2016). Effects of a ketogenic diet on ADHD-like behavior in dogs with idiopathic epilepsy. *Epilepsy and Behavior, 55,* 62-68.

[117] Pan, Y., Larson, B., Araujo, J. A., Lau, W., de Rivera, C., Santana, R., Gore, A., & Milgram, N. W. (2010). Dietary supplementation with medium chain TAG has long-lasting cognition-enhancing effects in aged dogs. *British Journal of Nutrition, 103,* 1746-1754.

Chapter Twelve

[118] Kar, U. K., & Joosten, L. A. B. (2020). Training the trainable cells of the immune system and beyond. *Nature Immunology, 21,* 115–119. https://doi.org/10.1038/s41590-019-0583-y

[119] Bray, E. E., Zheng, Z., Tolbert, M. K., McCoy, B. M., Dog Aging Project Consortium, Kaeberlein, M., & Kerr, K. F. (2022). Once-daily feeding is associated with better health in companion dogs: Results from the Dog Aging Project. *GeroScience, 44,* 1779-1790.

[120] Lin, T-Y., Liu, H-W., & Hung, T-M. (2021). The ketogenic effect of medium-chain triglycerides. *Frontiers in Nutrition.* https://doi.org/10.3389/fnut.2021.747284

Dr. Robert Silver, DVM

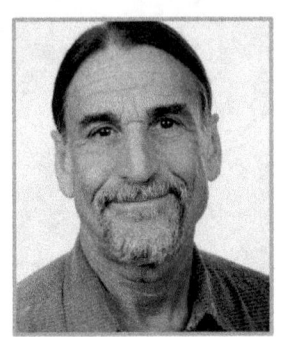 Dr. Robert Silver, a world-renowned holistic and integrative veterinarian, author, educator, and speaker, has spent the past four decades treating dogs, cats, horses, pocket pets, goats, llamas, birds, reptiles, and even a few circus animals.

An experienced veterinary mycologist, Dr. Silver is Chief Veterinary Officer for Real Mushrooms (www.realmushrooms.com), a Canadian functional mushroom company. As an experienced veterinary herbalist, he is former President of both the American College of Veterinary Botanical Medicine (www.ACVBM.org) and the Veterinary Botanical Medicine Association (www.VBMA.org).

Dr. Silver teaches a six-hour online course for veterinary continuing education titled "The Essentials of Medicinal Mushrooms" and sponsored by the College of Integrative Veterinary Therapies (www.CIVTedu.org). Dr. Silver also offers webinars, coaching, and live in-person events where he can work directly with pet parents to create healthy options for their four-legged family members.

Dr. Silver frequently speaks to large audiences, both domestically and internationally, and is the author of the 2015 book, Medical Marijuana and Your Pet. Dr. Silver has been formulating potent pet supplements for the past 30 years and owns and manages the Well-Pet Dispensary (www.wellpetdispensary.com), an online health supplement source for unique and highly potent nutraceuticals, herbs, and THC-free cannabinoid therapeutics for pets.

Well-Pet Dispensary also provides credible, scientifically established information to help guide pet parents in the safe and appropriate usage of these natural therapies.

Dr. Robert Silver graduated with his Doctor of Veterinary Medicine (DVM) from Colorado State University's College of Veterinary Medicine in 1982. He became certified in veterinary acupuncture in 1993 by the International Veterinary Acupuncture Society (www.IVAS.org). Dr. Silver taught the first course on Chinese Herbal Medicine for IVAS with Dr. Huisheng Xie, founder of the Chi University of Traditional Chinese Veterinary Medicine from 2001-2004 in Boulder, Colorado.

Currently, Dr. Silver shares his life with his partner of 30 years, Hannah, two Maine Coon kitties, Spencer and Rosie, who "rule the roost," and a sweet 10-year-old rescue Lab, Ollie.

www.ingramcontent.com/pod-product-compliance
Lightning Source LLC
Chambersburg PA
CBHW060851120626
46553CB00001B/47

GUNMEN, LAWMEN AND WILD MEN

OF EARLY GEORGIA

By R. Olin Jackson III
B.A., M.Ed.

Published by Whippoorwill Publications, LLC
Roswell, GA 30075

ISBNs: 979-8-9900211-2-9 (hc); 979-8-9900211-3-6 (pbk); 979-8-9900211-4-3(jkt)

Publisher's Cataloging-in-Publication Data
provided by Five Rainbows Cataloging Services
Names: Jackson, R. Olin, III, 1951- author.
Title: Gunmen, lawmen and wild men of early Georgia / R. Olin Jackson III.
Description: Roswell, GA : Whippoorwill Publications, 2024. | Includes bibliographical references and index. | Summary: This book is an account of gunmen, lawmen, and unusual characters in early Georgia history. | Also available in audiobook format.
Identifiers: LCCN 2024910835 (print) | ISBN 979-8-9900211-2-9 (hardcover) | ISBN 979-8-9900211-3-6 (paperback) | ISBN 979-8-9900211-4-3 (jacket)
Subjects: LCSH: Georgia—History. | Georgia—History—Civil War, 1861-1865. | Pioneers—Georgia. | Outlaws—Georgia. | Young adult nonfiction. | CYAC: Young adult literature. | BISAC: YOUNG ADULT NONFICTION / History / General. | YOUNG ADULT NONFICTION / History / United States / Civil War Period (1850-1877) | HISTORY / United States / State & Local / South (AL, AR, FL, GA, KY, LA, MS, NC, SC, TN, VA, WV)
Classification: LCC F289 .J33 2024 (print) | LCC F289 (ebook) | DDC 975.8/02—dc23.

Copies of Whippoorwill Publications, LLC books are available online at Amazon.com; BarnesandNoble.com; IngramSpark.com; and other fine booksellers.
Please visit www.georgiahistorytraveler.com for full details.